# Disordered Mind and Brain

## The Neural Basis of Mental Symptoms

Peter F. Liddle

To my parents, Jack and Nora; my wife, Elizabeth; and my son, Patrick.

# Contents

**Part II. Symptom clusters**

# Prologue

At the turn of the last century, Kraepelin (1896, 1919) laid the foundation for modern psychiatric diagnostic practice by distinguishing between schizophrenia and bipolar affective disorder. Kraepelin considered that these disorders were brain diseases. However, he and his contemporaries lacked anything but the most rudimentary techniques for examining the structure and function of the living human brain.

The century ended with the 'Decade of the Brain', a decade dedicated by the United States Congress and President to the enhancement of public awareness of the benefits derived from brain research. The human brain became the focus of studies by thousands of scientists and health care professionals with a mandate to conquer brain disease. By the end of the decade, and of the century, a vast wealth of data had accumulated. However, like many exciting scientific enterprises, the 'Decade of the Brain' has left us a legacy of challenging questions that overshadow the answers provided. We now know a great deal about both schizophrenia and bipolar affective disorder, yet we know neither the primary cause of these disorders nor the molecular mechanism by which their symptoms are generated.

None the less, the data have led us forward. The evidence demonstrates unequivocally that Kraepelin was right to regard schizophrenia as a brain disease. In the year 2000, the Nobel Prize in Physiology or Medicine was awarded to three neuroscientists, one of whom was Arvid Carlsson. He was awarded the prize for his work during the preceding decades, in which he had clarified the role of dopamine as a neurotransmitter. Carlsson's work provided the foundation for the hypothesis that the symptoms of schizophrenia arise from overactivity of dopamine. Recent studies have provided compelling evidence that dopaminergic neurons are hyper-responsive in schizophrenia (see Chapter 11), but meanwhile evidence for many other anomalies of brain structure and function in schizophrenia has accumulated. Furthermore, many of these anomalies are also discernible in bipolar affective disorder (see Chapter 12). Thus modern neuroscience has not yet succeeded in defining a clear boundary separating schizophrenia from bipolar affective disorder, and it remains uncertain whether or not the classification proposed by Kraepelin reflects a natural boundary between underlying pathological mechanisms.

This book draws together many of the strands of evidence that have been teased out by the techniques of modern neuroscience, with the purpose of assembling a conceptual framework for understanding the mechanisms by which mental symptoms are generated. Rather than starting with the disease entities defined by Kraepelin and his successors, we shall focus first on symptoms. In the field of chemistry, in the nineteenth century, it was the examination of the similarities and differences between chemical elements that revealed the pattern of properties that led to the construction of the periodic table. This in turn led to the delineation of the features of sub-atomic structure that account for the ways in which elements combine to form molecules. Similarly, examining the clinical characteristics of symptoms is a logical place to start the quest for an under-standing of the neural mechanisms by which symptoms are generated.

The challenge is to identify the most robust framework within which to classify and describe symptoms. A focus on symptoms, rather than diseases, reveals a striking feature. Certain groups of symptoms tend to coexist in a variety of different illnesses. For example, a set of symptoms that reflect diminution of mental and motor activity occur in schizophrenia, in affective disorders, in basal ganglion diseases such as progressive supranuclear palsy, and in certain dement-ing illnesses that are sometimes described as subcortical dementias. We shall examine (Chapter 8) the evidence indicating that this cluster of symptoms is associated with a similar pattern of cognitive deficits, and other anomalies of brain function, irrespective of the illness in which it occurs.

No individual mental symptom is confined uniquely to a single disease, and indeed virtually all the common symptoms of mental illness can occur in any of the currently recognised major mental illnesses. Closer inspection reveals that it is the norm rather than the exception to find that symptoms cluster in a similar manner in different diseases. Why should similar clusters of symptoms occur in diverse diseases? Perhaps the most plausible answer is that it is because these clusters of symptoms reveal something of the inner structure of the human mind, and of the organisation of the brain that supports it.

# The structure of the mind

The pattern of occurrence of symptoms in various mental illnesses suggests that there are five principal dimensions of psychopathology. Each dimension is associated with one or two characteristic clusters of symptoms, or syndromes (see Table P.1). Two of the dimensions are bipolar, such that patients at opposite poles of the bipolar continuum exhibit clusters of symptoms that are opposite in character. Thus, in total, there are seven clusters of symptoms. Each of the seven symptom clusters can occur in a variety of different illnesses, although certain clusters tend to be more common in a particular illness. For example, the disorganisation syndrome is most commonly seen in schizophrenia, although it can arise from traumatic brain injury and can also occur in the manic phase of manic–depressive psychosis. Similarly, the depression syndrome, although characteristic of major depressive illness, can also occur in traumatic brain injury and in schizophrenia.

Insofar as the clustering of symptoms indicates that they share features of their pathophysiology, examining symptom clusters is potentially an informative way to begin to delineate the relationships between symptoms and disordered neuronal function. By identifying the neural abnormalities that are common to several conditions in which a particular cluster of symptoms occurs, it is possible to distinguish the neural abnormality specific to that cluster of symptoms from other neural damage that is incidental to the symptoms of interest.

The inner structure of the mind is likely to be reflected in the structure and function of the brain. Recently developed functional imaging techniques, such as positron emission tomography and functional magnetic resonance imaging, offer the possibility of constructing images of human cerebral activity. These functional imaging techniques have provided direct and graphic evidence of the correspondence between patterns of brain activity and patterns of mental activity, in normal individuals and in patients with mental illness.

**Table P.1** The major clusters of mental symptoms

| Dimension | Syndrome | Symptom cluster |
|---|---|---|
| Reality distortion | Reality distortion | Delusions<br>Hallucinations |
| Disorganisation | Disorganisation | Formal thought disorder<br>Inappropriate affect<br>Disorganised or bizarre behaviour |
| Psychomotor | Psychomotor poverty | Flat affect<br>Poverty of speech<br>Decreased voluntary motor activity |
| | Psychomotor excitation | Labile affect<br>Pressure of speech<br>Motor agitation |
| Mood | Depression | Low mood<br>Low self-esteem<br>Hopelessness<br>Suicidality<br>Somatic symptoms |
| | Elation | Elevated mood<br>Elevated self-esteem<br>Decreased need for sleep |
| Anxiety | Anxiety | Feelings of unease, fear or dread<br>Overactivity of the sympathetic nervous system |

In this book, a cluster of symptoms is referred to as a syndrome, or as the expression of a dimension. A syndrome is a group of symptoms that tend to occur together. A dimension of an illness is a quantifiable aspect of the illness that can vary over a continuous range. A bipolar dimension is one in which deviations from normal can occur in either of two opposite directions.

While a focus on symptoms has proved to be a fruitful approach to delineating the relationship between the organisation of the brain and the organisation of the mind, specific pathological processes that damage neurons are likely to produce illnesses characterised by a particular symptom profile and time course. Hence, attempting to define diseases, as Kraepelin did, in terms of symptom profile and time course is likely to be relevant to an understanding of the relationship between mental disorders and pathological processes acting at the molecular level.

# The structure of this book

This book presents an examination of the evidence regarding the neural mechanisms of the seven major clusters of psychiatric symptoms, and then examines the way in which mental symptoms occur within several representative diseases, each characterised by a particular profile of symptoms and time course. The book is divided into three parts.

Part I assembles a description of the structure and function of the brain, with emphasis on the nature of the meaningful neural events associated with mental activity, particularly the neural processes that are implicated in mental disorders.

Part II provides a description of each of the major clusters of mental symptoms and delineates the neural circuits that are involved in the expression of those symptoms. The chapters of this section examine each of the five dimensions in turn. In each instance, the investigation begins with an examination of the nature of the symptoms and their interrelationships, with the object of defining the nature of the psychological processes involved. Then, various strands of evidence are drawn upon to identify the relevant neural systems implicated.

Part III examines three representative mental illnesses of early and middle adult life: schizophrenia, bipolar affective disorder and obsessive–compulsive disorder. It concludes with an examination of psychopathy, a personality disorder with a devastating impact on individuals and on society.

The book draws on studies employing the techniques of neuropsychology, cognitive psychology, electrophysiology, neuroimaging, neurochemistry and pharmacology. It attempts to integrate the diverse information from these fields into a coherent account of the cerebral processes by which symptoms are generated. It is intended for psychiatrists and psychologists with an interest in the origins of the symptoms they observe and treat, as well as for neuroscience students and researchers with an interest in the way that evidence gained in the laboratory may be related to the mental disorders that occur in clinical practice. Indeed, it is intended for anyone with a serious interest in how the mind works, and in how subtle disruptions of the brain can give rise to mental symptoms that cause personal devastation and great cost to society.

# Acknowledgements

The stimulus to write this book, and the ideas expressed within it, arose from countless discussions with my mentors, colleagues and students over a period of two decades. It was as a medical student, during an elective period spent working with Dr Tim Crow at Northwick Park Hospital, that I was inspired to devote my career to exploring the mechanisms of mental disorder, especially schizophrenia. While at Northwick Park, I was also influenced by the imagination and energy of Dr Eve Johnstone, Dr Chris Frith and Dr Bill Deakin. As a trainee psychiatrist in Oxford, I received rigorous mentoring from Dr Tamara Kowlakowska and Professor Michael Gelder. Subsequently, while working at Charing Cross and Westminster Medical School, my understanding of mental symptoms was sharpened by debate with Dr Thomas Barnes and Professor Steven Hirsch. The five years I spent at Hammersmith Hospital, where I was privileged to participate in exciting developments of the use of PET to map cerebral activity, was a period that transformed my approach to the brain. Professor Richard Frackowiak and Professor Terry Jones created an environment that encouraged imagination. Daily discussions with Dr Chris Frith and Dr Karl Friston led me to reformulate my understanding of neuroscience. More recently, my research students at the University of British Columbia have challenged and extended this understanding.

Above all, I am grateful to my wife, Elizabeth, who encouraged me to persist with writing when other demands on my time threatened to smother this book, and also provided many direct contributions. She not only offered frequent advice on stylistic issues, but also cast a shrewd lay person's eye over the scientific content.

*Peter Liddle*
*December 2000*

# Abbreviations

| | |
|---|---|
| ACTH | adrenocorticotrophic hormone |
| ATP | adenosine triphosphate |
| cAMP | cyclic 3,5-adenosine monophosphate |
| CBD | corticobasal degeneration |
| CCK | cholecystokinin |
| cGMP | cyclic guanosine monophosphate |
| CPT | continuous performance task |
| CREB | cAMP-responsive element-binding protein |
| CRF | corticotrophin-releasing factor |
| DAG | diacylglycerol |
| DSM–IV | *Diagnostic and Statistical Manual* (4th edn) |
| ERP | event-related potential |
| fMRI | functional magnetic resonance imaging |
| GABA | gamma-aminobutyric acid |
| GPe | globus pallidus externa |
| GPi | globus pallidus interna |
| GTP | guanosine triphosphate |
| 5-HIAA | 5-hydroxyindole acetic acid |
| HPA | hypothalamic–pituitary–adrenal [axis] |
| 5-HT | 5-hydroxytryptamine (serotonin) |
| HVA | homovanillic acid |
| IBZM | iodobenzamide |
| $IP_3$ | inositol triphosphate |
| LSD | lysergic acid diethylamide |
| $MAO_A$ | Monoamine oxidase A |
| m-CPP | m-chloro-phenyl-piperazine |
| MHPG | 3-methoxy-4-hydroxyphenylglycol |
| MRI | magnetic resonance imaging |
| MSA | multiple system atrophy |
| NMDA | N-methyl-D-aspartate |
| NO | nitric oxide |
| OCD | obsessional–compulsive disorder |
| PANSS | Positive and Negative Syndrome Scale |

| | |
|---|---|
| PCL–R | Psychopathy Checklist – Revised |
| PCP | phencyclidine |
| PET | positron emission tomography |
| PI | phosphatidyl inositol |
| PKC | protein kinase C |
| PSP | progressive supranuclear palsy |
| PTSD | post-traumatic stress disorder |
| PVN | paraventricular nucleus |
| rCBF | regional cerebral blood flow |
| SANS | Scale for the Assessment of Negative Symptoms |
| SAPS | Scale of the Assessment of Positive Symptoms |
| SMA | supplementary motor area |
| SNc | substantia nigra pars compacta |
| SNr | substantia nigra pars reticulata |
| SPET | single photon emission tomography |
| TDI | Thought Disorder Index |
| TLC | Thought, Language and Communication [assessment scale] |
| TLI | Thought and Language Index |
| VTA | ventral tegmental area |

# Part I

# Neuroanatomy and neurophysiology

**Chapter 1**

# The neural substrate of mental activity

## Introduction

The human brain synthesises information gleaned from a multiplicity of sensory systems, selects the most appropriate response and sends commands back to the periphery to mobilise skeletal muscles, visceral muscles, endocrine glands or the immune system. In this, it resembles the brain of other primates. However, a striking feature of much human behaviour is the looseness of the link between action and concurrent external circumstances. Not only is the information collected by sensory systems evaluated in the light of a vast and idiosyncratic compilation of information derived from previous experiences and a sophisticated estimation of future needs, but the motivation that governs the selection of action often appears to reflect a very abstract representation of the imperatives (self-defence, satisfaction of hunger and thirst, and reproduction) that govern animal behaviour.

Thus, while the human nervous system is indeed organised in a manner that allows the systematic processing of sensory information and the orderly execution of motor, endocrine and immunological responses, the dominant feature of the human brain is the mechanism that evaluates current information in light of a complex representation of past and future, and selects actions on a basis that transcends basic biological needs and enters a domain that might be described as aesthetic or spiritual. The delineation of the physical components of this sophisticated mechanism is far from complete. Its major elements are the thin crumpled layer of cortical grey matter that covers the cerebral hemispheres, the deep grey nuclei within the hemispheres, and the diencephalic structures, including the thalamus and hypothalamus, that connect the cerebral hemispheres to the brainstem, cerebellum, the peripheral nervous system and the endocrine system.

In this book we shall examine evidence leading to the conclusion that this extensive mesh of cortical and subcortical neurons acts as an integrated whole during the performance of mental activity. None the less, various subsystems can be identified within this neural system, based on both anatomical and functional considerations. It is convenient to divide the overall system into three overlapping components:

(1)   neocortical and palaeocortical association areas;
(2)   the limbic system;
(3)   cortico-subcortical loops, or feedback circuits.

This chapter provides an overview of the organisation of the entire system, with the object of constructing an outline of how it might support the motivational and supervisory aspects of human mental processing. The following three chapters will describe the three components of the system in greater detail.

Neocortical and palaeocortical association areas cover most of the lateral and much of the medial surfaces of the cerebral hemispheres (Plates 1–3). These areas combine information derived from the five external sensory systems – vision, hearing, smell, taste and somatic sensation – and supervise the execution of responses. They have a six-layered structure that is relatively uniform throughout, although there are regional differences in the ratio of pyramidal cells to granular cells, and in the presence or absence of certain neurochemical markers. There are also regional functional specialisations. The areas especially important for complex mental functions include the association cortex of the frontal, parietal and temporal lobes.

The limbic system consists of cortical and subcortical elements located on the medial aspect of the cerebral hemispheres. This system is especially involved in motivation and emotion. It facilitates the synthesis of information derived from sensory and cognitive processes in the cerebral hemispheres and from visceromotor centres at the base of the brain in a way that ensures that biological needs are met. In addition, the synthesised information is prepared for storage in memory. The structures of the limbic system include the hippocampus, amygdala, septal nuclei and part of the orbital cortex (Plate 4).

The limbic system can influence the function of the association cortex via directly projecting fibres and also by virtue of the ability of the hippocampus and amygdala to facilitate transmission through cortico-subcortical loops, which provide feedback to the frontal cortex. The cortico-subcortical loops follow paths through the deep grey matter of the cerebral hemispheres and the diencephalon. The deep grey nuclei comprise the basal ganglia, which include the corpus striatum and globus pallidus, and the thalamus. In its dorsal part, the corpus striatum is divided by the fibres of the internal capsule into the caudate nucleus and the putamen (Plate 5). These two grey masses are connected by strands of grey matter embedded in the internal capsule. The fibres of the internal capsule do not traverse the ventral part of the corpus striatum, and in this region the caudate and putamen cannot be distinguished.

Cortico-subcortical loops project from the cortex to the basal ganglia to the thalamus and back to the cortex. While the projections from the cortex to the basal ganglia are derived from widespread cortical areas, the loops largely project back to the frontal cortex. The architecture of the loops suggests that they modulate the activity in frontal cortical regions. Five parallel loops have been distinguished in the primate brain (Alexander *et al*, 1986). The extent to which there is interaction between these parallel loops remains an issue of debate, but evidence from animals suggests that information is transferred from the so-called 'limbic loop', which takes its origin in the ventromedial frontal cortex, to the other loops serving the prefrontal cortex, and finally converges on the motor loop, which serves the premotor cortex (Deutch *et al*, 1993). Such an architecture would support the transfer of information via a spiral path from the ventromedial prefrontal cortex towards the cortical regions engaged in the preparation of motor activity.

While this division of the brain into three major subdivisions resembles that specified by MacClean in his concept of the triune brain, the implied relationship between the three components is different. MacClean (1975) proposed three different types of mental processing, each controlled by one of three brain systems representing differing stages of evolution of the nervous system: the most primitive was the reptilian level, controlled by the brain-stem and basal ganglia, and assumed to be responsible for aggression and hostility; the second level was palaeomammalian processing, controlled by the limbic system and responsible for appetitive behaviour; the third level was neomammalian, characterised by neocortical control and responsible for objective cognition.

Some anatomical features provide partial support for the subdivision proposed by MacClean. In particular, the clearly layered isocortex (neo- and palaeocortex) forms a major part of the cerebrum of primates, especially man, while the less clearly layered allocortex (or archicortex) characteristic of the limbic system is relatively more prominent in supposedly primitive animals. However, the evidence we shall examine in subsequent chapters indicates that the three subdivisions are not self-contained systems that each serve a particular type of mental process, but rather groupings of elements that make a particular type of contribution to the collaborative execution of mental processes.

The view that the brain functions in an integrated manner is consistent with the dense connections found between anatomical elements from different subdivisions; and is supported by functional imaging studies of human subjects, which illustrate engagement of diverse cerebral areas during the performance of mental processes. Furthermore, a vast body of clinical evidence suggests an intimate link between cognition and emotion (Beck, 1976), and implies that the neural systems serving cognition and emotion do not function in isolation.

# Meaningful neural events

What is the nature of the meaningful neural events that correspond to specific mental events? In this context, the term 'mental event' could refer to a perception, thought, feeling, preparation for speech or motor activity, or memory. Penfield observed that stimulation by an electrode placed in the brain (during neuro-surgical exploration in a conscious patient) can evoke quite specific memories (Penfield & Rasmussen, 1950). This demonstrates that local electrical activity can trigger meaningful neural events. It is consistent with either of two types of neural process that might constitute a meaningful neural event. The first possibility is that a specific mental event corresponds to the generation of electrical action potentials in neurons located at a specific site. The second

**5**

possibility is that local electrical stimulation triggers a response in some distributed network of neurons connected to the site of stimulation.

## Barlow's cardinal neuron hypothesis

One influential attempt to describe meaningful neural events in terms of firing of neurons at a single location was the cardinal neuron hypothesis of Barlow (1972). According to Barlow's hypothesis, the majority of cortical neurons are cardinal neurons, each of which represents a particular facet of the perceived environment. At first sight, the cardinal neuron hypothesis is supported by the clinical evidence that patients with circumscribed focal brain lesions can suffer the isolated loss of the ability to identify a specific aspect of a sensory stimulus. For example, an individual might lose the capacity to recognise the face of a familiar person, while retaining the ability to recognise that person from their voice, or even from seeing their gait and posture. Thus it appears that the cues to the identification of the diverse attributes of a person are stored at multiple sites.

## The binding problem

Damasio *et al* (1990) have demonstrated that when a person can be recognised from any one of a variety of cues, each cue gives immediate access to the same set of attributes of that person. While the various components of the complete representation of the person may be distributed quite widely, these components must be bound together in some way. In it simplest form, the cardinal neuron hypothesis does not address this 'binding problem'. To make sense of a perception, it is necessary to know which features belong together.

One possibility is that the features of a single scene or event are bound together by synchronisation of the firing of the neurons representing different facets of that scene or event. Gray *et al* (1989) have demonstrated that pairs of neurons in the visual cortex with widely separated receptive fields exhibit synchronised firing when stimulated by a long bar that crosses both receptive fields. One way of promoting synchronicity would be a mechanism for establishing rhythmical firing such that all the neurons representing the same scene or event fire at the same frequency.

Regular rhythmic firing can be observed in the nervous system under many circumstances. For example, regular oscillations with a frequency of approximately 8–12 Hz (the alpha rhythm) can be recorded from the surface of the brain (or from the scalp) when a person is in a relaxed state with eyes closed. When the person is aroused by sensory stimulation or purposeful mental activity, the alpha rhythm gives way to high-frequency (25–80 Hz), lower-amplitude oscillations (Steriade & Amzica, 1996). The large amplitude of the alpha rhythm reflects coherence of the oscillations over extensive cortical areas. The lower amplitude of fast oscillations suggests less extensive coherence, but fast oscillations none the less exhibit coherence between widely separated cortical loci (Desmedt & Tomberg, 1994) and also between cortex and thalamus (Ribary *et al*, 1991).

There are several mechanisms by which cortical oscillations could be generated. One possibility is that some neurons have an intrinsic tendency to generate bursts of repetitive action potentials, which would induce trains of repetitive action potentials in the circuits containing these neurons. Another possibility is that oscillatory firing is a property of the circuits themselves. Mathematical modelling demonstrates that this is feasible. For example, Whittington *et al* (1995) have shown that a model system comprising groups of interneurons with realistic electrical characteristics exhibits oscillatory firing with a frequency of approximately 40 Hz as long as the interneurons are connected by inhibitory GABA-ergic synapses and also receive tonic excitation via glutamatergic synapses. Traub *et al* (1996) have demonstrated that groups of neurons that are locally interconnected in a manner similar to that modelled by Whittington *et al* (1995) can produce oscillations that are in phase over substantial distances.

If the predisposition to fire at a particular frequency was an established characteristic of a particular collection of neurons, it might facilitate the recruitment of that collection of neurons by the phenomenon of resonance. Oscillations in the gamma frequency band (around 40 Hz) in one region of the brain can induce gamma oscillations in a connected region. For example, Charpark *et al* (1995) demonstrated that in the guinea pig, production of gamma oscillations in the entorhinal cortex induced gamma oscillations in the CA1 region of the hippocampus. Thus, it is quite feasible that rhythmical firing would allow identification, and perhaps recruitment, of collections of neurons.

## Hippocampal theta waves in rodents

Theta waves are slow (4–10 Hz), rhythmical electrical waves detected in the vicinity of cell bodies in the CA1 area and in the dentate gyrus of the hippocampus during certain states of activity that correspond broadly to states of voluntary motor activity or, in some instances, responses to novel stimuli. The waves have large amplitude in rats and rabbits but much smaller amplitude in primates (Robinson, 1980) and, therefore, their relevance to humans is uncertain. However, the fact that they provide an illustration of neural activity that is temporally coordinated over an extensive area in association with purposeful, self-selected activity provides reason to consider them as a possible manifestation of supervisory mental activity.

Theta waves occur under a variety of circumstances. Typically, theta activity appears when an animal makes purposeful active movements. For example, Vanderwolf (1969) reported that hippocampal electrical activity in a rat was irregular while the rat was sitting nibbling fur on the right forepaw, became regular as the animal made a sudden postural shift to begin nibbling fur on the left forepaw, and then became irregular again during the renewed nibbling. The sensitivity of theta activity to pharmacological influence differs according to circumstance. Bland *et al* (1981) found that rhythmical firing in rabbit CA1 and dentate cells can be induced by a novel sensory stimulus while the rabbit remains motionless, and is also established during active hopping. Atropine, a muscarinic cholinergic receptor antagonist, abolishes the rhythmical firing induced by novel stimuli during immobility, but does not abolish the rhythmical firing associated with hopping. Destruction of the cholinergic input to the hippocampus from the nucleus of the diagonal band abolishes theta rhythms.

Evidence of coherent electrical oscillations in the hippocampus therefore supports the hypothesis that the concurrent activation of large numbers of neurons within a distributed network will be facilitated if the neurons comprising that network share a tendency to fire repetitively at a characteristic frequency. Neurons tending to fire repetitively at the characteristic frequency would readily become entrained as activation grew within the network.

## Gamma oscillations in humans

High-frequency oscillations (in the gamma band, 25–80 Hz) can be detected in the human brain under various circumstances. They appear to arise spontaneously in the alert brain, but can also be induced by various cognitive operations including calculation, thinking, reading, listening to music and the initiation of voluntary movements (Sheer, 1989). Gamma oscillations can also be induced by simple sensory stimuli, such as brief sounds, in which case the oscillations are time-locked to the stimuli (Pantev et al, 1991). Comparison of auditory and visual evoked potentials between the conscious and unconscious state in humans indicates that the presence of 30–40 Hz neural oscillatory activity in the mid-latency period, 20–120 ms after the stimulus, is a feature of the conscious state (Madler et al, 1991).

Ribary et al (1991) used magneto-encephalography to explore the possibility that gamma oscillations are generated by reverberation in thalamo-cortical circuits. Consistent with this hypothesis, they found well defined 40 Hz coherence between cortico-subcortical sites with a time shift that is consistent with thalamo-cortical conduction times. Synchronised gamma oscillations can be recorded from widely separated locations on the head when a person is required to choose a motor response on the basis of a sensory discrimination task. For example, Desmedt & Tomberg (1994) delivered weak electrical stimulation to one of four fingers and asked the subjects to move the corresponding toe to indicate which finger had been stimulated. Between the stimulus and response, synchronised gamma oscillations were recorded over contralateral parietal and prefrontal areas. The investigators interpreted their observations as evidence that gamma oscillations reflect the binding of neural activity at a widely distributed set of cortical sites so as to achieve a coordinated act.

## Organisation within networks

On the grounds of the evidence, such as that provided by Damasio et al (1990), that cues to the identification of a person are stored at multiple sites, together with consideration of the question of how the separate facets of a particular scene or event might be bound together, it appears that the representation of a particular meaningful event is unlikely to be represented by a single neuron (or local group of neurons), but rather by a network of neurons distributed across a variety of sites.

How might the proposed neural networks be organised? The two types of organisation might occur: hierarchical chains and distributed parallel networks. It appears that the preliminary stages of processing in sensory systems are mainly hierarchical. Sensory information is processed sequentially in chains of neurons extending from the peripheral sense organs into the cerebral cortex, with successive neurons in the chains gleaning information about increasingly abstract features of the stimulus.

In the visual system, there are two major processing streams. One stream, which projects from primary visual cortex to the parietal cortex, is concerned with identifying the location of a perceived object, while the other, which projects from the primary cortex to the inferior temporal cortex, is concerned with identifying what the object is. There are many distinguishable cerebral sites within each of these two processing streams, each of which has a specific role. In the macaque monkey, the identified locations on the pathway towards the inferior temporal cortex include the areas designated V1, V4 and IT. In area V1 (primary visual cortex), individual neurons respond to simple stimuli such as lines with a specific orientation. Area V4 is devoted to the perception of form. In this area, neurons respond to relatively complex non-rectilinear geometrical forms. Region IT (inferior temporal cortex) contains pattern-recognition neurons that fire when the perceived object matches the stored representation of an identifiable object. For example, individual neurons respond to a face or to a hand, irrespective of features such as spatial location or size (Van Essen *et al*, 1992).

Even within hierarchical sensory processing pathways, there are connections that allow 'top down' regulation of which aspects of a complex sensory stimulus are subject to attention. Many of the forward projections from processing sites early in the chain to later processing sites are matched with reciprocal projections in the reverse direction. In addition, each of the processing stages is subject to direct influence from the thalamus. For example, in the visual 'object recognition' pathway, areas V1, V4 and IT all receive direct projections from the pulvinar nucleus of the thalamus (Van Essen *et al*, 1992).

Sequential processing in a hierarchical (linear) chain of neurons is unlikely to be appropriate for complex mental processing because of the length of time it would require. It is more likely that the association cortex functions as a parallel distributed network, arranged so that the neural elements are connected via a network of multiple recursive paths connecting the individual elements, enabling concurrent processing at widely distributed sites.

The concept of such distributed, parallel processing has informed many recent attempts to describe cortical function associated with psychological processes (Rumelhart & McClelland, 1986). Mathematical models based on such an approach have even been used to simulate some of the cognitive processes presumed to underlie the symptoms of schizophrenia (Cohen & Servan-Schreiber, 1992).

## The strength of meaningful neural events

If we assume that meaningful neural events entail the firing of neurons in a distributed network that allows parallel processing, we must then address the issue of how the strength of a meaningful event might be represented. It appears that particular mental processes can be performed with continuously varying levels of intensity. At one extreme, mental processes can be subliminal: processing may occur at a level well outside conscious awareness, with minimal influence on current behaviour, yet the fruits of this subliminal processing emerge to influence behaviour at a later time. At the other extreme, a mental process can be sufficiently dominant to be experienced consciously and to play a major part in determining current behaviour.

Individual neurons typically have dendritic trees containing large numbers of synapses and the electrical state of each neuron is determined by the summation of many influences. None the less, the majority of neurons (apart from amacrine neurons) fire in an all-or-none manner. Therefore, gradations of strength are likely to be represented in either the frequency of firing of the neurons involved, or the number of neurons involved. As discussed above, there is reason to suppose that the frequency of firing serves as a identifier of neurons belonging to a particular assembly. It is therefore less likely that gradations in frequency of firing also represent gradations in strength.

The possibility that the strength of a particular meaningful neural event is reflected by the number of neurons recruited is supported by some approximate estimates of the relative abundance of different neuronal types and of the patterns of connections between neurons. The total number of neurons in the human neocortex is around 27 billion (Braengaard et al, 1990). In primate visual cortex, each cortical neuron receives about 4000 synapses (Beaulieu et al, 1992). Since a neuron usually makes only a few connections with any single target neuron, the input to a specific neuron reflects the converging influence from many neurons, and its output in turn diverges to influence a large number of neurons. Approximately 80% of cortical synapses are excitatory, mostly involving glutamate as the neurotransmitter, and 20% are inhibitory connections that involve the neurotransmitter gamma-aminobutyric acid (GABA). For example, in the visual cortex of primates, 20% of neurons are GABA-ergic (Beaulieu et al, 1992). While it is probable that every cortical neuron receives at least one GABA-ergic connection, allowing active inhibition of that neuron, the implications of a cortical architecture in which neurons are linked mainly by excitatory connections in a web-like structure, creating multiple pathways between neurons, is that positive feedback is a prevalent phenomenon. The potential significance of excitatory synapses in cortical function was appreciated by Hebb (1949) in his seminal proposal that a meaningful neural event might consist of the explosive ignition of an assembly of cells connected by excitatory synapses. Once ignited, the activity in such an assembly would be expected to persist for a period of time due to mutual excitation of its constituent neurons.

A more detailed examination of connections between cortical neurons (Chapter 2) leads to the conclusion that local excitatory interactions are dominant. In particular, there appear to be strong excitatory connections between pyramidal cells lying within columns of diameter of the order of 230 $\mu$m (oriented perpendicular to the cortical surface). In addition, there are excitatory connections extending over a horizontal distance of several millimetres, but in these longer-range connections a collateral axon of a presynaptic neuron makes contact with the branches of the dendritic tree distant from the cell body of the postsynaptic neuron. Such connections are unlikely to produce firing of the postsynaptic neuron unless it is coincident with some other excitatory input, such as input from thalamocortical projections.

As a consequence of this arrangement of local excitatory connections in the cortex, activation of pyramidal cells in an area that was receiving substantial concurrent excitatory input from thalamocortical projections would lead to a diffuse area of activation extending over a distance of several millimetres. As discussed in greater detail in Chapter 4, it appears that subcortical circuits providing feedback to the cortex via excitatory thalamocortical projections play a major role in moderating cortical function, especially in frontal association cortical areas.

Consequently, the pattern of activity comprising a meaningful neural event that is receiving reinforcement via subcortical feedback loops would be likely to include a diffuse area of neural activity at neocortical loci, especially in frontal areas. Thus it is likely that mental acts (thoughts and emotions) are associated with distributed neural activity that becomes less precisely localised as the strength of the neural activity grows. This arrangement offers several potential advantages. First, by virtue of recruitment of increasing numbers of neurons, it would allow graduated levels of strength of the pattern of neural activity associated with a particular mental act. Second, it would encourage overlap between the sets of neurons involved in different mental acts, thereby facilitating the emergence of novel patterns of mental activity when different mental acts occur simultaneously.

# Mapping meaningful neural events

Because of the inaccessibility of the living human brain, it is necessary to use indirect methods to glean the information required to map the neural events that underlie human mental activity. In this book we shall draw upon a variety of methods that between them provide information about the time course, cerebral location and neurotransmitters involved in mental activity. All of these methods have important limitations that must be taken into account when evaluating the evidence. Therefore, it is appropriate to review these various methods briefly at this point.

## Observations of performance and behaviour

Patterns of performance and behaviour under various circumstances provide important clues regarding the nature of underlying neural processes. The observation that the vast graduated range of colours that can be perceived by the human visual system are represented by various combinations of three primary colours indicates that there are three types of colour-sensitive neurons in the retina. Similarly, observations regarding more complex operations provide clues regarding the organisation of the neural systems that support such operations. For example, how does the brain manage to recognise objects irrespective of their orientation and location? It would scarcely be practical to have a stored representation of all familiar objects in every possible orientation and location. Cooper & Shephard (1973) devised a test of the ability to recognise letters of the alphabet in various orientations that provided part of the answer to this question. They presented letters or mirror images of letters in various orientations. The participants in their study were required to indicate whether the object was a letter or the mirror image of a letter. Cooper & Shephard found that the time taken to make the decision was proportional to the angular displacement of the presented letter from its usual upright orientation. This indicates that one step in the recognition of a familiar object is mental rotation to its usual orientation.

Of major importance with regard to understanding the mechanism of mental symptoms is the observation of consistent patterns of mental symptoms discernible in various different disorders; this provides clues about the organis-ation of the underlying neural processes. This observation is the foundation for the approach that we shall adopt in Part II of this book, in which we explore the patterns of neural activity associated with various clusters of mental symptoms. However, observation of behaviour alone only provides clues regarding the types of functional units that may exist in the human brain. It cannot provide information about the location of those units or the molecular mechanisms by which neurons execute the required tasks.

## The consequences of focal brain lesions

When a focal lesion destroys the ability to perform a specific task, we can conclude that the relevant brain site is likely to play a crucial role in that task and, furthermore, we can sometimes draw conclusions about the organisation of the underlying functional units. The confidence of our conclusion is even stronger if we observe a double dissociation. A double dissociation is a converse pattern of deficits in two patients who have suffered different brain injuries. For example, Etcoff et al (1991) described a patient who had previously suffered a head injury in a car accident who could recognise most familiar objects easily but was unable to recognise faces, even the faces of his wife and children. This defect is known as propagnosia. Behrman et al (1992) described a young man who suffered the converse deficit after a different type of head injury. He could not recognise most everyday objects but had no trouble identifying faces. These observations demonstrate that face recognition is achieved by a different mental mechanism than recognition of familiar objects with other geometrical characteristics. However clear-cut double dissociations are rare.

## Neuroendocrine measurements

In many instances, the administration of pharmacological agents that act on specific neurotransmitter systems, or that bind to hormone receptor sites in the central nervous system, leads to release of a hormone from the pituitary gland. For example, in Chapter 9, we shall examine evidence regarding the effects of agents that act at pre- and postsynaptic serotonin receptors on the release of prolactin and of cortisol. However, neuroendocrine studies alone cannot determine whether or not the observed effects reflects a generalised change in a particular type of neuroreceptor throughout the brain, or a localised change in a specific pathway that regulates the pituitary. In instances where neuroendocrine abnormalities are observed to be associated with mental symptoms, such as depression, it is often assumed that the abnormality reflects a generalised change in the relevant neuroreceptor. However, when such an interpretation is made, it is important to ask whether or not there are grounds for assuming a generalised change.

## Imaging neuroreceptors

Positron emission tomography (PET) and single photon emission tomography (SPET) can be used to measure the distribution of radioactively labelled tracers in the brain. When the tracer is a ligand for a specific neuroreceptor, the distribution of the labelled tracer provides a quantitative measure of the spatial distribution of accessible receptors. However, not only are there many technical difficulties in preparing a labelled tracer that binds with high specificity to the receptor of interest, and in executing the imaging procedure, but there are intrinsic uncertainties regarding the behaviour of ligands *in vivo* that complicate the interpretation of the observed binding of the administered ligand. In particular, the administered ligand must compete with any endogenous ligand that is present. A decrease in the amount of tracer that binds to receptors in a particular condition may reflect either a decrease in receptor number or an increase in the concentration of endogenous ligand occupying the receptors, thus making fewer available.

The situation is made even more complex by the fact that competition between endogenous ligand and administered ligand does not appear to obey the laws of equilibrium binding that are observed *in vitro*. If the administered radio-ligand is present at trace concentrations that occupy only a minute proportion of the available receptors, the number of available receptors should be determined by the total number of receptors and the concentration of endogenous ligand. The relative affinities of the endogenous ligand and the administered ligand for the receptor should have a negligible effect on the observed density of available receptors. The number of available receptors should be the total density of receptors minus the proportion occupied by the endogenous ligand, irrespective of the presence of trace amounts of the radio-ligand. However, that is not what is observed. The binding of administered ligands that bind very strongly to the receptor appears to be unaffected by the presence of endogenous ligand, whereas ligands that bind weakly are sensitive to the presence of endogenous ligand.

For example, the dopamine $D_2$ ligand N-methylspiperone, which binds very tightly to the $D_2$ receptor, is apparently insensitive to the presence of endogenous ligand, whereas raclopride, which binds relatively weakly, is affected by endogenous ligand, although less strongly than would be predicted. This has led to apparently contradictory findings regarding $D_2$ receptor density in the basal ganglia in schizophrenia, measured by different investigators using different tracers. Wong *et al* (1986), using N-methylspiperone, found an apparent increase in $D_2$ receptor density in previously unmedicated schizophrenic patients relative to healthy subjects, while Farde *et al* (1988), who employed raclopride, found no generalised increase, although they did find an increase in the left putamen relative to the right.

The reason for the anomalous competition between endogenous and administered ligands remains a subject of debate. None the less, if one accepts that administered ligands with a very high affinity are unaffected by endogenous ligands while those that are weakly bound are affected, it is possible to reconcile the apparently conflicting data regarding $D_2$ receptors in schizophrenia. Furthermore, by measuring available receptors using raclopride before and after a pharmacological procedure that depletes endogenous dopamine, it is in principle possible to estimate both the total $D_2$ receptor density and the baseline concentration of endogenous dopamine. In a series of experiments using iodobenzamide, a weakly binding SPET ligand which has similar affinity to that of raclopride, Abi-Dargham *et al* (2000) have obtained evidence indicating that schizophrenic patients have both an increase in their baseline level of endogenous dopamine in the synaptic cleft and also an increase in the total number of receptors, compared with healthy subjects. The potential significance of this is discussed Chapter 11.

In principle, using PET or SPET with a weakly binding radio-ligand, it is possible to measure the release of endogenous neurotransmitters associated with the performance of mental or motor tasks. Using PET with raclopride, Koepp *et al* (1998) measured the release of endogenous dopamine in the basal ganglia during performance of a game that was expected to be strongly motivating.

As long as the nature of the competition between administered ligands and endogenous ligands *in vivo* remains uncertain, the interpretation of *in vivo* ligand binding studies must be made with caution. While there is an emerging consensus that the binding of ligands that have a weak affinity for dopamine $D_2$ receptors is influenced by the presence of endogenous dopamine, for most other PET or SPET ligands it is unknown to what extent their binding is affected by the presence of endogenous neurotransmitter.


## Event-related electrical potentials

Following the presentation of many types of stimuli, event-related potentials (ERPs) can be recorded using scalp electrodes over a time scale of 0–1000 ms following the stimulus. One of the most intensively studied ERP paradigms is the oddball task, in which a series of rare (sparsely distributed) target stimuli are embedded in a train of frequent non-target stimuli. The potentials elicited by the target stimuli differ from those elicited by the non-target stimuli in several respects. The most prominent feature is a large positive potential, known as the P300 component, recorded approximately 300 ms after the stimulus. The amplitude, latency and scalp distribution of the P300 elicited by oddball stimuli is sensitive to processes involved in the allocation of attention and to processes involved in contextual updating, decision-making and response selection (Donchin & Coles, 1988; Alexander *et al*, 1995, 1996). A reduction in amplitude of the P300 is observed in schizophrenia (Chapter 11) and in other disorders, including psychopathy (Chapter 14).

The fact that the electrical currents generated in the brain following the presentation of simple stimuli are large enough to be detected at the scalp implies that a very large number of neurons, possibly numbering several millions, have been activated in a manner that is time-locked to the stimulus. This observation adds to the grounds for proposing that meaningful neural events entail the firing of large numbers of neurons. Indeed, intracerebral recording demonstrates that the presentation of oddball stimuli leads to time-locked neural activity at many cerebral sites (Halgren *et al*, 1998). While it is probable that activation at such a diverse array of sites is not essential for the execution of the simple response that the task demands, the occurrence of widespread activation suggests that the brain normally achieves potential flexibility in its responses by extensive activation. We shall re-examine this issue in Chapter 2, in the light of further evidence obtained employing functional magnetic resonance imaging (fMRI).

The major limitation of interpreting scalp ERPs is the difficulty of defining the anatomical location of the neural sources. The use of intracerebral electrodes is too invasive for use in all except special circumstances.

## Imaging regional cerebral blood flow

The evidence we have examined indicates that meaningful neural events may entail activity in a distributed network in such a manner that at each of the cortical loci involved there is coherent activation of neurons in an area extending over several millimetres. One corollary of this is that the patterns of activation are accessible to macroscopic imaging techniques that measure local changes in regional cerebral blood flow (rCBF) associated with changes in the metabolic requirements of active neurons. Techniques such as PET and fMRI can be used to provide images of rCBF with a spatial resolution of several millimetres. SPET provides images of rCBF with somewhat less sensitivity and resolution. It is likely that the demand for increased rCBF during neuronal firing will be greatest in the vicinity of the synapses, since synaptic processes consume a substantial amount of energy.

In principle, the activation of either excitatory neurons or inhibitory neurons can cause an increase in rCBF. In practice, it is likely that whenever neurons in a particular cortical location are engaged in meaningful processing, local circuits that include both excitatory and inhibitory neurons will be active, since a combination of excitatory and inhibitory neurotransmission would generally be required to produce meaningful temporal and spatial patterns of neural activity. None the less, because the major long-range fibres that bring specific information from a distant site to the local circuit are excitatory glutamatergic fibres, and these incoming fibres usually form synapses with many local neurons (Plates 6 and 7), it is reasonable to assume that an increase in local CBF reflects an increase in excitatory input to that location, while a decrease in local CBF reflects a decrease in excitatory input to that location.

Studies using PET confirm that mental processes are associated with activation at a distributed set of cerebral loci, with relatively extensive activation at each locus. For example, in studies of word generation carried out in collaboration with colleagues at Hammersmith Hospital (Frith *et al*, 1991a, 1991b), we found that during the internal generation of words beginning with a specified letter, there is activation of extensive regions in the left dorsolateral and medial frontal cortex, posterior cingulate and thalamus, while there is a diminution of activity in the superior temporal gyrus. The extent of activation in these regions was substantially greater than would be accounted for by smoothing arising from sources such as the limited spatial resolution of the PET camera. In these studies, the pattern of cerebral activity associated with the internal generation of words was determined by subtracting the pattern of activity during the articulation of a list of words provided by the experimenter from the pattern of activity during the articulation of words generated by the subject.

# Multiplex relationships between mental processes and neural elements

In the previous section we discussed evidence from imaging studies supporting the proposition that meaningful neural events entail the firing of neurons at diverse sites. Unlike the situation in those brain areas devoted to sensory perception or to the execution of motor acts, where each cerebral site has a very specialised role, the areas of the multimodal association cortex, limbic system and deep nuclei that are engaged during mental activity are likely to be called upon to engage in an open-ended range of activities. Does each site make its own unique contribution to the integrated action of the network during a given task? If that site is activated during a variety of tasks, does it play a similar role in each task?

In our studies of the internal generation of mental activity, we studied not only the internal generation of words, but also the internal generation of sequences of finger movements (Frith *et al*, 1991b). In the latter studies, cerebral activity during the execution of a random sequence of finger movements, in an order determined by the experimenter, was subtracted from cerebral activity during performance of a random sequence of similar movements determined by the subject. We found that the internal generation of finger movement engages the left dorsolateral and medial frontal cortex, while there is suppression of activity at a site in the left parietal cortex.

Comparison of similarities and differences between the patterns associated with the generation of words and finger movements suggests that the left dorsolateral and medial prefrontal cortex and anterior cingulate are implicated in the internal generation of verbal output and of motor actions. By comparing patterns of cerebral activity during two tasks that have common features, we were able to identify the sites that are likely to be engaged in the shared aspects of mental processing. By this process we have determined that several frontal sites are likely to be involved in generating diverse types of activity.

Do these different frontal sites activated during both word generation and movement generation make distinguishable contributions to the internal generation of action? To address this question, it is necessary first of all to dissect the task of generating activity into its various elements, and then to examine the findings of studies of cerebral activity recorded during other tasks that share some but not all of these elementary processes. Currently, there are many uncertainties regarding the roles of the various regions within the association cortex, limbic system and deep nuclei that are engaged during mental processes, and any conclusions must be regarded as tentative. None the less, it is informative to examine the findings from other relevant studies with the object of identifying the roles of the sites that we found to be engaged during the generation of words and finger movements.

What are the various processing elements common to the generation of words and finger movements? First, it is necessary to maintain a temporary memory trace of what one is doing. Not only is it necessary to remember the task instructions, but it is also necessary to remember what has been produced previously. In the word generation task, it is necessary to remember what words have already been produced, to avoid duplication. (The participant is instructed to produce as many different words within the specified category as possible.) In the finger movement task, production of a 'random' sequence of movements requires remembering the preceding few movements. Second, it is necessary to initiate the search for each new word or movement. In the case of word generation, this requires activation of the neural representations of words from a large store. In the case of finger movements, the repertoire of possible movements is much more limited. Third, it is necessary to select one item (word or finger movement) from among those items whose neural representation has been activated. In the case of word generation, this entails checking that the item belongs to the appropriate category and suppressing inappropriate responses. In the case of the generation of finger movements, it is necessary to ensure that a potential movement is not systematically related to the previous few movements in the sequence. It might be argued that selection of the appropriate action and suppressing inappropriate actions are two distinct steps performed by different neural assemblies; alternatively they may be two aspects of a single process. At this stage we shall leave this question open.

Subsequent steps in the execution of the selected response are not relevant to the interpretation of these studies, because these steps were also performed in the baseline comparison condition. Therefore, in summary, the three processes that are common to the two generation tasks are:

(1)  maintaining a memory trace of ongoing activity;
(2)  activating the neural representations of potential words or movements;
(3)  selecting an appropriate word or movement and rejecting inappropriate ones.

Maintaining a memory trace of ongoing activity is an aspect of working memory. Several studies have demonstrated that the left lateral frontal cortex is engaged during working memory tasks. For example, the left lateral frontal cortex is activated during the *N*-back task (Cohen *et al*, 1994; Awh *et al*, 1996), in which a series of stimuli are presented on a visual display unit and the participant is required to respond whenever the current stimulus is identical to that presented *N* items previously. It is noteworthy that this task does not require any internal generation of actions, as the required response is specified entirely by the rules of the task. It is therefore plausible that the left lateral frontal activation observed during the generation of both words and finger movements reflects the working memory aspects of the task.

A clue to the cerebral site engaged in initiating the activation of the neural representations of potential words or movements is provided by the observation that damage to the medial frontal cortex, for example as a consequence of stroke, can result in akinetic mutism, a condition in which the patient cannot speak or move (Barris & Schuman, 1953). More recently, in a PET study in which the participants indicated the occurrence of incidental thoughts that were unrelated to an identifiable stimulus, while engaged in various tasks, McGuire *et al* (1996) demonstrated that the occurrence of stimulus-independent thoughts was correlated with rCBF in the medial prefrontal region. Thus the medial prefrontal cortex is implicated in the initiation of both thought and action.

A variety of studies indicate that the anterior cingulate is involved in the selection of responses and suppression of inappropriate responses. Studies of cerebral activity during the Stroop task reveal activation of the anterior cingulate and adjacent medial prefrontal cortex (Pardo *et al*, 1990). In this task, colour names printed in an incongruent ink colour (e.g. RED in green ink) are presented and the participant is required to name the colour of the ink. Correct performance requires suppression of the dominant tendency to respond to the colour name. The studies of cerebral activity during the Stroop task do not establish whether the anterior cingulate is engaged in specifically suppressing an inappropriate response or in making a response in the face of competing responses.

In an event-related fMRI study of cerebral activity during a version of the continuous performance task, in which the participant was required to respond whenever a specified target stimulus was presented, Carter *et al* (1998) demonstrated that the anterior cingulate was activated not only during trials in which no responses were made, but also during trials in which correct responses were made, under conditions involving strong response competition. To clarify this issue further, my colleagues and I carried out an event-related fMRI study using a 'go/no go' task in which the probability of 'go' and 'no go' events was equal, thereby allowing an unbiased comparison of activity during 'go' and 'no go' trials (Liddle *et al*, 2001). We found that the anterior cingulate was equally engaged during 'go' and 'no go' trials, thus supporting the hypothesis that the anterior cingulate is engaged whenever there is competition between responses. The magnitude of this activation was similar irrespective of whether the appropriate action was a motor response or suppression of a response.

While our conclusions should be regarded as tentative, the available evidence indicates that each of the three frontal sites that were activated during the generation of both words and finger movements made a specific contribution to the achievement of the task. The left lateral frontal cortex is likely to have been engaged in maintaining a memory trace of ongoing activity. The medial prefrontal cortex is implicated in activating the neural representations of potential words or movements. The anterior cingulate is likely to have played a cardinal role in selecting an appropriate word or movement and rejecting inappropriate ones.

The more posterior areas in which rCBF was decreased during the internal generation of either words or sequences of finger movements, relative to the level of activity during the relevant control task, were more specific to the mode of activity. The superior temporal gyrus (corresponding approximately to Wernicke's area), in which activity was suppressed during the generation of words, plays a specialised role in processing words. It might be anticipated that this area would be activated when the neural representation of a word is activated, and hence activation of the area (relative to a hypothetical resting baseline) would be anticipated during word generation. However, in our studies, the cerebral activity during word generation was compared with that during articulation of words supplied by the experimenter. Hence, in both the conditions, representations of words were activated. Our observation of suppression during the internal generation of words relative to the comparison task suggests that in circumstances where the activation of the appropriate representation depends on information derived from the external world via the senses, Wernicke's area is more strongly activated.

Similarly, activity in the parietal cortex was less during the internal generation condition compared with the comparison condition, in which the required movement was specified by a touch on the dorsum of the appropriate finger (Frith *et al*, 1991b). The clinical observation that damage to the parietal cortex results in finger agnosia, in which the patient is unable to identify his/her fingers, indicates that activation of the parietal cortex might be expected when an individual identifies which finger he/she is about to move. Hence it would be anticipated that the parietal cortex would be activated (relative to a hypothetical resting baseline) during both the internal generation task and during the comparison condition. However, analogous to the situation with word generation, our findings indicate that activation in this area is greater when the required response depends on information derived from the external world via the senses.

The observation of relative suppression in the left superior temporal gyrus during internal generation of words, and in the left parietal cortex during internal generation of finger movements, suggests a 'top down' regulation of the amount of activation in the relevant areas of the sensory association cortex so as to minimise interference by extraneous information from the external world during the internal generation of action.

# Motivation

In the light of the observation that mental activity and behaviour are only loosely correlated with concurrent external circumstances, a cardinal issue in understanding human mental activity is the question of how a particular activity is selected from the array of possible activities potentially accessible at a particular time. What determines the selection? Human motivation has two striking characteristics: the ability to plan for the achievement of long-term goals and the diversity of the types of experience that provide motivation. Humans can be motivated not only by the importance of events to survival but also by the need to enhance self-esteem; curiosity; fulfilment of prediction; aesthetic appreciation; and hedonistic satisfaction.

The ability to postpone gratification, and the diversity of motivating experiences, is probably closely linked with the ability to employ language to formulate goals and plans for achieving them, in abstract terms, thereby facilitating the pursuit of goals that are independent of current sensory input. Although highly developed language is a human characteristic, motivational mechanisms in animals have some characteristics that allow the postponement of gratification, and the diversification of motivating experiences. Examination of these mechanisms in animals gives some insight into the way they may operate in humans.

For example, many animals hoard food at times of surplus. In rats, lesions of the mesolimbic dopaminergic cell bodies in the ventral tegmental area (VTA) of the midbrain abolish the tendency to collect and hoard surplus food. Lesioned animals simply attempt to eat the food in a poorly organised manner. Treatment with oral L-dopa, the metabolic precursor of dopamine, which indirectly promotes dopaminergic neurotransmission, completely restores normal hoarding behaviour (Kelley & Stinus, 1985).

A major mechanism by which dopaminergic neurotransmission regulates behaviour is modulation of the cortico-subcortical loops that provide feedback to the frontal cortex. The amount of feedback to the frontal cortex is determined by two major influences: gating by the limbic system, and modulation by mono-aminergic neurons, including dopaminergic neurons projecting from the midbrain. To understand the way in which dopamine could contribute to the regulation of behaviour, it is necessary first to examine the way in which the limbic system gates the cortico-subcortical loops.

The gating action of the limbic system is mediated via projections from hippocampus and amygdala, the principal components of the limbic system, to the striatum, which is the site of the first relay station in the feedback loops (Grace *et al*, 1998). Transmission in the fronto-subcortical loops can occur only while there is input from the hippocampus to the striatum. As we shall discuss in Chapter 3, there is evidence supporting the proposal that the hippocampus acts as a comparator, such that hippocampal neurons fire when they receive a combination of inputs that matches a previously reinforced pattern. When the current pattern of cortical activity is a good enough match to a previously reinforced pattern, hippocampal firing may open the striatal gate, thereby further enhancing the current pattern of cortical activity. Thus, the hippocampus has the characteristics of a comparator that can identify and promote patterns of cerebral activity that represent mental events consistent with the individual's goals. The amygdala exerts a gating influence complementary to that of the hippocampus. The evidence suggests that the amygdala identifies immediately threatening circumstances and facilitates an appropriate response.

Monoaminergic projections from the midbrain to the striatum modulate feedback mediated via the cortico-subcortical loops. For example, an increase in dopaminergic input to the striatum from the substantia nigra or the VTA in the midbrain tends to promote positive feedback to the cortex (Chapter 4), and thus promotes patterns of brain activity that have triggered hippocampal firing. Hence, adjustment of the level of dopaminergic activity can promote or inhibit the mental processing.

In both animals and humans, dopaminergic release in the striatum is increased by challenging circumstances (Thierry et al, 1976; Koepp et al, 1998). However, the processes by which dopamine release in the striatum is regulated are complex. Evidence from studies of animals indicates that projections from the frontal cortex to the midbrain normally act to control excessive rises in dopaminergic activity in the ventral striatum during stress. However, when the stress is too great, the regulation by the frontal cortex is insufficient, and there is a rise in ventral striatal dopaminergic activity that is manifest in overactivity and stereotyped behaviour (Thierry et al, 1976; Deutch et al, 1990). In contrast, when an animal is subjected to chronic mild stress, there is a compensatory decrease in dopamine $D_2$ receptor density in the ventral striatum that is associated with loss of interest in pleasurable activities (Willner et al, 1991).

Thus motivation appears to be mediated by modulatory monoaminergic neurotransmitters that regulate the level of activation of neural assemblies representing specific behaviours. Conversely, the action of neural assemblies responsible for processing information, especially stressful information, modify the activity of the monoaminergic systems, altering the strength of motivation.

# Generation of mental activity: a hypothesis

The processes by which mental activity is generated and monitored are central to understanding the neural mechanism of mental symptoms. The evidence reviewed briefly above, and discussed in greater detail in Chapters 2–5, provides a framework for understanding how mental activity may be generated and monitored. The cardinal tenets on which this framework is constructed are:

(1)   Mental activity, such as an idea or a plan to act, is represented by a distributed pattern of neural activity and the strength of this representation is increased by recruiting a larger number of neurons.

(2)   At any time, the neural representations of many mental events that have been salient in the recent past are active at a subliminal level. The plausibility of this hypothesis is demonstrated by the phenomenon of priming. For example, in a lexical decision task in which the participant is required to determine whether or not a sequence of letters constitutes a word, the speed of word recognition is increased by prior presentation of a semantically related word. For example, 'chair' is recognised more quickly if it is preceded by the word 'table'.

(3)  The neural representations of related mental events overlap. Study of priming reveals that the presentation of a word primes a hierarchical array of semantically related words. Thus activation of the representation of a particular mental event may spread so that the representation of related mental events are also activated.

(4)  Although the precise mechanism is unclear, there is accumulating evidence supporting the hypothesis that the hippocampus acts as a comparator of the existing pattern of neural activity in the brain with a representation of short- and long-term goals. Studies of regional cerebral activity during the performance of tasks that place high demands on the need to compare imagined speech with an internally maintained template (McGuire *et al*, 2000) or to compare actions with goals (Frith *et al*, 1992) have reported activation of the hippocampus and parahippocampal gyrus.

(5)  The output of the putative hippocampal comparator can amplify the represent-ation of a specific neural event, by virtue of the way that transmission through the striatum is gated by hippocampal output (Grace *et al*, 1998). The striatum is the first relay station in the cortico-subcortical loops that regulate frontal cortical activity, and so can allow the amplification of a specific pattern of cortical neural activity.

(6)  Once the strength of the representation of a particular mental event has become sufficiently strong, it may capture attention and trigger a motor response, prepared via neural activity in the supplementary motor area (SMA) and the lateral premotor cortex. The feedback loops that regulate the frontal cortex are not entirely segregated but tend to funnel information towards the loop that regulates the SMA and premotor cortex.

While these tenets are speculative, the existing evidence supports them. Together, they provide a mechanism by which mental and motor activity may be generated and monitored. In summary: at any point in time the representation of multiple recent events would be active; by virtue of the way in which activation could spread to the representation of related mental events, the representations of a range of related ideas or actions, including potentially novel combinations, might also be active. The hippocampal comparator would test emerging patterns against the representation of the individual's goals. Those neural representations consistent with goals might be amplified via the cortico-subcortical feedback loops, eventually reaching an intensity that captured attention. If the pattern of cerebral activity included activation of the premotor cortex, a voluntary motor response would ensue.

# Conclusions

The evidence indicates that the meaningful neural events associated with mental events consist of activity in an extensive neural network. While the firing of individual neurons or local groups of neurons makes a specific contribution to the overall pattern, the neural representation of a mental event entails the coordinated firing of neurons from many sites distributed through the association cortex, basal ganglia and limbic system. Groups of neurons can exhibit rhythmical firing patterns. Evidence suggests that the coordination of neural activity at distributed locations might be achieved through synchronisation of these rhythmical patterns via the phenomenon of resonance.

The strength of a mental event can vary from subliminal up to a level at which the event captures conscious attention. It is probable that the strength of the corresponding neural event is increased by the recruitment of more neurons. The observation that a rare, task-relevant stimulus activates an extensive array of cerebral sites suggests that the brain maintains the potential for flexible responding by activating areas that are superfluous to the minimum requirements. A characteristic feature of the human brain is the looseness of the link between action and external circumstances. The evidence that we have examined suggests a plausible hypothesis for the way in which the association cortex, limbic system and basal ganglia combine to generate action in the absence of an imperative external stimulus.

# Chapter 2

# The association cortex

## Introduction

The mantle of grey matter that covers the surface of the cerebral hemispheres can be divided into: the primary sensory areas; the association cortex; the primary motor cortex; and the limbic cortex (see Plates 2, 4 and 5). This chapter is concerned with the structure and function of the association cortex, which comprises the sensory association cortex, premotor cortex and multimodal cortex. The sensory association cortex is responsible for extracting specific aspects of information from sensory input. The premotor cortex (which includes both the premotor areas on the lateral surface of the hemispheres immediately anterior to the primary motor cortex and the supplementary motor area in the medial aspect of each hemisphere) is responsible for preparing motor acts. The multimodal association cortex receives information from diverse sources, and is characterised by rich interconnections between its various regions. These connections imply a role in integrating information of diverse kinds, although the mechanism by which this binding is achieved remains uncertain. Our principal focus will be on the multimodal association cortex, because of the major role that it plays in mental symptoms.

Much of the association cortex is neocortex – that is, of relatively recent evolutionary origin. It has a six-layered structure that reflects a fairly well ordered arrangement of cells of particular types, and of zones in which various types of association fibres terminate or take their origin. The cortex of the anterior cingulate on the medial aspect of each hemisphere is palaeocortex – that is, it originates from an earlier stage in the evolution of the brain. The palaeocortex is also six-layered. The palaeocortical areas have especially close functional links with the three-layered archicortex, which is found in the limbic structures on the medial aspect of the temporal lobe. The palaeocortical areas are therefore known as paralimbic areas. None the less, we consider them to be part of the association cortex because they have a six-layered structure, reflecting some similarity in organisational structure to neocortical association areas.

The first two sections of this chapter will examine the organisation of connections between areas of the association cortex and also the local connections within an area. The next two sections will examine evidence regarding the mechanism of several mental functions in which the association cortex plays a major role, and the way in which malfunction of the association cortex is involved in the generation of mental symptoms. It should be emphasised that the association cortex is a component of an integrated brain, and other brain areas, especially limbic structures and basal ganglia, also play a role in its function. The relationship between the association cortex and limbic structures will be described in Chapter 3, and the cortico-subcortical feedback circuits that appear to regulate the activity of the frontal cortex will be described in Chapter 4. The cerebellum also plays a significant role in many activities of the association cortex, and in our account of the functions of the association cortex we shall briefly outline some of the interactions between the cerebral cortex and cerebellum.

# Connections between cortical neurons

The majority of cortical connections are with other cortical neurons. Although all parts of the cortex receive an excitatory input from the thalamus, even in layer IV of the cortex, where the majority of fibres from the thalamus terminate, only 20% of excitatory connections are from the thalamus (Douglas & Martin, 1991). The intracortical connections are of two types: long-range cortico-cortical projections within the same hemisphere or to the opposite hemisphere; and locally spreading connections.

## Long-range cortico-cortical connections

Examination of the asymmetrical nature of the reciprocal connections between different cortical areas in the same hemisphere reveals an ordered hierarchy of cortical regions, directed from posterior towards anterior regions. Fibres feeding forward project from neurons in layers II or III in the region of origin and terminate in layer IV of the target area (Martin, 1984). Fibres feeding back project from neurons in layers V and VI, and terminate in the superficial cortical layers in the target region. The feedback projections are quite diffuse, such that the terminal field of a cortico-cortical feedback neuron often covers an area extending for several millimetres in layer I. This suggests that feed-forward projections convey relatively precisely addressed information towards executive and motor regions whereas feedback projections from the executive areas serve to provide a relatively unfocused modulation of activity in the more posteriorly located regions that serves to enhance or diminish further input from those regions. Long-range connections are mediated by excitatory, glutamatergic neurons.

## Local cortical connections

The circuits that mediate local spread of activity in the cortex are illustrated in Plates 6 and 7.

## Locally spreading excitatory connections

(1)  The terminal arborisation of incoming cortico-cortical fibres branch profusely after ascending to the upper cortical layers. They spread over an area extending for 6–8 mm in layers I and II and synapse richly with the apical dendritic arborisation of pyramidal cells.

(2)  Incoming excitatory fibres from the thalamus synapse with excitatory glutamatergic interneurons in layers IV and III. The axons from these spiny, non-pyramidal neurons project upwards through layers III and II to synapse with the dendrites of pyramidal neurons. They also synapse with inhibitory interneurons (not shown in Plates 6 and 7).

(3)  Branches from the axons of pyramidal cells split off from a cortical efferent axon before it leaves the cortex and spread laterally in layers III to VI for a distance of several millimetres. They form excitatory synapses with other pyramidal cells (Thomson & West, 1993), and with excitatory and inhibitory interneurons.

These connections permit local positive feedback. As emphasised by Hebb (1949), positive feedback leads to explosive amplification of signals and to coherent activation of extensive aggregates of neurons.

## Local inhibitory connections

(1)  Large basket cells exert an inhibitory influence via GABA-ergic synapses on the cell bodies of pyramidal neurons. Large basket cells receive excitatory input from incoming thalamocortical fibres (Mountcastle, 1998), as well as inhibitory input from double bouquet cells (Szentogothai, 1978).

(2)  Chandelier cells exert an inhibitory influence through synapses on the initial segment of the efferent pyramidal cells in layers II and III (the layers of origin of many cortico-cortical efferents) and thereby provide the potential for efficient control of cortico-cortical efferents.

(3)  GABA-ergic double bouquet cells occur in layers II and III, from where they send axons both upwards to synapse with the apical dendrites and downwards to synapse with the basal dendrites of pyramidal neurons.

(4)  Bi-tufted cells (also known as peptide cells), which are relatively few in number, exert an inhibitory influence on the synapses between the horizontal fibres and the apical dendritic arborisation of pyramidal cells.

These inhibitory connections allow the detailed sculpting of the output from a local cortical region. In addition, all types of cortical neurons, including pyramidal cells, excitatory interneurons and inhibitory interneurons, are subject to regulation by monoaminergic neurons projecting from the brain-stem. These diffuse monoaminergic projections produce generalised regulation of cortical output according to current needs (see Chapter 5).

## Studies of cell-to-cell interactions in local cortical circuits

Thomson and colleagues developed a painstaking technique for mapping the connections within local circuits (Thomson & West, 1993; Thomson et al, 1993; Deuchars et al, 1994). They inserted electrodes into pairs of nearby cortical neurons; established whether or not they were electrically connected; recorded the temporal characteristics of the electrical response elicited in the postsynaptic neuron by firing of the presynaptic neuron; and then injected dye into both neurons so that the morphology of the connection between the neurons could be visualised. They observed that synapses between adjacent pyramidal cells promote mutual facilitation. When a synapse is stimulated at rates of 1 Hz and above, the excitatory postsynaptic potentials increase in amplitude and duration, increasing the probability of eliciting an action potential. The action potentials generate excitatory postsynaptic potentials in closely neighbouring pyramidal neurons, resulting in reverberant excitatory activity within a pool of interconnected pyramidal cells. However, direct recruitment of one pyramidal cell by another appears mainly to occur between cells within a column of diameter of the order of several hundred microns.

When the two neurons are more widely separated horizontally, much smaller excitatory postsynaptic potentials are recorded, because the connections tend to be made in part of the dendritic tree of the postsynaptic neuron more distant from the cell body. Therefore, relatively distant connections are likely to elicit action potentials only if there is concurrent input from other afferents, such as thalamocortical afferents.

Firing of pyramidal cells can also recruit interneurons, which exert an inhibitory influence on pyramidal cells. The technique of recording from pairs of neurons demonstrates that the pattern of firing in the presynaptic pyramidal cell determines the relative probability of recruiting an inhibitory interneuron rather than another pyramidal cell. In general, random tonic activity is more likely to recruit another pyramidal cell, while burst firing is more likely to recruit an interneuron (Thomson et al, 1993). This pattern would favour the recruitment of surrounding columns when excitatory inputs are not too strong, but would tend to produce an area of inhibition surrounding a pyramidal cell that exhibited a very strong burst of firing.

# Association cortex afferents and efferents

## Connections with sensory areas

Multimodal association neocortical areas receive sensory information via unimodal sensory areas, and also send feedback projections to these sensory areas. These feedback projections presumably allow gating of sensory input according to priorities determined by a global synthesis of the individual's current situation. This is illustrated by the observation by Muller-Preuss (1978) that some neurons in the auditory cortex of the squirrel monkey respond to vocalisations relayed by loudspeaker but not to self-generated vocalisations. In humans articulating self-generated words, activity in auditory processing areas in the superior temporal gyrus is suppressed in comparison with activity in those areas during a control condition in which the individual articulates words provided from an external source (Frith et al, 1991a).

## Corticostriatal and thalamocortical connections

The connections between the association cortex, basal ganglia and thalamus serve two interlocking functions. The first is the provision of modulated feedback, via loops that feed back to the same cortical area from where they arose. (These feedback loops are described in detail in Chapter 4.) The feedback they provide is subject to modulation by midbrain monoaminergic nuclei, the limbic system and other cortical areas. The second function is the provision of an indirect route by which one cortical area can influence another.

The two functions are interlocking in the sense that the areas of striatum devoted to the two types of function are not distinct. Rather, it appears that one cortical area can influence another by interacting with the feedback loop that regulates the target cortical area. For example, corticostriatal projections from posterior areas such as the parietal and temporal cortex feed information into the loops that provide feedback to frontal areas. In contrast to direct cortico-cortical fibres, which transmit relatively precisely addressed information rapidly, it is probable that indirect transmission via subcortical structures exerts a more generalised modulatory influence.

Furthermore, corticostriatal fibres from a particular prefrontal area project not only to the striatal area involved in the loop that feeds back to that prefrontal area, but also into striatal regions serving other frontal areas. For example, Deutch *et al* (1993) report that anterograde tracer studies in the rat reveal that the ventral prefrontal area not only projects to the shell region of the nucleus accumbens (which is the first relay station in the feedback loop serving the ventromedial prefrontal cortex) but also sends less dense projections to the core area of the nucleus accumbens (which is the first relay station in the feedback loop serving the dorsal prefrontal cortex).

The interaction between cortico-subcortical connections serving different cortical areas is not confined to intermingling of corticostriatal projections. Deutch *et al* (1993) also present evidence that areas of the mediodorsal thalamus that participate in the feedback loop serving the ventral prefrontal cortex project not only back to the ventral prefrontal cortex, but also onwards to the dorsal prefrontal cortex. In general, the pattern of interaction between cortical areas via the subcortical channel serves to direct information from posterior areas towards anterior areas and, within the frontal lobe, from ventral towards dorsal areas. This pattern of information flow serves to channel information towards the primary motor cortex. It also serves to channel information from ventral areas that are implicated in emotional and motivational processing towards dorsal areas that are more strongly implicated in cognitive processing.

## Connections with the limbic system

The hippocampus and amygdala influence the association cortex not only by projections to the corpus striatum (which moderate activity in the cortico-subcortical feedback loops), especially the ventral striatum, but also by direct projections from the limbic output areas to the neocortex. The projections from the hippocampus pass via the entorhinal cortex to the parahippocampal gyrus and thence to the neocortex. It is probable that these projections from hippo-campus to neocortex enable the hippocampus to facilitate the storage of memories in the cortex, by promoting consolidation of the pattern of connections between cortical neurons that represents the memory (Rolls *et al*, 1989). Efferents from the amygdala pass to the cortex via the external capsule. It is probable that the efferents from the amygdala to the cortex act in concert with the efferents from the hippocampus to reinforce the consolidation of cortical memory traces according to their emotional significance.

### Afferents from midbrain aminergic nuclei

The midbrain aminergic nuclei influence neocortical activity not only by inter-acting with the cortico-subcortical loops, but also via direct projections to the neocortex. A more detailed account of these modulatory influences is provided in Chapter 5, but a brief outline is given here as part of our survey of cortical structure and function.

In the case of the dopaminergic system, the mesocortical fibres project mainly to the frontal cortex. Destruction of the dopaminergic input to the frontal cortex in animals produces behaviour deficits very similar to the effects of ablation of that same area of cortex. In schizophrenic patients, administration of the indirect dopamine agonist D-amphetamine partially alleviates their impaired ability to activate the prefrontal cortex (Daniel *et al*, 1991).

It appears that the dopaminergic projections from the VTA to the frontal cortex and the projections from the VTA to the ventral striatum are regulated in a complementary manner. For example, injection of 6-hydroxy-dopamine to inter-rupt dopaminergic transmission in the amygdala induces a decrease in dopamine utilisation in the prefrontal cortex and an increase in the ventral striatum (Simon *et al*, 1988). The evidence indicating complementary regulation of dopaminergic projections to the frontal cortex and ventral striatum is consistent with the evidence suggesting that cortical dopaminergic underactivity accompanies sub-cortical dopamine overactivity in schizophrenia (see Chapter 11).

The serotonergic projections from the midbrain raphe nuclei and the noradren-ergic fibres from the locus coeruleus project to widespread cortical areas. The serotonergic projections to the cortex play a role in regulating activities such as sleep and mood, while the noradrenergic projections play a major role in promoting arousal in response to potentially threatening circumstances (Chapter 5).

# Function of the association cortex

The association cortex plays a major role in many mental phenomena, including attention, language, supervisory functions and several aspects of memory. In this section we shall examine the mechanisms of working memory, selective attention and supervisory functions, because the circuits involved in these are implicated in the mechanisms that generate mental symptoms. Working memory is a mechanism that keeps a limited amount of information immediately accessible for current use or manipulation. Selective attention is a mechanism that facilitates the processing of information that is potentially especially salient to the current needs or goals of the individual. Supervisory functions are responsible for the planning, initiation, selection and monitoring of mental or motor acts, in situations where the circumstances leave a degree of ambiguity regarding the most appropriate course of action.

## Circuits supporting working memory in the rhesus monkey

Although our concern is with the function of the human neocortex, it is informative to begin with an examination of the circuits that support working memory in the rhesus monkey because these have been delineated in detail using techniques that are not feasible in humans. In particular, the technique of labelling two cortical areas that belong to a specific functional unit with two distinguishable anterograde tracer substances provides an elegant way of constructing a detailed map of areas that are linked to both the labelled areas (Selemon & Goldman-Rakic, 1985).

In monkeys, the neural substrate of working memory can be explored by measuring neural activity during various tasks that entail a delay of several seconds between the presentation of information and the requirement to make a response that utilises that information. For example, in a spatial delayed response task, the monkey observes the hiding of a reward under a cover at a particular spatial location, and then, after a delay, is allowed to retrieve the reward. Monkeys with lesions of the dorsolateral prefrontal cortex are impaired on such tasks. In normal monkeys, recordings of electrical activity from neurons in this area exhibit increased firing rates (Fuster, 1997). However, there is also increased activity in several other areas. The linkages between these areas have been explored in detail by Goldman-Rakic and colleagues using tracers.

In rhesus monkeys, circumscribed areas of the posterior parietal association cortex have reciprocal links with areas of the lateral prefrontal cortex. By concurrent injection of two distinguishable tracers into the posterior parietal cortex and lateral frontal cortex, Selemon & Goldman-Rakic (1985) demonstrated that these two areas are mutually interconnected to 15 other cortical areas. These other areas include the anterior cingulate, posterior cingulate, parahippocampal gyrus and superior temporal sulcus (Plate 8). These prefrontal, parietal, limbic and temporal areas all receive thalamocortical projections from the medial pulvinar nucleus of the thalamus. Thus they appear to comprise a closely integrated neural network, whose activity may be coordinated by virtue of the shared thalamic input (Goldman-Rakic, 1988).

Furthermore, the relationship between the terminals of the prefrontal and parietal projections within each particular mutual target area exhibits one of two characteristic patterns. One pattern is for the fibres from the two different areas to terminate in interdigitated, spatially distinct columns. Since pyramidal cell dendritic trees extend vertically within a column, the projections from the prefrontal and parietal cortex must make the majority of their synapses with different neurons. This pattern occurs in the cingulate cortex. The other pattern consists of terminations in complementary layers within a single column or cluster of columns. Such a pattern would allow fibres from the prefrontal and parietal cortex to make synapses with the same neuron in the mutual target area. This pattern occurs in the superior temporal sulcus. The existence of these two patterns of termination in mutual target areas implies that each target area performs one of two different types of synthesis of information from the prefrontal and parietal cortex.

More detailed examination of the network linking the lateral prefrontal cortex and posterior parietal cortex with other areas of the association cortex indicates that it is composed of several parallel networks, linking sub-regions within the broader areas identified. In particular, one network links the mutual targets of parietal area 7a and area 46 of the lateral prefrontal cortex, while an adjacent parallel network links the mutual targets of parietal area 7ip and prefrontal area 8 (Goldman-Rakic, 1987). Recording from electrodes in monkeys during the performance of spatial delayed response tasks demonstrates that prefrontal area 46 and parietal area 7a are involved in holding the information required to provide spatial guidance of hand movements in working memory (for periods of the order of 30 seconds). Prefrontal area 8 and parietal area 7ip are engaged when it is necessary to hold information for the guidance of eye movements in working memory.

Thus it appears that two adjacent, parallel networks are dedicated to maintaining separate aspects of spatial information in working memory. This observation raises the question of where or how information regarding separate aspects of a problem is integrated. The 'binding problem' which confronts attempts to ascribe the perception of each individual facet of a situation to a single 'cardinal neuron' (see Chapter 1) remains a problem for distributed networks too. However, there is in principle ample scope for interaction between parallel networks, either by means of local cortical connections in one or more of the cortical areas involved, or at the level of the thalamus.

In particular, the observation that many cortico-cortical feedback connections tend to terminate in a diffuse manner in the superficial layers of the cortex (Martin, 1984), together with the evidence from recordings in paired neurons in local cortical circuits that connections made in the superficial cortical layers are unlikely to trigger an action potential unless there is concurrent excitation, perhaps from thalamocortical input (Deuchars et al, 1994), suggests that 'binding' of distinguishable networks may be achieved by concurrent thalamic excitatory input at cortical sites where there are overlapping feedback projections involved in the distinguishable networks. As discussed in Chapter 1, it is possible that coherent gamma band oscillations mediate the identification of spatially separated neural activity associated with a particular mental event. The observations of Ribary et al (1991) support the hypothesis that gamma oscillations can be generated by reverberation in cortico-thalamic circuits.

Working memory for objects, which is tested in monkeys by paradigms in which a reward is associated with a specific object, rather than with a location in space, engages more ventral regions of the prefrontal cortex. Monkeys with ventrolateral lesions tend to be impaired on such tasks. Recordings from intracellular electrodes while monkeys engage in object recognition tasks have identified delay-sensitive 'object memory' neurons in the ventral prefrontal cortex (Wilson *et al*, 1993).

## Human working memory

The performance of virtually all of the tasks of everyday life requires the ability to synthesise and utilise current sensory input and relevant stored knowledge. The ability to keep the requisite information in mind and manipulate it is known as working memory. In the words of Patricia Goldman-Rakic (1992), "the ability to form and update an internal representation of the outside world is the cornerstone of the rational mind". The combination of moment-to-moment awareness and instant retrieval of archived information enables humans to string together thoughts and ideas, and to plan for the future.

The foundation for current understanding of the organisation of human working memory was laid by Baddeley & Hitch (1974). Previously, short-term memory had been regarded as a limited-capacity unitary store, capable of holding up to approximately seven items of information. For example, the number of digits that can be retained in this short-term store (known as the digit span) is approximately seven. Baddeley & Hitch carried out a series of experiments in which they examined the effects of loading a person with the task of temporarily remembering a string of digits while simultaneously performing another task, such as verbal reasoning. They observed that the amount of interference from near-span loads was much less than would be expected if there were a unitary working memory system holding all relevant information on-line. This prompted them to propose that working memory comprised a set of modules, each of limited capacity, specialised for handling different types of temporary storage. They proposed a central executive attentional system controlling several slave subsystems, including a speech-based articulatory loop for maintaining speech-based information, and a visuospatial 'scratch-pad' for maintaining visuospatial imagery.

In one of the first PET studies designed to investigate human working memory, Paulesu *et al* (1993) found activation of Broca's area (the left inferoposterior frontal cortex) and the left inferior parietal cortex, during a task that entailed holding a short string of words in memory. Furthermore, by comparing cerebral activation during a short-term memory task with that during a rhyming task that did not place demands on memory, they demonstrated that the inferior parietal activation occurs when the phonological store is activated. They concluded that Broca's area serves the inner articulation of verbal material, while the inferior parietal area provides the phonological store.

Petrides *et al* (1993) measured rCBF during a more demanding working memory task, in which nine of the ten integers one to ten were read aloud by the experimenter, and the participant was required to identify the omitted integer. This task entails not only holding a string of words in memory, but also the executive function of comparing it with a reference word string arranged in a different order. The mid-dorsolateral prefrontal cortex was active bilaterally during this task.

Thus, during tasks that entail working with words, a network of cortical regions, mainly left-sided, is activated. Different components of this network contribute differing aspects of processing to the integrated whole. In particular, the inferior parietal area contains the phonological store, Broca's area serves inner speech, while the left dorsolateral prefrontal cortex is called into play when executive functions are required.

The N-back task is a relatively simple task that can be employed to study the effects of increasing the demands made on working memory. A sequence of stimuli, such as letters of the alphabet, is presented on a visual display unit. The subject is required to respond whenever the current stimulus matches that presented N items previously. It is necessary for the subject to maintain a regularly updated memory of the N most recently presented items. In the one-back condition, the task entails only item recognition, and tests the ability to store information. In the two-back condition, it is necessary to continually update information about the temporal order of stimuli (an executive task), in addition to storing information. One-back tasks using verbal material engage Broca's area, the premotor cortex and the supplementary motor cortex, in addition to the parietal cortex (Jonides et al, 1997). Two-back tasks engage not only these areas, but also more anterior frontal areas, especially the dorsolateral prefrontal cortex (Cohen et al, 1994; Awh et al, 1996). Furthermore, during two-back tasks, not only the dorsolateral prefrontal cortex, but an extensive set of additional sites, including the thalamus, midbrain and cerebellum are engaged, suggesting that these sites comprise a circuit engaged in executive functions (Liddle et al, 1999).

In an fMRI experiment in which brain activity during the maintenance of a string of letters in working memory was compared with that during a similar task in which it was necessary not only to maintain but also to rearrange the order of the letters, D'Esposito and colleagues demonstrated a double dissociation between the sites involved in maintenance and manipulation of information (Postle et al, 1999). Simple maintenance activated the posterior lateral frontal cortex adjacent to the sylvian fissure, while manipulation engaged the dorsolateral prefrontal cortex.

Under some circumstances, the dorsolateral prefrontal cortex can be engaged during working memory tasks even when no manipulation of the information is required. For example, in a study using an event-related fMRI design that permitted identification of the time at which specific brain areas became active during the encoding and maintenance of a string of letters in working memory, Rypma & D'Esposito (1999) found that the dorsolateral prefrontal cortex became active when the memory load approached full capacity, even though no manipulation of information was required. However, they observed that the dorsolateral prefrontal cortex was mainly active during the initial encoding of information, rather than the maintenance phase.

As discussed above, in monkeys, working memory for object identity is mediated by a region of the frontal cortex ventral to that mediating working memory for spatial location. Functional imaging studies indicate that in humans, too, these aspects of working memory are mediated by different frontal areas. Smith *et al* (1995) employed a paradigm in which three faces were presented sequentially at three different locations on the screen of a visual display unit, followed by a probe face in a variable location. To test working memory for object identity, the participants were required to determine whether the identity of the probe face matched that of any of the three targets. To test working memory for spatial location, the participants were required to determine whether the position of the probe matched that of any of the targets. The object identity task activated regions in the right dorsolateral prefrontal cortex, while the spatial task activated the right premotor cortex. Thus, the emerging evidence from functional imaging studies supports the proposal by Baddeley & Hitch (1974) that working memory is supported by a modular system comprising several distinguishable components.

## Selective attention

The allocation of attention to a particular feature of the external environment, or to a particular aspect of mental processing, is not merely a matter of domination of awareness by the most prominent feature of the current situation. There are active processes that direct attention towards particular types of feature according to longer-term goals. This is illustrated by a wide variety of studies demonstrating that priming with an appropriate cue increases the speed of responding to a particular stimulus. Some features of the neural processes corresponding to such active directing of attention can be demonstrated by electrical recording from the scalp overlying the area where signals from a visual target stimulus are processed. If a priming signal comprising a white square is presented 80 ms before presentation of the target stimulus, the amplitude of the electrical signal elicited by the target stimulus is greater when the priming stimulus is presented at the same location as the target stimulus than when it is presented elsewhere in the visual field (Luck *et al*, 1993). Thus the priming stimulus initiates a neural process that can either enhance or diminish the amplitude of neural activation at the site which processes the subsequent target stimulus.

Studies of rCBF using PET (Corbetta *et al*, 1991) reveal that when a subject is instructed to attend to the colour of a subsequent stimulus, there is activation of the prestriate cortical area that specialises in the detection of colour. Similarly, when directed to attend to preparation for a motor act, there is activation in motor areas (Roland, 1985).

Posner & Dehaene (1994) have emphasised that the process of focusing attention involves both the suppression of irrelevant aspects of a situation and the amplification of relevant aspects. At the earliest stages in processing, in the primary sensory cortex, there is virtually full activation of neurons, which is independent of regulation by attentional mechanisms, while the late stages of processing occur only if the stimulus is actively attended to. Posner & Dehaene argue that the early stages of processing are largely devoted to suppression of irrelevant features, while the later stages entail amplification of the relevant features. Consistent with this, Luck (1995) demonstrated that in cued detection of a visual target, the first positive component (P1) of the evoked potential, which appears around 80 ms after stimulus presentation, was of the same amplitude for correctly cued and uncued stimuli, but was less for miscued stimuli. Thus, a correct cue did not enhance early processing of the stimulus relative to the situation in which the stimulus was not cued, but a false cue produced a reduction in early processing. This implies active suppression at the early stages of processing, but no active enhancement. However, the first negative component (N1), which appears around 150–200 ms after stimulus presentation, was increased after the correctly cued stimuli, compared with after either uncued or miscued stimuli.

When information concerning position in space is used to guide the selection of attention, the parietal cortex appears to play an especially important role. PET studies reveal that when attention is shifted from one location to another, there is increased activity in left and right superior parietal lobes (Corbetta *et al*, 1993). The involvement of the two hemispheres is not symmetrical. Left parietal activity increases only during right-field shifts, while right parietal activity occurs during shifts to either side. This is consistent with the clinical evidence that right-sided parietal lesions produce more extensive impairment of the ability to direct attention to a particular location. When aspects such as colour, form or motion are employed to guide attention, anterior areas, especially the anterior cingulate cortex, are active, but there is no parietal activation (Corbetta *et al*, 1991).

These findings from PET studies confirm the argument by Mesulam (1990), based on the observed effects of brain lesions, that there is a distributed neural network embracing the dorsolateral posterior parietal cortex, cingulate cortex and the frontal eye fields that serves the process of directing attention. These three areas are a subset of the larger number of cortical areas implicated in the parallel distributed circuit delineated by Goldman-Rakic (1987) that is related to the areas serving working memory in the rhesus monkey. Mesulam emphasises that each of the three cardinal cortical areas concerned with directing attention is connected with the medial pulvinar nucleus of the thalamus. Thus the anatomy of the network serving attention provides further circumstantial evidence for the hypothesis that the occurrence of excitatory thalamic input concurrently with cortico-cortical input plays an important part in the recruitment of cortical neurons representing a particular meaningful neural event.

## Supervisory functions

The supervisory mental processes are those that allow an individual to perform mental and motor actions that are not merely imperative responses to external circumstances. The extent to which supervisory mental processes are called into play depends on the degree to which external circumstances dictate the most appropriate response. Supervisory processes are most heavily involved in activity that is mainly driven by long-term goals that can be achieved only by the use of self-generated strategies. However, even quite simple tasks, such as responding to relatively rare 'oddball' stimuli, engage brain areas implicated in supervisory activity, possibly because it is advantageous to be prepared to respond flexibly when confronted by an odd stimulus.

The term 'supervisory function' is almost synonymous with executive function, although the latter term has somewhat broader connotations. Smith & Jonides (1999) list among the executive processes:

(1) focusing attention on relevant information and processes, while inhibiting irrelevant ones (*selection*);
(2) scheduling procedures in complex tasks that require switching between different procedures (*task management and initiation*);
(3) planning a sequence of procedures to achieve a goal (*planning*);
(4) updating and checking the contents of working memory (*monitoring*);
(5) coding representations in working memory for time and place of appearance (*contextual coding*).

All these executive processes are called into play in the supervision of mental activity. However, the feature that characterises supervisory function is the internal generation of activity when the external environment does not dictate a specific course of action. The core supervisory processes are: planning, initiating, selecting, and monitoring self-generated mental or motor activity.

Shallice (1988) introduced the term 'supervisory attentional system' to describe the mechanism by which an individual schedules activities when circumstances do not define the optimum course of action. As described by Shallice, the prefrontal cortex plays a dominant role in the activities of the supervisory attentional system. Recent functional imaging data support this hypothesis, but also demonstrate the involvement of many other areas of the association cortex. We shall now examine evidence for the localisation of various specific aspects of supervisory function.

## Planning

The Tower of London task is a well established test of planning ability. The subject is presented with a set of coloured rings stacked on one of three vertical rods, and also with a diagram illustrating a different arrangement of the coloured rings, which can be achieved by a sequence of steps in which the rings are moved, one at a time, to the other rods. The subject is required to move the rings so as to achieve the new arrangement in the minimum number of moves. Efficient performance requires planning. Using SPET, Andreasen *et al* (1992) demonstrated that healthy subjects activate the medial frontal cortex during this task. Furthermore, schizophrenic patients with negative symptoms, who have difficulty planning and initiating activities, fail to activate the medial frontal cortex during this task.

## Initiation of action

Prior to initiation of a movement, electrical signals can be detected over the frontal cortex (Deeke *et al*, 1969). The earliest of these signals, the readiness potential, typically begins 850 ms before the initiation of movement. If subjects are asked to estimate when they decide to make a movement (timed by reference to a clock displayed on an oscilloscope screen) while concurrent recordings of scalp electrical potentials are performed, the onset of the readiness potential is observed to precede conscious awareness of the decision to move by approximately 350 ms (Libet *et al*, 1983).

As discussed in Chapter 1, PET studies demonstrate that the medial prefrontal cortex is the cerebral region most heavily engaged during the generation of stimulus-independent thought (McGuire *et al*, 1996). Furthermore, patients who suffer damage to the inferomedial frontal cortex suffer a loss of ability to initiate movements, which, in its most marked form, presents as akinetic mutism (Barris & Schuman, 1953). It is therefore likely that the medial frontal cortex plays a cardinal role in the initiation of both thought and movement.

## Selection of action

Carter *et al* (1998) at the University of Pittsburgh have investigated the cerebral areas engaged in selecting action by employing fMRI to measure regional brain activity during the performance of tasks that entailed varying degrees of selection between competing responses. They concluded that the anterior cingulate cortex is activated under these conditions. In view of the observation that the ability to suppress inappropriate responses is impaired in certain disorders (including frontal lobe injury and schizophrenia – see Chapter 7), it is pertinent to ask whether there is a specific neural mechanism responsible for the suppression of inappropriate responses, or, alternatively, whether the suppression of inappropriate responses is an intrinsic consequence of the act of selecting an appropriate response. Carter *et al* (1998) argue for the latter.

None the less, in tasks in which participants are sometimes required to refrain from responding, the 'no go' trials engage cortical areas that are not engaged during 'go' trials. For example, in an event-related fMRI study in which participants were required to respond to the letter X and refrain from any response to the letter K, the anterior cingulate was engaged during both types of trial, consistent with the findings of Carter and colleagues, but in addition the dorsolateral and ventrolateral prefrontal cortex were engaged during 'no go' trials only, while the motor cortex, thalamus and cerebellum were engaged during 'go' trials only (Liddle *et al*, 2001). Thus the lateral prefrontal cortex appears to be specifically engaged in suppressing responses.

## Monitoring of action

The brain has an internal error-checking mechanism that can detect errors before feedback from the external world draws attention to the mistake. For example, when errors are made during a simple task that requires selection of an appropriate response to a stimulus, a large negative electrical potential can be recorded over the frontocentral areas of the scalp, commencing approximately 200 ms after the stimulus, but before the onset of muscle contraction that will execute the erroneous response. This error-related negativity can be localised to the anterior cingulate cortex. In an fMRI study in which the participants were required to respond to an X and inhibit responding to a K, false responses to the letter K were associated with increased cerebral activity in the anterior cingulate (Kiehl *et al*, 2000a).

Flagging errors is only one aspect of internal monitoring. Presumably the monitoring mechanism is engaged irrespective of whether or not the responses are appropriate. Other cerebral areas, in addition to the anterior cingulate, are implicated. For example, Frith *et al* (1992) devised a task designed to place heavy demands on internal monitoring of intended eye movements. The external ocular muscles have few proprioceptive receptors that provide feedback about the degree of muscle contraction, and hence it might be expected that the learning of a novel eye-movement task would require relatively intense internal monitoring. Frith and colleagues placed an electrode on the skin overlying the lateral rectus muscle, responsible for horizontal movements of the eye, and employed the electrical signal generated in the electrode by contraction of the lateral rectus to drive a diamond-shaped icon horizontally across the screen of a visual display unit. The connection was made in such a way that the diamond moved in the direction opposite to what was expected by the participant. The participant was instructed to attempt to make the diamond move smoothly to and fro across the screen at a rate of approximately one cycle every two seconds. PET was used to measure rCBF during six 2-minute periods. Comparison of rCBF during the early periods, in which there was a heavy demand on internal monitoring to overcome the confusing effect of the unanticipated external feedback, with that during later periods, when facility had been achieved, revealed greater activity in the left parahippocampal gyrus and in the visual association cortex during the early periods. Frith and colleagues interpreted the parahippocampal activity as a reflection of internal monitoring. The increased activity in the visual association cortex is likely to reflect greater attention to visual input.

The monitoring of self-generated speech is especially important. It might be expected that monitoring would occur at several stages in speech production. First, it is necessary to monitor the ideas to be expressed. Subsequently, the preparation of the speech motor programme requires monitoring. Finally, it might be predicted that the actual output would be subject to scrutiny. Several functional imaging studies have attempted to identify the cerebral sites involved in the internal monitoring of speech.

One strategy that has been employed to enhance the demands on internal monitoring of self-generated speech is to imagine speech spoken in the voice of another person. Incomplete sentences are presented and the participant is required to complete each sentence using inner speech, imagined in the voice of another person. McGuire *et al* (1995) used PET to measure rCBF during this task in healthy subjects and in schizophrenic patients. In healthy subjects, this task is associated with activation of the supplementary motor area and lateral temporal lobe. Schizophrenic patients with a tendency to suffer persistent hallucinations exhibited less activation at the temporal lobe site that was active in the healthy subjects, while schizophrenic patients who had never suffered hallucinations exhibited normal activation in this area.

In a subsequent study using fMRI to study cerebral activity during the same task, McGuire *et al* (2000) demonstrated activation in both the medial temporal lobe (hippocampus) and lateral temporal lobe (middle temporal gyrus) in healthy subjects. As in the previous study, schizophrenic patients with a tendency to suffer persistent hallucinations exhibited less activation at these temporal lobe sites, while patients who had never suffered hallucinations exhibited normal activation. Thus, it appears that patients prone to persistent hallucinations have an impaired mechanism for internal monitoring of speech production. Such a failure might lead to failure to recognise the source of internally generated speech.

Failures of the monitoring of internally generated mental activity might also be expected to contribute to other mental symptoms. For example, failure to detect errors might contribute to delusions. In this respect, it is potentially relevant to note that paranoid schizophrenic patients exhibit an abnormally small frontocentral negative scalp potential in response to errors (Kopp & Rist, 1999). Ford (1999) confirmed this observation and, in addition, found that schizophrenic patients are prone to exhibit inappropriately large frontocentral negativity during correct responses, implying an impaired mechanism for identifying errors.

## Oddball stimulus detection

In the oddball stimulus detection paradigm, an odd stimulus is interposed at irregular intervals within a series of identical stimuli. For example, the odd stimulus might be a 1500 Hz tone interposed within a sequence of regular 1000 Hz stimuli. The participant is usually required to respond to the oddball stimuli, either by a motor response or by counting the number of such stimuli. This simple task evokes a robust positive electrical potential (P300), detectable over much of the scalp, that reaches a peak 300–400 ms after presentation of the oddball stimulus. Intracerebral electrodes reveal that neural firing, time-locked to stimulus presentation, can be detected at many cerebral locations (Halgren et al, 1998). Using event-related fMRI, my colleagues and I (Kiehl et al, 2001) have demonstrated that many areas of the association cortex, including the lateral frontal cortex, anterior cingulate, lateral temporal lobe, inferior parietal lobule and superior parietal lobule are engaged during the detection of the oddball stimuli. The hippocampus and amygdala are also active. Apart from anticipated differences in activation of the primary sensory cortex, virtually identical sites are engaged in the auditory and visual modality.

The amplitude and latency of the P300 are influenced by various factors, including oddball stimulus probability, discrimination difficulty and task demands (Donchin & Coles, 1988). This has led to the suggestion that this electrical component reflects processes related to attention, decision-making and updating of memory. Although the psychological processes associated with the neural activity that generates the P300 component have not been fully delineated, the oddball paradigm is potentially of great value for probing cerebral function in psychiatric disorders. Patients with illnesses such as schizophrenia (McCarley et al, 1991; Ford, 1999) and personality disorders such as psychopathy (Kiehl et al, 1999b) demonstrate reduced amplitude of the P300 component, despite intact ability to perform the task. However, while both schizophrenic subjects and psychopaths exhibit reduced amplitude of the P300, the overall time course and spatial distribution of the electrical potentials detected at the scalp are quite different in the two conditions. In psychopaths, the electrical potential at frontal and central scalp sites exhibits a marked negative component during the period from 200 ms to 600 ms (Kiehl *et al*, 1999b), which is not seen in schizophrenia. Furthermore, fMRI demonstrates that psychopaths exhibit greater activity than healthy subjects in the lateral frontal cortex, and less activity at limbic sites (Kiehl & Liddle, unpublished data), whereas schizophrenic patients fail to activate most of the association cortex sites that are active in healthy individuals, despite exhibiting a normal level of activity in the motor cortex (Kiehl & Liddle, in press). The fact that schizophrenic patients fail to engage many association cortex sites, yet perform normally apart from a mild slowing of reaction time, indicates that much of the cerebral activity that occurs in healthy subjects is not essential for task performance.

These observations support two tentative conclusions of potential importance, one about the nature of healthy cerebral activity; the other about the nature of schizophrenia. The first conclusion is that, in some circumstances, healthy individuals systematically engage cerebral regions that are not essential for performance of the task in hand. In particular, the observations support the hypothesis that 'oddball' detection engages so many brain areas in healthy individuals because it is advantageous to be prepared to respond flexibly when confronted by an unexpected stimulus. The second conclusion is that schizo-phrenia is characterised by widespread, relatively subtle impairment of the function of the association cortex. In this chapter, we have noted several strands of evidence that support this conclusion, and we shall examine the issue in greater detail in Chapter 11.

# Association cortex and mental symptoms

In general, there are increases or decreases in neural activity (as revealed by changes in cerebral blood flow or metabolism) in multiple cerebral areas during the experience of mental symptoms. The patterns of activity associated with each of the major groups of mental symptoms are described in Part II of this book. This section provides an overview, with the object of illustrating some of the general phenomena worth bearing in mind when interpreting the patterns of cerebral activity associated with a specific group of symptoms.

There are several possible types of relationship between the observed changes in cerebral activity and the mechanism of symptom production. In some instances, the evidence indicates underactivity in several mutually connected areas, implying reduced neurotransmission in the circuit connecting these areas. For example, the left dorsolateral prefrontal cortex and inferior parietal lobule are relatively underactive in patients with poverty of speech, in both major depression and schizophrenia (Liddle *et al*, 1992; Dolan *et al*, 1993). The circuit connecting these areas is normally engaged during word generation.

Such underactivity could, in principle, reflect either reversible processes, such as abnormal activity of a modulatory neurotransmitter (see Chapter 5), or loss of cerebral tissue, which would be less readily reversible. For example, using magnetic resonance imaging (MRI) to estimate the thickness of cortical grey matter in a group of chronic schizophrenic patients, Chua *et al* (1997) demonstrated that severity of psychomotor poverty was correlated with decreased thickness of the cortical grey matter in left frontal cortex, in an area where Liddle *et al* (1992) had observed an association between psychomotor poverty and decreased rCBF. However, it is important to note that this group of patients had been selected on the basis of having severe persistent illness, and the findings should not be assumed to apply to less severely ill people. The question as to which neural elements are reduced in those areas where grey matter volume is reduced remains a subject for speculation. There is little evidence for substantial loss of cell bodies in schizophrenia, which suggests that the loss of tissue may reflect a decrease in neuropil. Neuropil includes dendrites, axons and the synapses between them (Selemon & Goldman-Rakic, 1999).

In other instances, related cerebral areas exhibit changes in opposite directions. For example, Mayberg *et al* (1999) reported that during the induction of sad mood, healthy subjects exhibit increased activity in the paralimbic cortex, especially in the part of the anterior cingulate lying inferior to the genu of the corpus callosum, together with decreased activity in the lateral frontal cortex and parietal cortex. Conversely, during symptom resolution in patients with major depression, they found that activity in the paralimbic cortex decreased, while that in the lateral frontal cortex increased. These observations indicate that depressed mood is associated with increased activity in the paralimbic cortex and decreased activity in lateral neocortex. In contrast, during the processing of emotionally laden words, psychopaths, who characteristically lack normal emotional responses, exhibit reduced activation in the paralimbic cortex and increased activity in the lateral frontal cortex and temporal pole, compared with healthy subjects (Kiehl *et al*, 2000c). Such reciprocal relationships between cerebral areas suggest that the change in one region is a compensatory response to the change in the other.

In the case of several types of symptoms, there is indirect evidence indicating that predisposition to suffer the symptoms is associated with underactivity in that cerebral area, while the actual experience of symptoms is associated with an increase in activity in that area relative to baseline. For example, Drevets *et al* (1997) observed diminished tissue volume and reduced cerebral metabolism in the subgenual anterior cingulate in depressed patients. However, as discussed above, Mayberg *et al* (1999) observed that the actual experience of depression is associated with overactivity in this region. These findings suggest that neural damage can lead to impaired ability to produce normal activity in an area, and also a propensity to suffer pathological overactivity in that same area.

# Chapter 3

# The limbic system

## Introduction

The term 'limbic lobe' was introduced in the 19th century by Broca (1861) to describe an extensive ring of cortex on the medial aspect of each hemisphere and related subcortical structures. The elements of this limbic lobe include the hippocampal formation, amygdala, septal nuclei and parts of the frontal cortex and cingulate gyrus.

The developmental history of the forebrain illuminates both the structural organisation and the functional role of Broca's *grand lobe limbique*. During the sixth week of human embryonic development, when the embryo is approximately 14 mm long, the cerebral hemispheres are discernible as vesicles that balloon outwards from the diencephalon at the rostral end of the developing central nervous system. The diencephalon, which is composed principally of the thalamus and hypothalamus, provides the connection between the hemispheres and the rest of the brain. The developing hemispheres expand rapidly and eventually engulf the diencephalon. The structures that comprise Broca's limbic lobe are on the medial aspect of each hemisphere, and form in a ring around the open neck of each of these two hollow hemispheres.

The initially simple structure of each hemisphere, comprising a globe connected to the diencephalon via a neck, becomes distorted by differential development of its various regions and also by the intrusion through the neck of the massive sheet of callosal fibres connecting the two hemispheres. None the less, it requires only a little imagination to visualise each hippocampal formation as a folded collar extending part of the way around the neck of each hemisphere (Plate 4). The hippocampal formation comprises strips of cortex including the fimbria, dentate gyrus, hippocampus proper and subiculum, aligned side by side, parallel to the long axis of the formation (Plate 9). The hippocampus proper is divided into four sectors, designated CA1 to CA4, on the basis of their cellular architecture. The folding generates a tight S-shaped curve transverse to the long axis which itself curves in a C shape around the neck.

The tail of each hippocampal formation is split apart by the intruding corpus callosum. Consequently, a remnant of the hippocampus, the indusium griseum, passes over the upper surface of the corpus callosum, while the most prominent hippocampal outflow tract, the fornix, follows an arched trajectory below the under-surface of the corpus callosum, to the septal area, and ultimately to the hypothalamus and other structures within the diencephalon (Plate 4). The septal area is a collection of grey matter at the base of the septum pellucidum, a sheet of tissue lying in the midline between the anterior horns of the lateral ventricles. The nuclei of the septal area and the hippocampus are together known as the septohippocampal system.

Similarly, in each hemisphere, the amygdala develops from a ring of tissue encircling the neck of the bulging globe that develops into the cerebral hemisphere. In the fully developed brain, the main mass of the amygdala lies in the anteromedial part of the temporal lobe, anterior to the hippocampus. However, a remnant, known as the stria terminalis, arches over the thalamus, beneath the corpus callosum. It is composed predominantly of fibres projecting from the amygdala to the hypothalamus and nearby mesial basal forebrain structures. Along its length, it contains scattered patches of grey matter, known as the bed nucleus of the stria terminalis. The main mass of the bed nucleus lies in the mesial basal forebrain adjacent to the lateral septal nuclei in the inferior part of the septum pellucidum. The amygdala together with the bed nucleus of the stria terminalis is known as the extended amygdala. The ring of amygdala-related tissue is completed by a direct connection, known as the ventral amygdalofugal system, extending from the amygdala via the uncus to the mesial basal forebrain and hypothalamus.

This consideration of developmental anatomy suggests that one major role of the limbic lobe is to link the sensory and cognitive processing in the cortex of the cerebral hemispheres with the visceromotor control centres, especially the hypothalamus, which influence the rest of the body through the endocrine and autonomic systems. Because the hypothalamus regulates essential functions such as nutrition, fluid balance and reproductive activity, limbic structures might be expected to play an important role in mediating cerebral influence on the appetites that help ensure that these bodily needs are met. The hippocampus and amygdala form the main link between cerebrum and the hypothalamic–pituitary–adrenal (HPA) axis, which regulates many of the interactions between the brain and the rest of the body, and in particular mediates the hormonal response to stress (see Chapter 5). Furthermore, by virtue of its role as the major link between the cerebral hemispheres and regulatory centres in the diencephalon and brain-stem, evolution has endowed the limbic structures with a special role in motivation and emotion. In addition, by virtue of its developmental origin as a collar around the neck of the cerebral vesicle, the limbic system communicates directly with virtually all cerebral regions, and plays a cardinal role in mediating the storage of converging information from throughout the hemispheres in memory.

While Broca included the cingulate gyrus in his definition of the limbic lobe, as discussed in Chapter 2, it is probably more logical to regard it as paralimbic cortex, rather than a part of the limbic system proper. From the evolutionary perspective, the cingulate cortex is palaeocortex, which is intermediate between the primitive archicortex found in the hippocampus and amygdala, and the more recently evolved neocortex, which comprises the remainder of the cortex. Archicortex has a three-layered allocortical structure, while palaeocortex and neocortex have a six-layered isocortical structure. Allocortex lacks the outer cortical layers (layers I to III) that mediate associative links between adjacent areas of isocortex. Possibly this difference between allocortex and isocortex reflects the dominant role that projection to other brain structures plays in the function of the limbic cortex, whereas local connectivity is a relatively more important aspect of the function of isocortical association areas.

If the cingulate cortex is excluded, the principal components of the limbic system are the hippocampal formation and septal nuclei, the extended amygdala, including the bed nucleus of the stria terminalis, and the allocortical part of the orbital cortex. It might be argued that the ventral striatum should also be included in the limbic system, since it is a subcortical structure that not only receives major input from the amygdala and hippocampus, but also receives major input from the orbitomedial frontal cortex, and sends efferents to the hypothalamus. However, the ventral striatum grades continuously into those parts of the corpus striatum that are structurally and functionally linked closely with neocortical regions of the frontal cortex. It is more convenient to regard the entire corpus striatum as a brain structure that provides one of the routes via which the hippocampus and amygdala influence the function of frontal cortex. The way in which striatum participates in the feedback loops that regulate the frontal cortex is discussed in detail in Chapter 4.

In the light of the fact that the above definition of the limbic system gives it a relatively clearly defined role within the integrated functions of the brain, it is reasonable to ask to what extent the major elements of this narrowly defined limbic system have distinct roles. While in humans the phenomena elicited by direct electrical stimulation of the hippocampus are very similar to those elicited by stimulation of the amygdala (Halgren *et al*, 1978), more discriminative techniques possible in animals reveal differences in function. The projections from the hippocampal formation and amygdala to the ventral striatum appear to function in a complementary manner. In rats, both structures exert a gating influence on the transmission of neural signals from the frontal cortex to the thalamus via the ventral striatum. In the absence of input from the hippocampus, the spiny neurons of the ventral striatum are hyperpolarised, and transmission from the frontal cortex is blocked (Grace *et al*, 1998). In the presence of input from the hippocampal formation, the resting membrane potential of the striatal neurons is less polarised, so they are capable of firing in response to input from the frontal cortex. Projections from the hippocampal formation and from the amygdala to the ventral striatum have opposite effects on the hyperactivity induced by systemic administration of amphetamine in rats. The projections from the hippocampal formation enhance the hyperactivity, while the gluta-matergic projections from the amygdala decrease it (Cools *et al*, 1991).

Studies in animals such as rats suggest that the amygdala and hippocampus are involved in different types of learning. For example, the amygdala is involved in the acquisition of conditioned fear (Kapp *et al*, 1984), while the hippocampus is engaged in the learning of spatial information required for navigation (O'Keefe & Nadel, 1978).

In contrast to the hippocampus, which receives input from all parts of the association cortex, but not from the sensory cortex, the amygdala receives direct input from unimodal sensory areas. Furthermore, as discussed in greater detail below, the organisation of the local connections of pyramidal neurons in the hippocampus imply that it engages in precisely focused processing of information, whereas the local connections in the amygdala are more diffuse. Overall, the evidence suggests that the amygdala is designed to respond to imperative external stimuli by arresting concurrent cognitive processing and mobilising a 'fight or flight' response, whereas the hippocampus participates in a more considered evaluation of the current situation.

# Hippocampal afferents and efferents

Afferent fibres reach the hippocampus from widespread cerebral areas via the entorhinal cortex. The entorhinal cortex forms the anterior part of the parahippo-campal gyrus, while the parahippocampal area forms the posterior part of the parahippocampal gyrus, and although these two regions are contiguous regions of a single gyrus, they are distinguished by having different connections, and can even be distinguished by the naked eye, on account of the 'verrucae' on the surface of the entorhinal cortex that correspond to islands in cortical layer II (Gloor, 1997).

The entorhinal cortex projects to the granule cells of the dentate gyrus, which in turn project via mossy fibres to pyramidal cells in the CA3 area (Plate 10). The efferents from CA3 divide: efferent fibres leave the hippocampus via the fimbria to join the fornix, which travels caudally on the medial wall of the temporal horn to the hippocampal commissure (which allows communication with the opposite hemisphere). From the hippocampal commissure, the fornix arches upwards and forwards in the roof of the third ventricle, before descending to the mamillary body and hypothalamus. The remaining CA3 fibres, the Schaffer collaterals, do not leave the hippocampus at this stage, but project to the pyramidal cells of the CA1 area. From CA1, efferents leave the hippocampus via the subiculum. Fibres from the subiculum project back to the entorhinal cortex, and thence to the parahippocampal area, and eventually to more distant neocortical areas. The projections from the hippocampal formation to the ventral striatum travel via the fimbria and fornix.

# Function of the hippocampus

## Role of the hippocampus in memory

The role of the hippocampus in memory is illustrated dramatically by the well known case of the patient HM, who had a bilateral temporal resection that involved the removal of both the hippocampus and amygdala, for the treatment of epilepsy. HM suffered a severe loss of the ability to acquire new declarative memories (Scoville & Milner, 1957). Declarative memories are concerned with 'knowing that', in contrast to procedural memories, which are concerned with 'knowing how'. Declarative memories include episodic memories, which are those for particular events, and also semantic memories, which are those for facts. In HM, the deficit included a loss of the ability to lay down new memories and to retrieve recent memories. The amnesia extended for one to three years before the surgery (Milner, 1966).

Subsequent attempts to establish the relative importance of the hippocampus and amygdala in memory impairment by producing bilateral medial temporal lobe lesions in monkeys led to conflicting findings, but, on balance, the evidence indicates that hippocampal damage alone is sufficient to produce memory deficit (Mahut et al, 1982; Squire & Zola-Morgan, 1983).

There has also been debate regarding the degree to which the hippocampus is engaged in laying down new memories or in the retrieval of memories. Studies using functional imaging techniques have provided uncertain findings, probably because activation of the hippocampus is relatively difficult to detect, as the hippocampal cortex lacks layers corresponding to layers I to III in isocortex. In isocortex, layer I contains horizontally spreading fibres that mediate the local spread of activation. In the absence of layer I, neural activation is likely to be more focused and less likely to produce a large change in blood flow that could be detected easily using functional imaging techniques. Early PET studies of memory demonstrated prominent frontal lobe activation during the acquisition and retrieval of memories, but relatively little evidence of hippocampal activation (Tulving et al, 1994). More recent studies have confirmed frontal lobe involvement but also demonstrated that the hippocampal formation is active during both the encoding and retrieval of memories. By 1999, over 40 functional imaging studies had reported activation of the medial temporal lobe during memory tasks, and in many of these studies the location of activation was within the hippocampal formation (see reviews by Lepage et al, 1998; Schacter & Wagner, 1999).

On the basis of their review of PET studies on memory, Lepage et al (1998) concluded that the anterior hippocampus is engaged during the encoding of memories, while the posterior hippocampus is engaged during retrieval. However, in a more comprehensive review, including additional PET studies, and also studies employing fMRI, Schacter & Wagner (1999) demonstrated that most fMRI studies have reported posterior hippocampal activation during encoding, while approximately 60% of sites of activation reported in PET studies of encoding were located anteriorly. The tendency for a difference between fMRI and PET studies in the reported location of activation during encoding may reflect differences in the nature of the memory tasks in the various studies. At this stage, the balance of evidence indicates that both the anterior and posterior hippocampal formation are engaged during encoding. The majority of studies of retrieval have revealed posterior activation, but any interpretation of this observation must be tempered with caution, because factors such as the nature of the material that is being processed may also affect the location of activation.

In accord with the evidence that the hippocampus is involved in spatial learning in rats (O'Keefe & Nadel, 1978), imaging studies demonstrate that this is also the case in humans. Maguire *et al* (1998) demonstrated, using PET, that during navigation through a complex, virtual-reality town, activation of the right hippocampus was associated with knowing accurately where places were located and navigating accurately between them. More recently, she and her colleagues have demonstrated, using structural MRI, that taxi drivers with extensive navigation experience have enlargement of the posterior hippocampus, bilaterally, compared with control subjects (Maguire *et al*, 2000).

The evidence indicates that both the right and left hippocampus are engaged during encoding and retrieval of figurative (i.e. non-verbal) material. The majority of studies of the encoding of verbal information report left medial temporal activation, whereas both the left and right medial temporal lobes are implicated in the retrieval of verbal memories (Lepage *et al*, 1998).

A further issue of debate has been whether the hippocampus plays a role only in consciously accessible memories (i.e. declarative memories), or whether it is also involved in non-conscious memory for the associations between features of a complex situation. A study by Chun & Phelps (1999) provides compelling evidence that the hippocampus is involved in memory for contextual information, irrespective of conscious recollection. Chun & Phelps demonstrated that patients with hippocampal lesions were unable to benefit from background contextual information, whereas healthy subjects did benefit from this information irrespective of conscious awareness. The involvement of the hippocampus in the utilisation of contextual information suggests that a major feature of the role of the hippocampus in memory is the integration of information received simultaneously from diverse sources. One of the defining features of episodic declarative memories is the attachment of the remembered item of information to the context in which it occurred. Attachment to context not only makes it possible for contextual prompting to facilitate retrieval, but also enables validation of the remembered information.

In summary, studies of the role of the hippocampus in human memory demonstrate that it plays a cardinal role in declarative episodic memories. In conjunction with the frontal cortex and other areas, it is involved in both laying down and retrieving memories. As in animals, the human hippocampus is involved in spatial learning. It also facilitates the use of contextual information, irrespective of conscious awareness.

It is possible that the essential contribution of the hippocampus to memory is the consolidation of the association between the multiple features of a complex stimulus. By recording electrical activity in hippocampal neurons of rhesus monkeys, Cahusac *et al* (1989) demonstrated that some hippocampal neurons fire during the learning of a new association between visual stimuli and spatial responses and, furthermore, that the activity of these neurons is modified during the learning. Monkeys with hippocampal damage have an impaired ability to perform object–place memory tasks, in which they have to remember not only what was seen but also where it was seen (Gaffan, 1994). On the basis of a review of the role of the hippocampus in memory in rats, monkeys and humans, Squire (1993) concluded that the feature of hippocampal function common to these three species is a role in paired-associate learning.

Inputs from diverse cortical areas are focused on a relatively small number of pyramidal neurons in the CA3 region of the hippocampus. Furthermore, the output of each CA3 pyramidal neuron is fed via recurrent collateral fibres to the dendritic trees of many other CA3 pyramidal neurons (Rolls, 1989). Assuming that these recurrent connections between CA3 neurons are strengthened in proportion to the frequency of their activation, Rolls (1989) has shown, by mathematical modelling, that the CA3 region could act as an auto-association memory device. An auto-association memory device is a neural network in which memories are stored by strengthening the connections between the neurons in the network in such a manner that re-exposure of the network to a fragment of a previously presented pattern of inputs reactivates the entire pattern of neural activity evoked by the previous pattern of inputs. According to Rolls' hypothesis, the excitation of a combination of CA3 neurons during initial exposure to a particular combination of features of a complex stimulus would strengthen the connections between these neurons in such a way that subsequent firing in a small subset of these neurons would recreate the initial firing pattern throughout the network. In other words, subsequent stimulation of a subset of neurons in the network would reactivate the memory.

Not only does the CA3 region receive highly convergent input from widespread cortical areas, but it also projects back to these cortical areas (Rolls, 1989). As a consequence, the activation of a memory trace in the CA3 region would be expected to re-create a pattern of cortical activity similar to that which existed during the initial exposure to the remembered event. Assuming that activation of the cortex according to a particular pattern strengthens synaptic connections so as to reinforce that pattern, the re-creation of the initial pattern of cortical activity would consolidate that pattern. Eventually, the cortical representation of the memory might become sufficiently strong that hippocampal activity would no longer be required for the reactivation of that pattern of activity. By that stage, the memory would have been transformed from an episodic memory (information related to a specific event) to an item of semantic memory (something that is known as a fact possessing generalised validity).

## The hippocampus and monitoring

In Chapter 2, we examined evidence from functional imaging studies demonstrating that the parahippocampal gyrus and the hippocampus are active during the performance of tasks that make heavy demands on the mechanism for internal monitoring of self-generated activity. This was the case for a demanding eye-movement task (Frith *et al*, 1992) and also for the generation of 'alien' internal speech, imagined in the voice of another person (McGuire *et al*, 2000).

If the CA3 region of the hippocampus acts as an auto-association memory device, as proposed by Rolls (1989), it would also have the potential to adjust the pattern of cortical activity during the generation of a motor or speech act so as to match the intended pattern of cortical activity. The preparation for a motor act entails activation of the motor areas that will be engaged during performance of the act (Roland, 1985). During this preparatory stage, the CA3 region would be expected to store a representation of the intended pattern of cerebral activity. As the execution of the act proceeds, provided any part of the intended pattern was being achieved, the entire representation would be activated in the CA3 region, and projected back to the cortical regions involved, thereby reinforcing those components of the current pattern that match the intended pattern, and tending to correct any deviations from the intended pattern.

# Anatomy of the amygdala

## Cortex-like and non-cortex-like nuclei

The amygdala is an accumulation of grey matter structures interspersed with several prominent fibre bundles. The accumulations of grey matter can be divided into two major types: those that resemble cerebral cortex in having pyramidal cells as a prominent element, and those that do not have pyramidal cells. The cortex-like cell masses include the lateral nucleus, basal nucleus, accessory basal nucleus and the peri-amygdaloid cortex (Plate 11). The principal non-cortex-like nuclei are the central nucleus and the medial nucleus, which lie adjacent to each other on the dorsal aspect of the amygdala. Although these two nuclei are separated by the medial fibre bundle, there is some overlap of the dendritic trees of their constituent cells.

## Internal connections

A simplified representation of the multiplex internal connections within the amygdala is given in Plate 11. In general, there are strong interconnections between the cortex-like nuclei. In addition, the cortex-like nuclei project to the non-cortex-like nuclei but there are relatively few fibres projecting back from non-cortex-like nuclei to cortex-like nuclei (McDonald, 1992). The more lateral of the cortex-like nuclei project heavily to the central nucleus, while the more medial cortex-like nuclei project to the medial nucleus.

## External connections

In primates, the amygdala, especially its cortex-like part, has extensive connections with the neocortex (Amaral et al, 1992). The amygdala receives input from unimodal sensory areas engaged in relatively high-level processing of the sensory input, and sends fibres in return to both higher- and lower-level processing areas in the sensory cortex, which suggests that the amygdala has the capacity to modify many levels of sensory processing. The amygdala also has strong reciprocal connections with the frontal, insular and cingulate cortex. The reciprocal connections with the frontal lobe tend to be concentrated in the medial, orbital and

**49**

lateral regions, rather than with the dorsolateral frontal cortex. The fibres of the extensive amygdalocortical projections travel in the external capsule, which lies adjacent to the lateral and ventral aspects of the amygdaloid formation. In addition to direct amygdalocortical projections, the amygdala can also influence frontal cortical areas via projections from the amygdala to the dorsomedial nucleus of the thalamus, which in turn projects to the frontal cortex. The basal and accessory basal nuclei of the amygdala project to the corpus striatum, especially the ventral striatum.

In addition to the connections to the cortex, dorsomedial thalamus and striatum, the amygdala has major connections with basal forebrain cholinergic nuclei, such as the nucleus basalis of Meynert; with the entorhinal cortex and hippocampus; and with the midline thalamic nuclei, the hypothalamus and the brain-stem. The central and medial (non-cortex-like) nuclei of the amygdala are the major source of the strong projections that travel via either the stria terminalis or the ventral amygdalo-fugal pathway to the hypothalamus, making it possible for the amygdala to exert a strong influence on visceral functions that are under hypothalamic control.

In summary, the amygdala receives a major input from sensory processing areas and from the frontal cortex, in addition to lesser inputs from a multitude of sites, including basal cholinergic nuclei, midline thalamus and hypothalamus. After the input is processed, which apparently entails interaction between the various nuclei within the amygdala, the output is transmitted via efferent fibres back to sensory areas reflecting diverse levels of processing, and to the frontal cortex and related subcortical structures, such as the striatum and dorsomedial thalamus. In addition, there are projections from the central and medial nuclei of the amygdala to the thalamus, hypothalamus and brain-stem.

Thus the connections of the amygdala indicate a capacity to support mediation between cortical processes and hypothalamic control of visceromotor and hormonal processes. Such mediation could entail learning to associate perceived objects with visceral responses. Although the internal structure of the amygdala does not have the regularity of the hippocampus, and perhaps does not lend itself so readily to the precise response to complex patterns, such a capacity for precise response may be irrelevant in the sphere of visceral responses. The extensive projections from the amygdala to the cortex may indicate an ability not only to transmit information concerning sensory perception to visceromotor centres, but also to reflect to the cortex an evaluation of perceived object with regard to the satisfaction of basic bodily needs.

# Role of the amygdala in motivation and fear in animals

The multiplicity of connections of the amygdala provide it with the information necessary for complex evaluation of the motivational significance of a situation. Such an evaluation is illustrated by Nishijo's identification of amygdala neurons that fire when a monkey is presented with a watermelon, but not when presented with a watermelon salted to make it unpalatable (Nishijo *et al*, 1988).

Projections from the amygdala to the ventral striatum interact with dopaminergic influences ascending from the substantia nigra and VTA in the midbrain, to regulate flow through the feedback loops that regulate activity in the prefrontal cortex. Cador *et al* (1989) showed that excitotoxic lesions in the basolateral part of the amygdala decreased the rate of responding in rats presented with a conditioned reinforcer (a dipper noise that the rats had been trained to associate with the delivery of water). On the basis of comparison with relevant control conditions, they concluded that the lesions of the amygdala diminished the rewarding property of the conditioned stimulus, without impairment of the discriminative properties of the stimulus. Amphetamine infused to the ventral striatum amplified the residual ability to respond to the conditioned stimulus that remained after the amygdala lesion.

As mentioned above, the amygdala plays a crucial role in conditioned fear in animals. Kapp *et al* (1984) demonstrated that lesions of the central nucleus of the amygdala obstruct the acquisition of conditioned fear reactions. Conversely, a conditioned aversive tone triggers neural firing in the amygdala. Evidence indicates that extinction of learned fear is mediated by projections from the medial prefrontal area to the amygdala (Morgan *et al*, 1993).

Bilateral removal of the amygdala, together with the adjacent temporal isocortex, produces the Kluver–Bucy syndrome in rhesus monkeys (Kluver & Bucy, 1937). This includes a form of psychic blindness, together with changes in emotional and sexual behaviour. The monkeys approach objects, animate or inanimate, without fear, and examine them by oral contact or sniffing. The psychic blindness is a form of visual agnosia, mainly due to the loss of the temporal isocortex, which forms part of the pathway for object identification. The decrease in fear and other emotional changes are attributable to loss of the amygdala.

# Function of the human amygdala

Circumscribed damage to the amygdala is rare, but in the few reported cases of patients with such lesions, there are emotional deficits. For example, a patient with Urbach–Wiethe disease, which causes bilateral destruction of the amygdala but preserves the hippocampus and neocortex, suffered from impaired ability to recognise emotion in facial expressions (Adolphs *et al*, 1994). She was most markedly impaired in recognising fearful expressions, despite a well preserved ability to recognise the identity of faces. Such impairment leads to subtle social consequences. Adolphs *et al* (1998) examined the ability of three patients with bilateral amygdala damage to judge the faces of unfamiliar people with respect to attributes important in real-life social encounters: approachability and trustworthiness. All three patients judged unfamiliar individuals to be more approachable and trustworthy than did healthy subjects.

The consequences of electrical stimulation of the human amygdala indicate that its activation can generate powerful emotional experiences, but that these are very dependent on circumstances (Halgren *et al*, 1978; Gloor *et al*, 1982). In general, the elicited phenomena are reproducible within a session, but variable between sessions, depending on circumstances, and also between individuals, depending on personality.

Functional imaging studies demonstrate that the amygdala is active during the perception of fearful faces (Morris *et al*, 1996). In an fMRI study of cerebral activity during the learning of words, my colleagues and I found that the amygdala, together with the ventral striatum and anterior cingulate cortex, were active during the processing of emotional words, compared with the processing of emotionally neutral words (Kiehl *et al*, 1998).

Despite this evidence that the amygdala plays a role in emotion, especially fear, the consequences of amygdala lesions in humans are less dramatic than in animals. This may indicate that, in the human, alternative methods of motivation have rendered limbic mechanisms less dominant. For example, it is possible that behaviour that is guided by plans formulated in linguistic terms is adequately supported by neocortical language areas. While a person whose behaviour was guided entirely by plans formulated linguistically would be deprived of subtle subjective experiences, the behaviour of that individual might not be overtly abnormal in the eyes of an observer.

# Limbic system and mental symptoms

In the light of the evidence that the limbic system is involved in emotional and motivational processing, it might be expected that the limbic system would be involved in anxiety and depression. In particular, the evidence that the amygdala is involved in conditioned fear in animals, and in responses to fearful situations in humans, suggests that aberrant overactivity in the amygdala is likely to play an important role in anxiety disorders. In accord with this expectation, the majority of functional imaging studies of anxiety disorders reveal limbic overactivity in anxiety disorders (e.g. Rauch *et al*, 1996), although paradoxically, the studies by Frederickson and colleagues (Wik *et al*, 1993; Fischer *et al*, 1998) report limbic underactivity. This issue is discussed further in Chapter 10.

In Chapter 2 we discussed evidence indicating that the predisposition to depression is associated with underactivity in the paralimbic association cortex, while the actual experience of depression can be associated with overactivity in these areas. The limited available evidence regarding core limbic structures indicates that the amygdala is overactive in both the depressed and remitted state, at least in patients with familial depression. Drevets *et al* (1992) used PET to study patients with familial depression, both during a depressive episode and during remission. They found increased activity in the left amygdala in the depressed and in the remitted state, but the degree of increase was statistically significant only during the depressed state. In addition, they observed activation in the ventral striatum and anterior cingulate during the depressed state. The authors concluded that the abnormal overactivity in the left amygdala may represent a trait marker of familial pure depressive disease, although they acknowledged that further assessment with a larger sample is necessary to establish this. The complex body of evidence regarding activity of the limbic and paralimbic cortex in depression is discussed in greater detail in Chapter 9.

There is also evidence that the hippocampus is involved in depression, possibly by virtue of its susceptibility to damage by excessive levels of corticosteroids. Sheline *et al* (1999) found that elderly patients with a long history of depressive illness had decreased hippocampal volume. The potential role of the hippocampus in channelling information from the cerebral cortex to the HPA axis also raises the possibility that the hippocampus may not merely be damaged by depression, but may also play an active part in the mechanism through which stress precipitates depression. This issue is also discussed further in Chapter 9.

There is substantial evidence, which we shall review in detail in Chapter 6, indicating that hippocampal overactivity plays an important role in the mechanism of reality distortion. In particular, we shall explore the evidence that aberrant firing within the hippocampus leads to false attribution of contextual support for ideas and internally generated perceptions, which leads to delusions and hallucinations. In addition, the evidence from the study of generation of 'alien' internal speech by McGuire *et al* (2000), discussed above, indicates that hippocampal malfunction may contribute to a diminished ability to monitor the source of self-generated speech, which could predispose the sufferer to auditory verbal hallucinations.

# Chapter 4

# Cortico-subcortical circuits

## Introduction

The level of neural activity in the frontal cortex is subject to modulation by feedback loops that project from the cortex to the basal ganglia to the thalamus and back to the cortex. In primates, five major bundles of loops have been distinguished (Alexander *et al*, 1986; Alexander & Crutcher, 1990a), serving, respectively:

(1)  the motor areas (comprising the primary motor cortex, supplementary motor area and premotor cortex);
(2)  the oculomotor areas (the frontal eye field and supplementary eye field);
(3)  the medial frontal cortex (the medial orbital frontal cortex and anterior cingulate cortex);
(4)  the dorsolateral prefrontal cortex;
(5)  the lateral orbital frontal cortex.

The motor and oculomotor loops are concerned with the planning and execution of limb and eye movements respectively, while the other three loops, which serve limbic and prefrontal areas, play a role in the maintenance and switching of more complex behavioural patterns.

## Basic loop circuitry

The general structure of these loops is shown in Plate 12. The first step is a monosynaptic excitatory glutamatergic projection from the cortex to the corpus striatum, which functions as the input terminal to the basal ganglia.

The second step connects the striatum to the output terminal of the basal ganglia, located in either the globus pallidus interna (GPi) or the substantia nigra pars reticulata (SNr). This second step can follow either a direct monosynaptic route or an indirect route involving two or three synapses. The direct pathway is a GABA-ergic projection from the striatum to the GPi/SNr that exerts an inhibitory effect on the output from the basal ganglia. The GABA-ergic striatal neurons of the direct pathway employ substance P as a co-transmitter. The striatal neurons projecting via indirect routes employ enkephalin as a co-transmitter. The two-synaptic indirect route comprises a GABA-ergic projection from the striatum to the globus pallidus externa (GPe) and, thence, a second GABA-ergic projection to the output neuron in GPi or SNr. The three-synaptic route comprises a GABA-ergic projection from the striatum to the GPe, followed by a GABA-ergic projection to the subthalamic nucleus, which sends an excitatory projection to the output neuron in the GPi/SNr. In both instances, the indirect path includes two inhibitory synapses within the basal ganglia, so the net effect of activity in this pathway is an excitatory influence on the output terminal in the GPi/SNr.

The third step is an inhibitory GABA-ergic projection from the GPi/SNr to the thalamus. The fourth step is an excitatory glutamatergic projection from the thalamus back to the cortical region where the loop began.

The GPi/SNr output neurons have a high tonic rate of spontaneous firing that exerts a tonic inhibitory effect on the thalamus. Therefore, when the inhibitory direct pathway between the striatum and the GPi/SNr is activated, the thalamic inhibition is diminished and the loop provides positive feedback to the cortical area of origin. Conversely, when the indirect pathway is activated, the tonic inhibition of the thalamus by the GPi/SNr is enhanced and the loop provides negative feedback to the cortical area of origin.

The five major bundles of feedback loops are at least partially segregated. At the basal ganglion input stage, the motor and oculomotor cortex project to different parts of the putamen (that part of the striatum lying lateral to the internal capsule), while the dorsal and ventrolateral prefrontal cortex projects to different parts of the caudate nucleus (which lies medial to the internal capsule), and the limbic frontal cortex projects to the ventral striatum (which lies below the level of the internal capsule). At the basal ganglion output stage, the motor and oculomotor loops project to ventrolateral thalamic nuclei and to the pars magnocellularis and the pars parvocellularis of the ventroanterior nucleus, while in the prefrontal and limbic loops, the basal ganglia output neurons project mainly to the thalamic mediodorsal nucleus.

The motor loop has been most comprehensively investigated, and hence understanding of the other loops is guided by these findings. As further knowledge accumulates, it is likely that unique features characteristic of each individual type of loop will emerge, although the general architecture of the loops is similar. The only loop to show a discernible difference in general structure is that serving the limbic cortex, which differs insofar as both the direct and indirect pathways in this loop project from the striatum to a region of the globus pallidus in which internal and external pallidum cannot be distinguished. None the less, the direct and indirect pathways can be distinguished by the fact that the striatal efferents of the direct loop contain substance P as co-transmitter while the striatal efferents of the indirect loop contain enkephalin as co-transmitter.

# External influence on the loops

Although the loops are closed, they are not isolated from influences derived from other regions. The striatum receives moderating dopaminergic influences from the substantia nigra pars compacta (SNc), and also noradrenergic influences from the locus coeruleus and serotonergic influences from the raphe nuclei. These monoaminergic influences are of vital importance in setting the tone for activity in each of the loops. The modulatory effects of monoamines on the loops provide them with the potential to play a key role in the amplification or diminution of the level of activity in the neural assemblies that represent meaningful neural events.

## Dopaminergic modulation

The modulation of the loops by dopaminergic projections from the SNc is complex. The evidence suggests that increased dopaminergic activity inhibits activity in the indirect pathway while enhancing activity in the direct pathway (Alexander & Crutcher, 1990a). Because activation of the indirect pathway achieves a net reduction of thalamic activation of the cortex, while activation of the direct pathway enhances thalamocortical activation, increased dopaminergic activity tends to enhance positive feedback to the cortex, while decreased dopaminergic activity has the opposite effect.

Within the dopaminergic system there are compensatory mechanisms, such as an increased synthesis of dopamine and a decreased rate of dopamine inactivation, that restore function after neuronal loss, to the extent that virtually complete destruction of SNc neurons is required before sustained, clinically significant effects become apparent (Zigmond *et al*, 1990). Furthermore, in the light of evidence that dopaminergic nigrostriatal fibres exert their inhibitory effects in the striatum by means of a presynaptic inhibitory influence on glutamatergic corticostriatal neurons, it would also be possible, at least in principle, to compensate for decreased dopaminergic activity by a reduction in strength of glutamatergic transmission (Carlsson & Carlsson, 1990). As a corollary, a pathological reduction in corticostriatal glutamatergic activity in the presence of normal levels of dopaminergic activity would mimic a hyperdopaminergic state.

## Limbic gating

As discussed in Chapter 3, projections from the limbic structures of the medial temporal lobe probably play a major role in the deployment of contextual or motivational information to regulate the feedback that the loops provide to the prefrontal cortex (Kelley & Domesick, 1982). Grace *et al* (1998) have demonstrated in studies of rats that in the absence of input from the hippocampus, the spiny neurons in the ventral striatum are hyperpolarised, and therefore unable to fire in response to input from the prefrontal cortex. Sustained input from the hippocampus via the glutamatergic projections to the striatum relieves the hyperpolarisation, so that the spiny neurons are able to fire in response to input from the prefrontal cortex. Thus the hippocampal input has a gating action on transmission in the cortico-subcortical loops.

## Non-frontal cortical input

In addition to the frontal cortical area that receives the feedback from the loops, other cortical areas, including sensory cortical areas, send efferents to the input stage of the basal ganglia.

# Parallel processing

There has been substantial debate regarding the extent to which the basal ganglia act as a funnel for information from different cortical areas. For example, funnelling would be anticipated if the role of the basal ganglia was to produce convergence of cortical neural activity into a small number of integratory units at a late processing stage in the execution of behaviour. While a degree of funnelling is implicit in the observation that the posterior sensory cortex and medial temporal limbic cortex project to the loops that serve the frontal cortex, the loops serving different frontal areas appear to be fairly well segregated within the basal ganglia.

Selemon & Goldman-Rakic (1988) have argued for essentially segregated pathways on the basis of the evidence that different cortical areas project to distinguishable, although adjacent, areas of the striatum. Within each major loop, the available evidence suggests that the various subdivisions also remain segregated. For example, in the motor loop, there are separate somatotopic channels for the control of leg, arm and orofacial movements (Alexander *et al*, 1990). Furthermore, at each stage of the loop, different neurons are involved in different levels of processing, such as defining the target, determining the trajectory and activation of specific muscles (Alexander & Crutcher, 1990b).

On the other hand, Hazrati & Parent (1992) have demonstrated that neurons from the striatum and subthalamic nucleus have multiple representations in the globus pallidus and SNr, implying diversification of the influence of striatal and subthalamic nuclear neurons upon thalamocortical neurons. In a review of the roles of the anatomically distinct core and shell regions of the ventral striatum in rats, Deutch *et al* (1993) argue that the shell region is part of a loop that has its origin in the inferomedial prefrontal cortex, but the output of this loop projects not only back to the cortex of origin, but also to more dorsal regions of the prefrontal cortex, which in turn project to the core region of the ventral striatum, from where projections eventually reach premotor areas. Thus, in addition to the strictly circular loop pathway, there is a spiral pathway that allows information to be transmitted from one loop to an adjacent loop serving cortex nearer to the motor cortex.

On balance, while much evidence indicates that the loops are essentially parallel, there is also evidence for interaction between loops, including a tendency for information to converge towards cortical areas that are nearer to premotor and motor areas. The essentially parallel organisation suggests that the main role of the basal ganglia is to provide modulated feedback to localised cortical areas. In addition, it is probable that they play a part in collecting information from diverse areas, and funnelling it towards the motor cortex.

## Sequential and parallel processing within loops

Recording of electrical potential in monkeys indicates that when the onset of a movement is triggered by a stimulus, neuronal firing can be detected in cortical areas before it can be detected in the subcortical components of the motor loop, which indicates that the initiation of processing by the loop follows a sequential pattern beginning in the cortex. None the less, for most of the duration of the response, electrical activity can be detected in all components of the circuit, which implies concurrent processing at all stages of the loop (Crutcher & Alexander, 1990).

# Striatal matrix and patch structure

On the basis of histochemical characteristics and connections, it is possible to distinguish demarcated patches from the matrix of the corpus striatum. The striatal neurons that participate in the loops that feed back to the cortex via the thalamus are located in the matrix. The cortical afferents to these neurons derive from the more superficial layers of the cortex. The neurons in the patches receive cortical afferents from deeper parts of the cortex – layers V and VI (Gerfen, 1989) – and project largely to the dopaminergic neurons of the substantia nigra and also to other deep nuclei, such as the acetylcholinergic basal nucleus of Meynert. Thus the connections of the neurons in the patches indicate that they have the potential to transmit information from the cortex to nuclei containing modulatory neurotransmitters. This is an essential component of the reciprocal flow of information between the cortex and brain structures specialised for mediating motivation.

Within the corpus striatum, the density of patches is least in the regions serving the motor loops and greatest in the ventral striatum, which serves the limbic loop (Alheid & Heimer, 1988). This is consistent with the expectation that the limbic loop is much more heavily involved in the regulation of the motivational processes that govern the selection and initiation of meaningful neural events.

# Cortico-subcortical loops and supervisory processes

The architecture of the loops implies a potential capacity to support the supervisory mental functions, such as initiation, selection and monitoring of mental activity, that are implicated in the mechanisms of mental symptoms. If a monkey is provided with a priming stimulus that indicates the direction of a subsequent movement that is to follow a triggering stimulus, electrical activity can be detected in the precentral motor areas, including the premotor cortex and SMA, and the globus pallidus during the preparatory phase between the priming stimulus and the triggering stimulus, which implies that the motor loop is engaged in the establishing 'motor set' (Alexander & Crutcher, 1990c). There are several specific types of processing for which the loops appear well suited, which are relevant to their potential role in supervisory mental functions.

## Modulating the amplitude of neural events

The structure of the loops indicates that they may either enhance or diminish a signal arising in the cortex. It would be predicted that, in conditions such as Parkinson's disease, a reduction in dopaminergic tone would produce a hypokinetic state by shifting the balance of activity from the direct to the indirect pathway from the striatum to the GPi/SNr. This prediction is supported by the observed effects of the destruction of nigrostriatal dopaminergic projections in monkeys by the toxin MPTP, which produces hypokinesia resembling that in Parkinson's disease. In particular, the hypokinetic state following MPTP administration is accompanied by increased tonic firing of neurons in the GPi and subthalamic nucleus, and a decrease in tonic firing of GPe neurons, as would be expected if the indirect pathway was more active (DeLong, 1990). Conversely, disorders such as L-dopa-induced dyskinesia, which entail reduced striatopallidal influences mediated via the indirect pathway, produce hyperkinetic motor disorders (DeLong, 1990). Thus, at least within the motor loop, shifting the balance towards the indirect pathway produces hypokinesia, and shifting the balance away from the indirect pathway causes hyperkinesia. Similarly, decreased dopaminergic tone in the loops serving prefrontal areas would be expected to producing a slowing or a diminished amount of thought, while increased dopaminergic tone would be expected to be associated with pressure of thought.

In hyperkinetic motor disorders, such as L-dopa-induced movement disorders and Huntington's chorea, involuntary tics and grimaces occur. This suggests that in a state of marked imbalance in favour of the direct pathway, motor acts that have not been selected on the basis of either contextual or motivational relevance tend to intrude. In the case of Tourette syndrome, which also entails dopamin-ergic hyperactivity, and hence is likely to lead to imbalance in favour of the direct pathway, involuntary vocalisations can occur.

The repetitive nature of the tics or grimaces in hyperkinetic motor disorders, and the verbalisations in Tourette syndrome, is consistent with the hypothesis, proposed in Chapter 1, that the initiation of actions entails the emergence of the neural representation of a specific act from among a multitude of neural representations that are at least subliminally active at any one time. By virtue of multiple repetitions, the patterns of neural activity representing a rehearsed act would be expected to be relatively strongly represented among the multitude of neural patterns present at any time, and hence would be prone to amplification by positive feedback, irrespective of contextual or motivational relevance.

## Focusing on a specific activity

In monkeys rendered Parkinsonian by the dopaminergic neurotoxin MPTP, there are problems not only with the level of motor activity but also the selectivity of activity. The phasic signals in the GPi associated with proprioceptive feedback concerning limb position are decreased in selectivity, and so tend to produce coarse adjustments involving more muscle groups than necessary. This failure of focusing in states of dopamine depletion implies that, at least in the prefrontal motor loops, appropriately regulated dopaminergic tone helps maintain focus on the currently salient activity.

The focus produced by the well balanced functioning of the cortico-subcortical loops does not merely entail enhancement of a single act at the expense of all other acts. It appears that optimum dopaminergic tone facilitates the concurrent execution of several separate actions. Patients with Parkinson's disease are slower at performing each of two motor acts when the acts are performed either concurrently or sequentially than when they are performed at quite different times, even in instances where the actions are sufficiently simple that a normal individual might perform the two together without noticeable interference (De Long, 1990).

## Monitoring of activity

The loops also appear to play a role in the monitoring of continuing activity to ensure that it follows a predetermined plan. For example, the triggering of proprioceptive neurons by passive movement of limbs generates phasic discharge in the globus pallidus (De Long, 1990). When taken together with the observation that there is activity in the globus pallidus during the establishment of 'set' prior to a motor act (Alexander & Crutcher, 1990a), this raises the possibility that the loops play a role in monitoring the execution of internally generated plans for action.

# Relevance of cortico-subcortical loops to mental symptoms

The specific patterns of cerebral activity associated with the various syndromes of psychiatric symptoms (which we shall consider in greater detail in Part II) include either excessive or diminished activity in subcortical structures. For example, studies using PET indicate excessive positive feedback to the frontal cortex, mediated via the cortico-subcortical loops, in both the disorganisation syndrome (formal thought disorder, inappropriate affect) and the reality distortion syndrome (delusions and hallucinations). In the disorganisation syndrome, there is overactivity in the medial frontal cortex and in the thalamus (Liddle *et al*, 1992). In the reality distortion syndrome there is overactivity in the frontal cortex, medial temporal lobe and ventral striatum (Liddle *et al*, 1992; Silbersweig *et al*, 1995). Treatment with antipsychotic drugs produces a reduction in metabolism in the ventral striatum, thalamus and frontal cortex (Liddle *et al*, 2000). This observation is consistent with the hypothesis that antipsychotic drugs, which block dopamine, act by alleviating excessive positive feedback via the cortico-subcortical loops.

The role of the cortico-subcortical feedback loops in psychomotor poverty (poverty of speech, flat affect, decreased spontaneous movement) is less clear. In a study of patients with severe persistent schizophrenia, my colleagues and I observed that psychomotor poverty is associated with underactivity in the frontal cortex and overactivity in the basal ganglia, especially in the corpus striatum (Liddle *et al*, 1992). The association of psychomotor poverty with frontal underactivity and subcortical overactivity was confirmed by Yuasa *et al* (1995).

The combination of frontal underactivity and striatal overactivity is paradoxical, since frontal underactivity might be expected to be associated with striatal underactivity. It should be noted that in our study (Liddle *et al*, 1992), the observed region of overactivity in the basal ganglia apparently embraced both the caudate nucleus and the globus pallidus. Given the limited spatial resolution of PET, it is possible that the observed increase might in fact have reflected overactivity in the globus pallidus rather than the caudate nucleus. Because the striatum exerts an inhibitory action on the globus pallidus, decreased neural firing in the striatum would be expected to lead to increased firing in the globus pallidus.

This speculation is consistent with the observation by Porrino *et al* (1987) that lesions produced in monkeys by MPTP lead to decreased metabolism in the frontal cortex and increased metabolism in the globus pallidus (detected by postmortem autoradiography several months after the administration of MPTP). Consistent with the fact that the lesions were produced by damage to dopamine neurons, Porrino also observed decreased metabolism in the substantia nigra and VTA, where the cell bodies of dopaminergic neurons are located. The resemblance

**61**

between the pattern of cerebral activity in psychomotor poverty in schizophrenia, and that produced by destruction of dopamine neurons in monkeys, supports the hypothesis that chronic dopaminergic hypoactivity plays a role in psychomotor poverty in schizophrenia.

In conclusion, the cortico-subcortical circuits appear to play a major role in regulating those frontal regions that are strongly implicated in the mechanism of psychiatric symptoms. The available evidence from functional imaging studies supports this hypothesis, although the limitations of the imaging techniques employed hitherto make it necessary to be cautious in attempting to identify the precise pathways involved.

# Chapter 5

# Neurotransmission and humoral influences

## Introduction

There are several characteristics of cerebral neurotransmission that are important for understanding the neural processes associated with high-level cognitive processing, motivated acts and the experience of emotion.

(1) Several types of neurotransmitter molecules, especially the amine transmitters, serve a predominantly modulatory role. That is, they act to adjust the level of activity in an assembly of neurons, rather than transmitting discrete items of information to specific postsynaptic neurons. Thus, in contrast to a digital electronic computer, the neural network supporting human mental activity is subject to continuous adjustment of the tone of processing.

(2) There is a variety of mechanisms by which activity in a neural system can produce enduring change in the structure of that neural system. In other words, the human nervous system exhibits plasticity. The molecular composition of the neurons changes in response to activity, which allows both adaptation and memory.

(3) Each individual mental act involves interaction between a number of different neurotransmitter systems. Just as the individual anatomical elements in the cerebrum make their own specific contribution to the collaborative activity of a distributed assembly of elements, so too do the different neurotransmitter systems make distinctive contributions to the activity of an integrated system involving various neurotransmitters and receptor types. Each mental act is likely to involve long-distance point-to-point information transfer via excitatory glutamatergic neurons; regulation by inhibitory GABA-ergic local circuit neurons; and modulation by several interacting aminergic systems. In addition, other modulators, such as neuropeptides, may also play a part. Meaningful neural events are unlikely to be fully understood by focusing on a single neurotransmitter system.

# Actions of neurotransmitters

Neurotransmitters are molecules that are released from a nerve terminal (the presynaptic terminal) in response to an electrical action potential, and bind to a specific receptor on an adjacent neuron (the postsynaptic neuron), producing an effect on the electrical and/or metabolic state of that neuron. Information transfer in the nervous system entails both electrical and metabolic processes. As a consequence of the metabolic processes, the transfer of information can produce enduring changes in the composition and structure of the participating neurons.

There are two major classes of neuroreceptor: ionotropic receptors (ligand-gated ion channels) and metabotropic receptors (ligand-gated metabolic transducers). The former have a structure specialised for the production of rapid changes in postsynaptic transmembrane electrical potential. The latter produce a diverse range of metabolic effects. None the less, binding of a neurotransmitter at either type of receptor can produce both electrical and metabolic changes.

## Ionotropic receptors

Ionotropic receptors are multi-subunit proteins embedded in the cell membrane so as to frame an ion channel. The receptor has a site shaped to match that of a corresponding neurotransmitter molecule, and this allows the selective binding of the neurotransmitter at this recognition site. The binding of the neurotransmitter alters the conformation of the receptor protein in such as way as to permit the passage of a particular type of ion through the channel. Thus the binding of the neurotransmitter opens the ion channel, leading to a change in transmembrane electrical potential.

This class of receptor includes several types of glutamate receptor (see Table 5.1) and two types of GABA receptor – $GABA_A$ and $GABA_C$. Serotonergic 5-HT$_3$ receptors and the nicotinic class of cholinergic receptor are also ionotropic receptors.

Ionotropic receptors can be either excitatory, as in the case of glutamate receptors, or inhibitory, as in the case of GABA receptors. In general, at excitatory ionotropic receptors, binding of the neurotransmitter causes the opening of ion channels that allow the flow of potassium and sodium ions. Because intracellular potassium concentration is high and intracellular sodium is low, relative to the extracellular concentrations of these ions, opening of the channel results in the efflux of potassium ions and the influx of sodium ions, which causes a depolarisation of the transmembrane potential, thereby generating an excitatory postsynaptic potential. At inhibitory ionotropic receptors, binding of neurotransmitter leads to the opening of chloride ion channels, which allows influx of chloride ions; this causes hyperpolarisation of the membrane, thereby generating an inhibitory postsynaptic potential.

The ability of ionotropic receptors rapidly to generate a postsynaptic excitatory or inhibitory potential makes this type of receptor suited to the transmission of information that is sharply focused in time and location. Ionotropic excitatory glutamatergic receptors are the major type of receptor mediating long-distance point-to-point information transfer, while GABA receptors are the major type of receptor mediating spatially precise inhibition of local neural activity. In contrast, 5-HT$_3$ serotonergic receptors and nicotinic cholinergic receptors, although ionotropic, appear to play a predominantly modulatory role.

While the primary event mediated by an ionotropic receptor is the opening of an ion channel, leading to a rapid change in transmembrane potential, the activation of such receptors can also produce metabolic changes that may lead to plastic changes in the postsynaptic neuron. For example, activation of glutamate receptors of the N-methyl-D-aspartate (NMDA) class can lead to changes in intracellular calcium ion concentration that mobilise enzymes such as proteases, phospholipases and protein kinase C (PKC). These enzymes catalyse a variety of metabolic changes in the cell.

## Metabotropic receptors

Binding of the relevant neurotransmitter to a metabotropic receptor sets in train a series of biochemical steps, mediated by intracellular molecules known as

**Table 5.1** The principal types of neuroreceptor

| | Ionotropic | | Metabotropic |
|---|---|---|---|
| | **Excitatory** | **Inhibitory** | |
| Glutamate | NMDA Kainate Quisqualate | | Metabotropic glutamate receptors |
| GABA | | GABA$_A$ GABA$_C$ | GABA$_B$ |
| Acetylcholine | Nicotinic | | M$_1$, M$_2$, M$_3$, M$_4$ (muscarinic) |
| Dopamine | | | D$_1$, D$_5$ (activate cAMP system) D$_2$, D$_3$, D$_4$ (inhibit cAMP system) |
| Noradrenaline | | | Alpha$_1$ Alpha$_2$ (autoreceptors) Beta$_1$ Beta$_2$ |
| Serotonin | | 5-HT$_3$ | 5-HT$_{1A-E}$ (activate cAMP system) 5-HT$_{2A-C}$ (activate PI system) 5-HT$_4$ 5-HT$_5$ 5-HT$_6$ 5-HT$_7$ |

cAMP system, cyclic AMP second messenger system.
PI system, phosphatidyl inositol second messenger system.

second messengers, that leads to a cascade of different metabolic responses in the neuron. Metabotropic receptors are linked to G proteins, which are membrane proteins that bind guanosine triphosphate (GTP). The G protein can couple the receptor either to membrane-bound enzymes that produce second messengers or, in some circumstances, to an ion channel, allowing relatively direct effects on transmembrane electrical potential.

The second messengers generate a cascade of biochemical changes, which in most cases lead ultimately to the activation of intracellular proteins by phosphory-lation. Virtually all active intracellular neuronal proteins are subject to regulation by phosphorylation. Phosphorylated proteins are responsible for processes such as energy metabolism, neurotransmitter synthesis and release, changes in receptor sensitivity, and also the expression of genes, thereby producing poten-tially long-term changes in the composition of the neuron. In addition, protein kinases can phosphorylate ion channels, which leads to either the activation or inhibition of these channels. The changes in transmembrane potential resulting from the phosphorylation of ion channels are slow in comparison with the electrical potentials generated at ionotropic receptors.

In general, metabotropic receptors are suited to the task of exerting a modulatory influence that is relatively diffuse in duration of action. The majority of aminergic receptors are metabotropic receptors, including the alpha and beta classes of adrenoreceptors, the $D_1$ and $D_2$ families of dopamine receptor, the 5-$HT_1$ and 5-$HT_2$ families of serotonergic receptor, and all four types of muscarinic cholinergic receptor. Because aminergic neuronal systems fan out widely from a few localised points of origin at the base of the brain or in the brain-stem, the aminergic neurotransmitters tend to have an effect that is diffuse in location as well in duration. While several types of glutamate receptors, such as the NMDA receptor, are ionotropic, it should be noted that there are also metabotropic glutamate receptors. Table 5.1 summarises the mechanisms of each of the main receptor types.

## Metabotropic receptor structure

Metabotropic receptors belong to a family of protein molecules with a common structure, in which the protein chain is folded so as to cross the cell membrane seven times. Thus the protein is a chain with seven transmembrane domains, with intervening segments that form extracellular or cytoplasmic loops. The transmembrane domains contain the binding site for the neurotransmitter, while the cytoplasmic loops are coupled to a membrane-bound G protein. G proteins couple receptors to one of two enzymes: adenylate cyclase or phospholipase C. These membrane-bound enzymes in turn activate second messenger systems.

## Second messengers

Adenylate cyclase catalyses the conversion of adenosine triphosphate (ATP) to the labile high-energy compound cyclic 3,5-adenosine monophosphate (cyclic AMP, or cAMP), which acts as a second messenger and activates protein kinases that in turn phosphorylate intracellular proteins (Plate 13). This produces a diverse range of effects. Metabotropic receptors can either activate or inhibit the adenylate cyclase. For example, dopamine $D_1$ receptors are linked to G proteins that activate adenylate cyclase, while $D_2$ receptors are linked to G proteins that inhibit it.

Among the diverse consequences of activation of cAMP is the triggering of gene expression. An important mediator of gene expression is cAMP-responsive element-binding protein (CREB). Abnormalities related to CREB are potentially relevant to a number of mental disorders. For example, Kawanishi *et al* (1999) have reported an association between the occurrence of two specific variants of the gene for CREB and schizophrenia. Cyclic AMP and CREB have also been implicated in the action of mood stabilisers and antidepressants. Mood-stabilising drugs tend to decrease cAMP signalling in the brain. For example, the long-term administration of the mood stabiliser lithium inhibits the induction of phosphory-lation of CREB and the binding of CREB to DNA by the adenyl cyclase activator forskolin, in human neuroblastoma SH-SY5Y cells (Wang *et al*, 1999). These results support the hypothesis that lithium blunts the cAMP signal transduction pathway. Chen *et al* (1999) demonstrated that long-term treatment with lithium decreases CREB phosphorylation in rat cerebral cortex and hippocampus. However, long-term treatment with valproic acid, another mood stabiliser, did not achieve this same effect, indicating that other mechanisms may also be involved in mood stabilisation. We shall return to a discussion of this issue after introducing the phosphatidyl inositol second messenger system.

The other main second messenger system is the phosphatidyl inositol (PI) system (Plate 14), which is activated by the enzyme phospholipase C. This enzyme degrades an inositol lipid, PI biphosphate, producing two major products: inositol triphosphate ($IP_3$) and diacylglycerol (DAG). $IP_3$ acts to release calcium from intracellular stores, thereby initiating a series of calcium-dependent metabolic processes. DAG activates PKC, which regulates a wide range of intracellular processes by phosphorylation of proteins. Furthermore, DAG itself is hydrolysed to arachidonic acid with the subsequent formation of prostaglandins that regulate a range of metabolic processes.

One of the most influential hypotheses regarding the mechanism underlying lithium's therapeutic efficacy in bipolar affective disorder in the 1990s was the inositol depletion hypothesis, which postulated that lithium produces a thera-peutic lowering of myo-inositol in critical areas of the brain. To test this hypothesis, Moore *et al* (1999) measured regional brain myo-inositol levels by means of quantitative proton magnetic resonance spectroscopy at three time points: at baseline and after short-term (5–7 days) and long-term (3–4 weeks) lithium administration, in depressed bipolar patients. They found that both short-term and long-term administration of lithium reduced myo-inositol levels in the right frontal lobe of patients. The acute myo-inositol reduction occurred at a time when the patient's clinical state was unchanged. They concluded that the short-term reduction of myo-inositol was not associated directly with therapeutic response and therefore their findings did not support the inositol depletion hypothesis in its original form. They proposed instead that a short-term lowering of myo-inositol results in a cascade of secondary changes in signalling and gene expression within the central nervous system that are ultimately associated with lithium's therapeutic efficacy.

This hypothesis is supported by substantial evidence that not only lithium but also sodium valproate inhibit PKC, one of the major mediators in the PI signal transduction pathway. Sodium valproate is an anticonvulsant with a complex molecular structure quite different from the simple ionic structure of lithium. Manji & Lenox (1999) have reviewed evidence obtained in their own laboratory, and confirmed by others, that indicates that the family of PKC isozymes is a shared target in the brain for the long-term action of both lithium and valproate. In rats chronically treated with lithium, the expression of two protein kinase isozymes, alpha and epsilon, is reduced in the hippocampus. In addition, chronic treatment with lithium leads to a reduction in the expression of a major PKC substrate, MARCKS, which has been implicated in long-term neuroplastic events in the developing and adult brain. Further support for the hypothesis that PKC inhibition plays a role in mood stabilisation comes from data indicating that tamoxifen, an anti-oestrogen used in treating breast cancer, which also inhibits PKC, has antimanic properties.

Manji *et al* (1999b) have also demonstrated that chronic lithium treatment markedly increases the levels of the major neuroprotective protein bcl-2 in rat frontal cortex, hippocampus and striatum. Consistent with the increases in bcl-2 levels, lithium exhibits robust protective effects against diverse insults, both *in vitro* and *in vivo*.

Thus, at this stage, there is converging evidence that mood stabilisers achieve their therapeutic effects via effects on second messenger systems. However, in the light of the many effects that these agents have on signal transduction and gene expression mechanisms, the identity of the specific action that is responsible for the therapeutic effect remains uncertain. Furthermore, it should be noted that, under some circumstances, mood stabilisers have an acute antimanic effect that may be accounted for by the direct effects of receptor blockade itself. For example, several studies have demonstrated that valproate achieves an antimanic effect within a day of achieving an adequate serum concentration (approximately 350 $\mu$g/ml) (Keck *et al*, 1993). In view of the fact that valproate is an agonist at GABA$_A$ receptors, it is plausible that enhancement of the action of the inhibitory neurotransmitter, GABA, has an immediate antimanic effect.

# Neuromodulation via axonal receptors

Classical neurotransmission involves the summation of the concurrent excitatory and inhibitory postsynaptic potentials generated in the spines distributed along the spreading branches of the dendritic tree. An action potential is generated when a threshold for firing is achieved. The action potential is transmitted along an axon to a remote site where that axon synapses with the dendrite of another neuron. The arrival of the action potential triggers the release of neurotransmitter molecules into the synaptic cleft, and the subsequent binding of neurotransmitter to postsynaptic receptors on the dendrite leads to electrical and chemical changes in the postsynaptic neuron, which can in turn promote or inhibit firing of that neuron. However, the transmission of information is subject to modulation at many sites. In particular, modulatory neurotransmitters can bind to receptors on the axon in the vicinity of the presynaptic terminal in a way that either promotes or inhibits the release of transmitter into the synaptic cleft.

It is probable that modulatory effects mediated by these receptors play a central role in the generation of mental symptoms. Many psychotropic drugs act at these neuromodulatory receptor sites. The fact that these sites allow interaction between different types of neurotransmitter creates the potential for subtle influence on the function of a particular neural pathway without the complete paralysis of information transmission that would result from simple blockade of the pathway.

## Presynaptic heteroreceptors

In some instances, presynaptic receptors are specific for a neurotransmitter other than the neuron's own transmitter. Such heteroreceptors allow one neuro-transmitter to modulate the release of a different neurotransmitter. For example, serotonin acts at $5\text{-HT}_3$ receptors on presynaptic dopaminergic terminals to inhibit dopamine release, and at $5\text{-HT}_3$ receptors on presynaptic cholinergic terminals to inhibit the release of acetylcholine. Serotonin can also inhibit dopamine release via presynaptic $5\text{-HT}_{2A}$ receptors. The existence of different types of heteroreceptor modulating a particular neurotransmitter in different brain regions offers scope for regionally specific modulation of that neuro-transmitter. Noradrenergic neurons interact with the dopaminergic system, both at the level of the brain-stem dopaminergic nuclei and in the cortex (Tassin, 1992). In rats, noradrenergic activity in the VTA promotes dopaminergic activity in the frontal cortex but not in the ventral striatum (Herve *et al*, 1982).

## The mechanism of atypical antipsychotic action

A substantial body of evidence indicates that typical antipsychotic drugs act by blocking dopamine $D_2$ receptors. In Chapter 6 we shall examine evidence indicating that blockade of $D_2$ receptors in the ventral striatum plays a cardinal role in the antipsychotic effect. However, simple blockade of $D_2$ receptors throughout the brain produces not only an antipsychotic effect but also undesir-able side-effects, such as extrapyramidal movement disorders, through blockade of $D_2$ receptors in the dorsal striatum, and elevation of prolactin as a consequence of blockade of dopamine in the hypothalamus. The discovery that clozapine, which blocks many neuroreceptors, including serotonin $5\text{-HT}_{2A}$ and alpha adrenoceptors, in addition to $D_2$ receptors, can achieve superior antipsychotic effects to those achieved by typical antipsychotics without causing significant extrapyramidal movement disorders or sustained elevation of prolactin raises the possibility that blockade of other neurotransmitters can enhance the antipsychotic effect while minimising undesirable side-effects.

The mechanism or mechanisms by which clozapine achieves its atypical effects remain a subject of debate. However, a potentially important clue is provided by the observation that several drugs that block both $D_2$ receptors and $5\text{-HT}_{2A}$ receptors have atypical antipsychotic effects (Meltzer *et al*, 1989). There are several sites at which serotonin and dopamine interact that may be relevant to understanding atypical antipsychotic action. For example, in the striatum, there are $5\text{-HT}_{2A}$ receptors on the presynaptic terminals of dopamine fibres that project from the substantia nigra to the striatum. Occupation of these receptors by serotonin can inhibit dopamine release (Kapur & Remington, 1996). Hence the simultaneous blockade of $5\text{-HT}_2$ receptors and $D_2$ receptors would be expected to produce a compensatory increase in dopamine release into the synaptic cleft that might minimise the adverse effects of dopamine blockade in the dorsal striatum.

However, there are alternative possibilities. One important issue is the possibility that many of the undesirable side-effects of typical antipsychotics are due to sustained blockade of dopaminergic neurotransmission, while antipsychotic action requires only the blockade of transient surges of dopamine release. In a study using microdialysis to measure dopamine levels in the striatum in freely moving rats, Lucas & Spampinato (2000) found that pharmaceuticals that selectively block $5\text{-HT}_{2A}$ receptors do not alter basal levels of dopamine release but reduce the compensatory transient dopamine increase produced by administration of the typical antipsychotic haloperidol. This observation suggests that blockade of $5\text{-HT}_2$ receptors concurrently with blockade of $D_2$ receptors would provide protection against the effects of surges of dopamine at relatively lower levels of $D_2$ receptor blockade. However, the $5\text{-HT}_2$ receptor blockade would not be expected to produce an undesirable reduction in the baseline level of dopamine release.

It should be noted that interactions between serotonin and dopamine also occur in the frontal cortex. The reported therapeutic effects of atypical antipsychotics in the treatment of the negative symptoms of schizophrenia may arise from an interaction whereby serotonin blockade acts to promote dopaminergic activity in the frontal cortex (Kapur & Remington, 1996).

## Autoreceptors

Many neurons have inhibitory receptors that bind the same neurotransmitter as that produced by the neuron itself. These are known as autoreceptors. Because these autoreceptors are inhibitory, they can provide negative feedback by which a neurotransmitter can regulate its own release. Autoreceptors can be located either on the presynaptic surface or on the cell body and adjacent dendrites, in which case they are referred to as somatodendritic receptors. As a result of the existence of autoreceptors, pharmacological agents that might have been expected to enhance the action of a particular transmitter (by acting as either a direct or indirect agonist, or by inhibiting reuptake of the neurotransmitter) can sometimes produce a reduction in the release of that neurotransmitter.

In the cerebral noradrenergic system, alpha$_2$ adrenoceptors act as autoreceptors, and hence alpha$_2$ agonists such as idazoxan tend to diminish the release of noradrenaline. In other aminergic systems, a particular receptor type can be postsynaptic in one brain area and presynaptic in another or, in some instances, in the same area. For example, in the brain-stem raphe nuclei, 5-HT$_{1A}$ receptors act as somatodendritic autoreceptors and 5-HT$_{1A}$ agonists are potent inhibitors of the firing of raphe neurons. However, in the hippocampus, 5-HT$_{1A}$ receptors are postsynaptic, so the administration of a 5-HT$_{1A}$ agonist would be expected to mimic serotonergic firing in the hippocampus despite inhibiting serotonergic neurons projecting from the raphe.

In the dopaminergic system, D$_1$ and D$_2$ receptors are located presynaptically as well as postsynaptically in the basal ganglia, whereas in the cortex there are postsynaptic D$_1$ receptors but no presynaptic autoreceptors. Since autoreceptors tend to be preferentially activated at low doses of an agonist, administration of a low dose of a non-specific dopaminergic agonist, such as apomorphine, would be expected to enhance cortical dopaminergic function and inhibit subcortical release, while a larger dose might produce enhanced dopaminergic activity in both the cortex and basal ganglia.

## Reuptake sites

One of the major ways in which neurotransmitters that have been released into the synaptic cleft as a consequence of neural firing are removed from it is via active reuptake into the presynaptic terminal via transporter molecules embedded in the cell membrane. Inhibition of reuptake leads to accumulation of the transmitter in the synaptic cleft and thereby increases the effect of that neurotransmitter. Tricyclic antidepressants and the more recently introduced selective serotonin reuptake inhibitors and noradrenaline reuptake inhibitors apparently achieve their therapeutic effect via inhibition of the reuptake of monoamine neurotransmitters.

# Major cerebral neurotransmitter systems

## Glutamatergic neurotransmission

As discussed above, glutamate is the transmitter mainly responsible for the long-distance transmission of temporally and spatially focused information in the brain and therefore it is probable that glutamate plays a cardinal role in all mental acts. Glutamatergic fibres project from the thalamus to the cortex; from the cortex to the basal ganglia; from one cortical area to another; and also provide the excitatory component of transmission in the local circuits that coordinate neural activity within a cortical region. As shown in Table 5.1, there are three types of ionotropic glutamatergic receptor: the NMDA, kainate and quisqualate receptors, each named for the pharmacological agent for which it has a specific affinity. In addition, there are metabotropic glutamate receptors.

The NMDA receptor is of particular interest because it is a complex protein with separate binding sites for various molecules in addition to glutamate itself;

this gives it the scope for relatively subtle pharmacological regulation of glutamatergic neurotransmission. In particular, there is a specific binding site for the amino acid glycine, distinct from the site for glutamate. The recreational psychotomimetic drug phencyclidine (PCP), more commonly known as 'angel dust', binds at a site within the ion channel itself, thereby acting as a glutamatergic antagonist. PCP and other drugs binding at the same site, including dizocilpine (MK801) and the anaesthetic drug ketamine, produce a psychosis with clinical features similar to schizophrenia, including not only the delusions but also disorganisation of mental activity and core negative symptoms. This observation has led to the proposal that the glutamatergic system plays a special role in the pathophysiology of schizophrenia, an issue we shall return to in Chapter 11.

The NMDA receptors are also of special interest because their activation can, under some circumstances, lead to the death of the postsynaptic neuron. This provides a potential mechanism by which neural activity might actually lead to loss of cerebral neurons. Such a process might account for the observation that progressive damage to neurons occurs in at least a minority of patients with schizophrenia.

## GABA-ergic neurotransmission

GABA is the neurotransmitter employed by the interneurons exerting an inhibitory influence in the local circuits that coordinate neural activity within the cerebral cortex. In addition, a series of GABA neurons in the basal ganglia provide the links extending from the caudate nucleus to the thalamus within the cortico-striato-thalamo-cortical feedback loops that regulate cortical activity.

There are three types of GABA receptor, $GABA_A$, $GABA_B$ and $GABA_C$. The $GABA_A$ and $GABA_C$ receptors are ionotropic. At these receptors, binding of the transmitter leads to opening of the chloride channels and hyperpolarisation of the transmembrane potential. The $GABA_A$ receptor has a distinct site at which benzodiazepines bind. Benzodiazepines enhance the effect of GABA, possibly by blocking binding of a putative endogenous ligand that acts as a non-competitive antagonist of GABA. The $GABA_B$ receptor is metabotropic and can be negatively coupled to adenylate cyclase via a G protein. In postsynaptic terminals, its actions include the activation of potassium channels, thereby generating slow inhibitory postsynaptic potentials.

## Cholinergic neurotransmission

Cholinergic neurons are located in a diffuse collection of nuclei at the base of the brain, including the basal nucleus of Meynert, medial septum and adjacent diagonal band. The cholinergic fibres from these neurons project widely, but especially to limbic areas and to the basal ganglia. In general, acetylcholine increases the likelihood of neuronal firing in response to other inputs (McCormick & Prince, 1985). None the less, an increase in cholinergic tone tends to produce a state of psychomotor retardation characterised by apathy, withdrawal, decreased energy, slowed or diminished amount of thought, reduced affective responsivity and anhedonia (Risch *et al*, 1981). Mesulam (1988) suggests that its major role is channelling relevant sensory information towards the limbic system. In view of the importance of the hippocampus for the laying down of declarative memories, such a proposal is consistent with the impairment of memory that results from cholinergic blockade.

Nicotinic cholinergic receptors are responsible for activation of interneurons in the hippocampus and in other forebrain areas. A deficit in nicotinic receptor activity can result in defective gating of sensory input. For example, the positively directed change in scalp electrical potential that occurs at approximately 50 ms after an auditory signal (P50) is normally inhibited following the second of two closely spaced signals. Cholinerigic neurons play a cardinal role in the circuit that mediates this gating of the P50 potential. In schizophrenia, P50 gating tends to be attenuated by virtue of a deficit in nicotinic receptor activity (Freedman *et al*, 1997; see also Chapter 11).

## Dopaminergic neurotransmission

Dopaminergic pathways extend from the substantia nigra and VTA in the midbrain to the basal ganglia, limbic structures and frontal cortex. They play a crucial role in adjusting the tone of mental and motor activity, thereby facilitating the transformation of motivation into action. Molecular biological techniques for identifying genes have demonstrated a rich diversity of dopamine receptor types. There are there are at least five distinct types of receptor, each specified by a different gene. Some of these exist in long and short forms, where the short form has a chunk missing from the amino acid chain specified by the gene. Despite this diversity, similarities in pharmacological characteristics justify the grouping of the five different types of dopamine receptor into two families, the $D_1$ family, which includes the $D_1$ and $D_5$ receptor, and the $D_2$ family, which includes $D_2$, $D_3$ and $D_4$ receptors.

The different types of dopamine receptor tend to be coupled to different effector mechanisms and also to exhibit differences in their relative abundance in different cerebral areas. For example, $D_1$ receptors stimulate adenylate cyclase, and are found principally in the basal ganglia and frontal cortex. The $D_2$ receptors inhibit adenylate cyclase, and are abundant in the basal ganglia but present only at very low concentrations in the cerebral cortex. Despite these differences in biochemical effect and anatomical distribution, pharmacological agents that act as agonists at either $D_1$ or $D_2$ receptors tend to produce increased locomotor activity in animals. Evidence suggests that this similarity of overall effect might be because $D_1$ receptors act mainly to promote transmission via the direct pathway from the caudate nucleus to the thalamus, thereby enhancing cortico-striato-thalamico-cortical positive feedback, while $D_2$ receptors have an inhibitory effect on the indirect pathway that forms part of a negative feedback loop (Alexander & Crutcher, 1990a).

Dopamine $D_3$ receptors are especially abundant in the limbic cortex. In contrast to either $D_1$ or $D_2$ receptors, $D_3$ receptors exert an inhibitory influence on locomotor activity in animals.

The effects of binding at $D_4$ and $D_5$ receptors are less clearly established.

It is traditional to subdivide the dopaminergic pathways projecting from the midbrain into three systems on an anatomical basis: the nigrostriatal system projects from the substantia nigra to the corpus striatum; the mesolimbic system projects from the VTA to limbic structures and the ventral striatum (homologous with the nucleus accumbens in rodents); and the mesocortical system projects from the VTA to the frontal cortex.

However, in the light of the concept of cortico-striato-thalamo-cortical loops considered in Chapter 4, it is perhaps more rational, from a functional point of view, to divide the dopaminergic pathways into two major divisions, the motor division and the psychomotor division, each of which involves both cortical and subcortical projections. According to such a scheme, the motor division comprises the dopaminergic projections from the midbrain (mainly the substantia nigra) to the dorsal striatum and also the projections from the midbrain to the premotor and supplementary motor cortex. This division of the dopaminergic system is predominantly concerned with the execution of motor activity. The psychomotor division comprises the projections from the midbrain (mainly the VTA) to the ventral striatum, limbic cortex and prefrontal cortex. This division is primarily concerned with motivation and other aspects of linkage between emotion and voluntary action. Furthermore, prefrontal dopaminergic projections are strongly implicated in regulating responses to stress.

There is substantial evidence suggesting that prefrontal and subcortical dopaminergic activity are regulated so that they change in a reciprocal manner under many circumstances. In an influential early study, Pycock et al (1980) showed that lesion of the prefrontal dopaminergic terminals in rats led to increased levels of dopamine in the nucleus accumbens (the analogue of the human ventral striatum) and also the dorsal striatum. Although this precise finding has not been replicated, many subsequent studies have demonstrated reciprocal interactions between prefrontal and striatal dopaminergic activity. For example, Louilot et al (1989) showed that blockade of dopamine transmission in the prefrontal cortex by a dopamine receptor blocker leads to increased dopaminergic transmission in the nucleus accumbens. The injection of an indirect dopamine agonist, such as amphetamine, into the nucleus accumbens produces increased levels of motor activity. When amphetamine is injected into the prefrontal cortex alone, there are no significant locomotor effects. However, when amphetamine is injected simultaneously into both the prefrontal cortex and the nucleus accumbens, the amount of hyperactivity is substantially less than that produced by injection into the nucleus accumbens alone (Tassin et al, 1988).

Dopaminergic systems are implicated in a number of aspects of the response to stress. In rats, mild stresses produce an increase in prefrontal dopaminergic activity but relatively little increase in striatal dopaminergic activity (Thierry et al, 1976). Deutch et al (1990) found that stress produced substantial increases in subcortical dopaminergic activity in animals that had lesions of the prefrontal dopaminergic terminals, but not in animals without such lesions, which suggests that the prefrontal dopaminergic system acts to buffer subcortical dopaminergic activity so as to avoid overreaction in stressful circumstances. More severe stresses produce increased dopaminergic utilisation in the nucleus accumbens despite intact prefrontal dopamine terminals.

Overall, the evidence indicates that the prefrontal dopaminergic system acts to regulate dopaminergic activity in the accumbens whenever there is a tendency for that activity to rise towards the level at which behavioural disturbances become manifest. This suggests that the prefrontal dopamine system normally acts to control responses to stress, but when the stress is too great (or when the prefrontal dopaminergic system is impaired) there is an increase in accumbens dopamine activity, which is manifest in overt behavioural signs of stress, such as overactivity and stereotyped behaviour.

Chronic stress results in loss of interest in activities. If rats are subjected to chronic mild stresses, such as changes in cage mates, overnight illumination or tilting of the cage, they exhibit a decrease in their spontaneous consumption of sweetened water (Willner *et al*, 1992). This apparent anhedonia is associated with evidence of decreased $D_2$ receptor numbers in the ventral striatum (but not in the caudate nucleus). Such a down-regulation of $D_2$ receptors might arise as a compensatory consequence of episodic increases in dopaminergic activity induced by stress. The overall effect of the $D_2$ receptor down-regulation would be a decrease in the background level of the postsynaptic effects of dopamine in the nucleus accumbens. In general, responses that lead to inhibition of dopamine activity in the accumbens diminish responsiveness to motivational stimuli.

## Noradrenergic neurotransmission

The cell bodies of the neurons comprising the major noradrenergic system in the brain are located within the locus coeruleus and nearby areas in the brain-stem. These noradrenergic neurons project, via the ventral noradrenergic bundle, to the thalamus, hypothalamus and hippocampus and, via a dorsal bundle, to wide-spread areas of the cerebral cortex. The different types of adrenergic receptors include $alpha_1$ and $alpha_2$, and $beta_1$ and $beta_2$. As discussed above, $alpha_2$ receptors are often located on presynaptic cell membranes and act to suppress further release of noradrenaline.

As with the other monoamine neurotransmitters, noradrenaline appears to play an important role in responses to aversive stimuli and other stressors. Aversive stimuli increase firing of locus coeruleus neurons in rats (Abercrombie *et al*, 1986). In animals, even mild stress results in increased utilisation of noradrenaline in many brain areas but especially the hypothalamus (Tanaka *et al*, 1982). The ventral noradrenergic bundle plays a role in mediating the neuro-endocrine responses, including the stress-induced release of adrenocorticotrophic hormone (ACTH) from the pituitary (Checkley, 1992). Evidence from animal studies suggests that the dorsal noradrenergic bundle pays a part in maintaining arousal and, in particular, produces a focusing of attention in response to potentially threatening situations (Maier, 1991).

## Serotonergic neurotransmission

The cell bodies of serotonergic neurons in the central nervous system are located in several clusters in the raphe area of the brain-stem. Those located in the medulla oblongata project to the spinal cord and are involved in processes such as the gating of pain and in motor activity. Those located in the midbrain project widely to the cerebrum, innervating the cortex, hippocampus, amygdala, striatum, substantia nigra and hypothalamus.

The number of different recognised types of serotonin (5-HT) receptor increased dramatically with the advent of techniques for identifying genes. By the mid-1990s, seven major classes, most of which comprised a multiplicity of subtypes each specified by distinct genes, were recognised. For example, there are at least five different types of $5\text{-HT}_1$ receptor, while there are three types of $5\text{-HT}_2$ receptor. As shown in Table 5.1, $5\text{-HT}_1$ receptors are coupled to adenylate cyclase, $5\text{-HT}_2$ receptors are coupled to the PI system, while $5\text{-HT}_3$ receptors form ion channels.

The serotonergic system is implicated in a range of different functions of the central nervous system, including the regulation of sleep and wakefulness, appetite, sexual behaviour and mood. A substantial body of evidence suggests that, in the realm of higher mental processing, serotonin plays a cardinal role in impulse control, as it tends to inhibit many types of behaviour. The enhancement of serotonergic transmission by the administration of a serotonin reuptake inhibitor reduces impulsiveness in animals (Thiebot *et al*, 1992), while a number of indicators of harmful impulsiveness, including suicide and some forms of violence, are associated with low levels of the serotonin metabolite 5-hydroxy-indole-acetic acid in the cerebrospinal fluid (Linnolia *et al*, 1983).

Serotonin is also involved in responses to stress. Substantial stress causes a decrease in serotonin levels in the hippocampus, neocortex and in parts of the hypothalamus in rats (Hellhamer *et al*, 1983), presumably indicating increased serotonergic turnover during times of stress. Acute and chronic stress produce a variety of changes in serotonin receptors. For example, in rats, acute stress leads to an increase in $5\text{-HT}_{2C}$ receptor mRNA, while chronic stress leads to decreased expression of $5\text{-HT}_{2C}$ receptor mRNA in the hippocampus (Holmes *et al*, 1995). Chronic stress increases cortical $5\text{-HT}_{2A}$ receptors and decreases hippocampal $5\text{-HT}_{1A}$ and $5\text{-HT}_{1B}$ receptors (Lopez *et al*, 1997). It is especially noteworthy that there are pronounced changes in the hippocampus, in view of the cardinal role that the hippocampus plays in regulating the HPA axis.

## Peptide and enkephalin co-transmitters

A large number of peptides are found in neurons and many of them have been shown to have the properties of neurotransmitters. In many instances they exist as co-transmitters in either monoaminergic or GABA-ergic neurons. For example, in the corpus striatum, the neurons in the direct pathway from the striatum to GPi have the peptide substance P as a co-transmitter, while the neurons of the indirect pathway have enkephalins (endogenous opiates) as co-transmitters.

Up-regulation of enkephalin neurotransmission in rats appears to be a compensatory response to a diminution of dopaminergic transmission (Churchill *et al*, 1992). The administration of psychostimulants such as amphetamine that promote dopaminergic activity can result in a sensitisation such that the behavioural consequences of subsequent administration of the same drug are enhanced. Opiates such as morphine can cross-sensitise for amphetamine. Thus, in a number of respects, circumstantial evidence suggests that enkephalins reinforce the effects of dopamine. However, the markedly different properties of amphetamine, which is a stimulant, and opiates, which tend to depress brain activity, suggest that dopamine and enkephalins have substantially different roles. Belluzzi & Stein (1977) concluded that drive-inducing reward mechanisms, which promote the pursuit of goals, are likely to be mediated by catecholamines (such as dopamine), while drive-reducing reward mechanisms, which produce satiety, may be mediated by enkephalins.

# Hormones acting on the central nervous system

In general, hormones interact with neurons by one of two types of process: binding to receptors on membranes; or binding to receptors that can attach to DNA, leading to the modulation of gene transcription. The steroid hormones and also thyroid hormones can act by both types of mechanism. The receptors for these hormones belong to a superclass that include within them a particular sequence of 15 amino acids that appears to enable binding to DNA in a way that modifies gene transcription (Beato, 1989; Checkley, 1992). They are likely to play a role not only in medium- and long-term responses to environmental stimuli in adulthood, but also in the development of the central nervous system.

## The HPA axis

Corticosteroid and mineralocorticoid hormones, which are released from the adrenal cortex in response to stress, play a role in mediating the medium- and long-term consequences of stress on the brain. As with the effects of steroids on other tissues of the body, these effects can be either protective or destructive (McEwan *et al*, 1992).

The release of the major stress-related hormone, cortisol, from the adrenal cortex is promoted by ACTH produced in the pituitary, at the base of the brain. Release of ACTH from the pituitary is in turn promoted by corticotrophin-releasing factor (CRF) produced in the paraventricular nucleus (PVN) of the hypothalamus, and secreted into the blood supplying the anterior lobe of the pituitary. Circulating cortisol can act at the level of both the pituitary, to reduce ACTH production, and at the hypothalamus, to reduce CRF production, thereby providing regulation through negative feedback.

Several neural systems, of which the hippocampus and brain-stem noradrenergic systems are the most important, act on the hypothalamus to stimulate the production of CRF at times of stress. The hippocampus plays a major role when the stressful stimulus is interpreted in the light of previous experience, whereas direct influence from the brain-stem noradrenergic system probably plays a larger role in the case of marked somatic stresses, such as hypoglycaemia (Herman *et al*, 1996).

Noradrenergic fibres that travel in the ventral noradrenergic bundle from the brain-stem to the PVN have the potential to activate postsynaptic alpha$_1$ adrenoceptors on PVN cells containing CRF or vasopressin. This noradrenergic mechanism for activating the HPA axis is apparently inactive under resting conditions in humans, but can be activated by various stressful circumstances. In particular, blockade of alpha$_1$ receptors has no effect on the normal circadian rhythm of cortisol release, but does inhibit cortisol responses to hypoglycaemia (Checkley, 1992). Immobilisation of animals dramatically increases the rates of synthesis, release and metabolism of noradrenaline in the hypothalamus, which supports the hypothesis that noradrenergic projections to the PVN stimulate release of CRF (Pacak *et al*, 1995).

The ventral subicular region of the hippocampus exerts a strong inhibitory influence on the release of CRF from the PVN. Fibres from the hippocampus travelling in the lateral fimbria and fornix form synapses in the hypothalamus with GABA-ergic interneurons that inhibit the release of CRF from the PVN (Herman *et al*, 1992, 1995). Rats with lesions of the ventral subiculum do not show changes in basal corticosteroid secretion at either circadian peak or nadir, when compared with rats with sham lesions. However, rats with lesions of the ventral subiculum exhibit a prolonged glucocorticoid stress response (Herman *et al*, 1995).

Although circulating corticosteriods exert negative feedback to the HPA axis via receptors in the pituitary and hypothalamus, they can exert an even more powerful regulatory influence by binding to receptors in the hippocampus. Of all brain regions, the hippocampus has the highest concentration of both glucocorticoid and mineralocorticoid receptors. It is also rich in CRF receptors. The high density of corticosteroid receptors not only facilitates the cardinal role of the hippocampus in regulating the HPA axis, but also makes it extremely vulnerable to damage by sustained levels of corticosteroid hormones. High levels of corticosteroids produce memory impairment in laboratory animals and in humans (Lupien *et al*, 1999). Uno *et al* (1989) demonstrated that vervet monkeys with low social dominance and high social stress have adrenal gland hyperplasia and hippocampal degeneration. Pyramidal neurons in the CA3 region of the hippocampus were shrunken and diminished in number. In contrast, the monkeys exhibited only minimal evidence of neuronal damage elsewhere in the brain. Subordinate tree shrews exposed to 28 days of psychosocial stress, which produces constant hyperactivity of the HPA axis, exhibit apical dendrite atrophy in the CA3 region (Magarinos *et al*, 1996). Furthermore, elderly depressed patients exhibit diminished hippocampal volume, and this is more marked in those who have a longer history of depression (Sheline *et al*, 1999). Depression is associated with elevated cortisol levels and adrenal hyperplasia.

Not only does the evidence demonstrate that sustained increases in cortisol can damage the hippocampus but, in particular, the ability of the hippocampus to regulate the HPA axis can be damaged. For example, Fuchs & Flugge (1995) showed that in subordinate tree shrews, chronic stress significantly reduced the number of binding sites for CRF in the anterior lobe of the pituitary and in the dentate gyrus and the CA1–CA3 areas of the hippocampal formation. There is substantial evidence that exposure to stress at an early stage in development can produce sustained impairment of HPA axis regulation, which predisposes to excessive cortisol release on subsequent exposure to stress. For example, monkeys subjected to erratic maternal care in infancy have elevated levels of CRF in the cerebrospinal fluid that persist into adult life (Coplan *et al*, 1996). This abnormality is associated with low sociability and decreased tolerance of emotional challenges.

## Sex steroid hormones

The increased risk of mental disorder at times when there are rapid changes in the levels of the sex steroid hormones suggests that these hormones influence neural activity. Perhaps the most dramatic temporal association between changes in levels of sex steroids and mental disorder is the relationship between childbirth and post-partum psychosis. In view of the evidence that oestrogens modulate the sensitivity of dopaminergic receptors, it is tempting to speculate that post-partum psychosis arises from an enhancement of dopaminergic activity as a result of rapid decreases in oestrogen in the post-partum period. This speculation is consistent with evidence indicating that dopaminergic hyper-responsivity four days after childbirth, at which time oestrogen levels are falling precipitously, is associated with the subsequent development of post-partum psychosis in women whose history indicates a high risk of psychosis. Kumar *et al* (1993) assessed the responsivity of the dopaminergic system by measuring the growth hormone response to the dopamine agonist apomorphine, four days after delivery, in a group of women with a previous psychotic illness. Those who developed psychosis in the six months after childbirth had increased growth hormone response compared with those who did not.

Conversely, high levels of oestrogens appear to protect against symptom exacerbations in women with schizophrenia (Seeman, 1996). Symptoms are more severe during the low-oestrogen phase of the menstrual cycle, and exacerbations often occur at menopause.

# Locally acting humoral influences

Cells within the central nervous system can communicate by means other than classical neurotransmission. One mechanism is communication by the diffusible gas nitric oxide (NO). NO is produced in neurons by the enzyme nitric oxide synthase (which is identical to NADPH diaphorase). It can diffuse readily across cell membranes and stimulates the enzyme guanylate cyclase, which produces the nucleotide cyclic guanosine monophosphate (cGMP). Like the second messengers in classical neurotransmitter systems, cGMP can regulate protein kinases, phosphodiesterases and ion channels.

Nitric oxide synthase is located widely in the central nervous system, especially in the cerebellum and olfactory system, but also in the cerebral cortex, hippocampus and striatum. Its role in the function of the brain is a subject of debate (Vincent & Hope, 1992). It almost certainly plays some part in regulating the changes in local cerebral perfusion when neurons become active, a response which incidentally allows the detection of local neural activity by imaging of cerebral blood flow using PET, SPET or fMRI. NO has been considered a candidate for mediating long-term potentiation, and also the processes of natural cell death. NO may also be involved in guiding the migration of neurons during early development, a process potentially of importance in the genesis of the predisposition to major mental illnesses such as schizophrenia.

# Summary

Neurotransmitter systems employing ionotropic receptors allow the rapid transfer of information that is sharply focused in time and place. However, the rich diversity of receptor type, the multiplicity of interactions between different modulatory neurotransmitters, and the array of hormonal and local neurohumoral factors that act on neurons allow subtle regulation of the processes of information transmission in the brain.

The nature of modulatory neurotransmission makes pharmacological therapy for mental disorders feasible. Although the specific content of a thought might be expected to depend on the firing of a specific set of neurons, the symptoms of mental disorder appear to reflect disorder of the processes responsible for the initiation, selection and evaluation of thoughts and emotions. These aspects of mental processing are likely to depend strongly on the level of activity in modulatory neurotransmitter systems. Because these systems set the tone in an assembly of neurons, it is potentially feasible to produce a beneficial effect with pharmacological agents that act in a manner that is diffuse in time and location.

The fact that activity in the nervous system can produce enduring changes in neural structure and function makes it possible for psychological processes to produce long-term effects that may be either beneficial or harmful. In particular, the neurohumoral processes involved in the response to stress can produce long-term changes that may generate psychiatric symptoms and also increase susceptibility to the adverse effects of subsequent stressful events.

# Part II

# Symptom clusters

# Chapter 6

# Reality distortion

## Nature of hallucinations and delusions

Hallucinations and delusions, the phenomena that lie at the heart of psychosis, are perhaps the most enigmatic of all mental symptoms. Both entail a mismatch between a compelling representation of reality produced by the individual's own mind and the representation supported by objective evidence. In many psychotic illnesses they tend to occur together; they tend to follow a similar time course; and they respond similarly to antipsychotic medication. This suggests that they share major aspects of their pathophysiology irrespective of the illness in which they occur. Studies employing factor analysis to examine the relationships between symptoms confirm that delusions and hallucinations usually load on a single factor in various psychotic illnesses, including schizophrenia (Liddle, 1987a; Malla *et al*, 1993) and affective psychosis (Maziade *et al*, 1995). This chapter examines the evidence regarding the nature of the pathological processes that give rise to these two core psychotic phenomena.

A hallucination can be defined as a perception with the quality of a sensory perception but not derived from stimulation of a sense organ. Typically, a psychotic patient assumes falsely that the origin of the perception lies in the external world. In those instances where the patient recognises that the perception arises from within his/her mind, the experience may strictly be described as a pseudo-hallucination. During the acute phase of illness, it is quite common for hallucinations to be perceived as arising in the external world. As the acute episode resolves and insight returns, some patients recognise that it arises from within, while none the less still experiencing the abnormal perception. In this book we shall follow the *Diagnostic and Statistical Manual* (DSM–IV) of the American Psychiatric Association (1994) in using the term 'hallucination' for both 'real' and 'pseudo-hallucinations'. However, the fact that this distinction can be made emphasises that a fully fledged hallucination involves both aberrant perception *and* impaired recognition of the origin of the experience.

A delusion can be defined as a firmly fixed belief that is derived by erroneous inference or unjustified assumption, and that cannot be accounted for on the basis of culture or religion. It is usually, but not necessarily, false. The essential issue is not the falsity of the belief but rather the lack of rational grounds for holding it. The classic illustration of a situation in which a belief may in fact be true, but none the less delusional, is provided by the Othello syndrome, in which the patient vehemently maintains that his/her spouse has been unfaithful on the basis of irrational argument. The belief is sometimes held with such blind passion that the spouse's life is in danger. The condition is diagnosed on the basis of the irrationality of the argument rather than the question of whether or not the spouse has in fact been unfaithful.

Some delusions appear to arise via an unreasonable extrapolation from evidence, such as 'I know the security services are spying on me because a stranger looked at me in the street'. Such instances, at first sight, suggest that the essential issue in delusional thinking is a faulty process of logical deduction. However, a psychotic individual does not exhibit a generalised failure of the processes of logical inference. As we shall discuss in greater detail in the section below concerned with neuropsychological correlates of reality distortion, logical thinking is intact under many circumstances. In psychosis, it appears that a few ideas are mentally labelled in a way that makes them immune to the normal process of evidential evaluation.

In an attempt to define the nature of the mental processes that underlie delusions and hallucinations, it is instructive to compare the distortion of reality that is characteristic of psychotic illness with the distortions of thought and perception that can occur in non-psychotic illnesses. In many instances, a clear basis for the distinction between psychosis and neurosis can be formulated, although in clinical practice the boundaries often become blurred. An adequate account of the mechanism of psychosis must be able to account not only for the distinguishing features but also for the frequency with which the boundaries become blurred.

# Comparison of psychotic and non-psychotic distortions of reality

In principle, a delusion can be clearly distinguished from the distorted thinking that occurs in neurotic conditions, such as obsessional disorder and non-psychotic depression, on the grounds that the neurotic patient recognises the irrationality of the belief, and the idea is at least partially amenable to examination by rational argument.

## Obsessional ruminations

Obsessional ruminations are intrusive thoughts that the patient experiences as alien, in the sense of being contrary to his/her own values or intentions, but which the patient none the less recognises as arising from within his/her own mind. The content of the ruminations can be quite bizarre in some instances. None the less, the patient recognises them as an unwanted intrusion and usually resists them.

For example, a conscientious young woman, whom we shall call Jane, became preoccupied by the fear that if she bought new clothes for herself she would become possessed by the devil. She had been brought up as a strict Christian, with a strong sense of right and wrong. In her childhood she believed that evil ideas arose from the prompting of the devil. In early adulthood, she had rejected the simple piety of her childhood, and no longer attended church regularly. At a superficial level, she no longer believed in the devil. However, she retained a strong sense that self-indulgence was wrong, and it is scarcely surprising that the temptation to spend money on clothes for herself rekindled her childhood conviction that such temptations came from the devil. However, even she recognised that the fear that she would become possessed by the devil was far beyond the scope of her childhood beliefs. None the less, despite recognising that this was a 'silly idea' that arose from her own mind, she developed a state of overwhelming panic if she attempted to go into any sort of shop, even if only to make quite mundane purchases. Avoidance of shops seemed to be the only way to keep the panic at bay. Ironically, her recognition of the irrationality of the idea caused her to question her own sanity and she became intensely agitated by the prospect that she was going mad.

In contrast to a deluded patient, Jane was able to identify the intrusive idea as a product of her own mind. She was even able to ascribe it, quite reasonably, to an interaction between her overconscientious nature and puritanical aspects of her upbringing, but such rationalisation provided her with little consolation. Her rumination intruded with such force as to dictate her behaviour and dominate her life. In a state of torment, she eventually went to see a psychiatrist. The fact that much of her torment arose from the fear of being eventually overwhelmed and unable to resist the idea of possession by the devil pointed to a diagnosis of obsessional neurosis rather than psychosis. Treatment with the serotonin reuptake inhibiter sertraline, augmented by cognitive–behaviour strategies, directed at restoring her confidence in her ability to go shopping, led to a gradual resolution of her symptoms.

Despite the difference in principle between obsessional ruminations and delusions, the ability to recognise that an obsessional idea is unreasonable varies between individuals. In some instances an idea may be resisted at early phases of the illness but eventually the ability to discern what is real is lost. In a survey of 475 patients with obsessive–compulsive disorder (OCD), Eisen & Rasmussen (1993) found that 14% had psychotic symptoms and 4% met the full diagnostic criteria for schizophrenia. According to DSM–IV, an additional diagnosis of delusional disorder, or psychotic disorder not otherwise specified, should be made in cases of OCD with psychotic symptoms.

Conversely, in a substantial number of cases of schizophrenia, the patient experiences unwanted, persistently intrusive ideas, and recognises them to be unreasonable. For example, between psychotic episodes, a conscientious young man with schizophrenia was tormented by the fear that he might sexually molest the child of a member of the congregation at the church he attended. Understandably, this thought led him to question the nature of his own sexuality, but he was quite able to distinguish his fear of molesting a child from reality. However, subsequently, at a time when the newspapers were dominated by accounts of a sexually motivated murder, he suffered a psychotic relapse and turned himself in to the police, confessing to the murder. The police had no difficulty in establishing that he could not have been the murderer, and brought him to hospital.

Such cases imply that delusion formation involves both the mental (and neural) mechanisms by which ideas are generated and the mechanisms by which they are evaluated, but the essential characteristic of delusional thinking is a failure of the mechanism for evaluating ideas. In OCD, compelling, unreasonable ideas can arise, but the individual none the less correctly recognises that they are unreasonable. When the ability to evaluate these ideas is lost, the borderline that separates OCD from psychosis is crossed.

## Depression

Even in non-psychotic depression, evaluation of oneself and the world is usually distorted. Depressed people tend to see themselves as worthless and the future as bleak. As Beck *et al* (1979) have emphasised, there is often an 'all-or-nothing' character to such depressive thoughts. However, a person with non-psychotic depression can be engaged in debate about the basis for their beliefs. Confrontational debate rarely alters the depressed person's evaluation of the evidence, but Socratic dialogue can produce a shift in that evaluation (Beck *et al*, 1979). The problem appears to be a bias in attending to perceptions and in the generation of ideas; there is also evidence of a disorder of the evaluation of ideas, insofar as a depressed person finds a negative interpretation of the evidence more compelling than a positive interpretation. None the less, the patient with a milder form of depression is usually able to recognise that perceptions and ideas must pass a test of their plausibility before they can be accepted. With increasing severity, however, depressive thinking can become psychotic and no longer amenable to reason. Typically in depressive psychosis, the content of delusions is an exaggeration of the self-devaluing or guilty thoughts characteristic of non-psychotic depression. The individual may also experience derogatory auditory hallucinations. Less commonly, the content of delusions and hallucinations can be non-congruent with the depressive mood.

As in the case of the relationship between obsessional thinking and delusions, the relationship between depressive cognitions and delusions implies that the mechanism involved in the generation of ideas and also that involved in the evaluation of ideas are implicated in the formation of delusions. In non-psychotic depression, the mechanism of evaluation operates, but with a pronounced bias towards negative evaluation. However, when the evaluation mechanism no longer operates, the depression becomes psychotic. It is the failure of evaluation that defines it as psychosis.

# Reality distortion in psychosis

Delusions and hallucinations commonly occur in schizophrenia, mania, psychotic depression and in psychosis arising from overt brain injury or degeneration. It is an intriguing fact that the majority of delusions and hallucinations express ideas drawn from a limited set of approximately a dozen themes related to relationships with others; self-identity and worth; and supernatural or existential issues. These themes include persecution; alien control of thoughts, feelings or actions; religion; grandiosity; and guilt. The themes tend to differ between conditions. For example, delusions of guilt are especially common in depressive psychosis. Delusions of reference, which entail the belief that the conversation or behaviour of nearby people, objects in the environment, or events, has a specific significance for oneself, are also common. The specific content of a delusion or hallucination is influenced by contemporary cultural issues, but similar themes can be identified across time and culture, and this suggests that they reflect universal features of mental structure.

## Schizophrenia

A diverse range of types of delusion and hallucination occur in schizophrenia. For example, in the International Pilot Study of Schizophrenia conducted by the World Health Organization (1978), second-person auditory hallucinations occurred in 35.6% of subjects; persecutory delusions in 51.8%; and delusions of reference in 49.6%. Furthermore, relatively rare delusional themes, such as delusional misidentification, delusions of parasitic infestation, and erotomania, occur in schizophrenia, even though they are perhaps more typically seen in instances of overt brain injury or other special circumstances. The overall diversity of types of reality distortion occurring in schizophrenia is consistent with the evidence, discussed in greater detail in Chapter 11, that the pathophysiology of schizophrenia entails a subtle maldevelopment affecting virtually all areas of the cerebral cortex, resulting in the disruption of an extensive range of aspects of mental processing.

A particular type of delusion that is characteristic of schizophrenia, and which illustrates an important aspect of reality distortion, is the autochthonous delusion, a delusional belief that arises without any identifiable mental antecedents. The belief arises as a fully formed notion that has not been inferred in any discernible way from evidence. In particular, it is not possible to identify a fault in logical deduction; rather, there appears to be a failure to recognise that the idea demands logical justification. For example, a schizophrenic patient maintained that his head had been split by an axe. He denied that this was in any way a figurative expression and insisted that it had really happened, despite his lack of ability to produce any grounds for his belief. The occurrence of autochthonous delusions suggests that the process of delusion formation can bypass logic rather than distort it.

Further evidence that delusions entail exemption from logic rather than faulty logical deduction is provided by the clinical observation that, in many instances, schizophrenic patients can discern the logical inconsistency in their belief, and acknowledge that others would not accept it, but none the less continue to believe it.

For example, an intelligent young man suffering from schizophrenia was admitted to hospital after stabbing himself. He reported that he had been stabbed by an evil person named Michael, although he himself had been the only person present at the time, and he admitted that he had held the knife. He maintained that the act was none the less the act of Michael. He spoke of Michael as of a real person who controlled his actions. Several months later, when he had recovered from the episode of acute psychosis, he still claimed that he had been stabbed by Michael. When presented with the evidence that he had been alone and had held the knife himself, he readily acknowledged that, in light of this evidence, others might conclude that he had stabbed himself; this demonstrates that his capacity for rational evaluation of the relevant evidence was intact. None the less, he appeared to assume that his explanation of the origin of his experience was exempt from logical re-evaluation.

One of the clearest illustrations of the way in which the delusional beliefs of schizophrenic patients appear to be exempt from logic is provided by the historic case of Daniel Schreber, a high-ranking judge from Leipzig who suffered a late-onset schizophrenic illness. Schreber's account (Schreber, 1955; see also Spitzer *et al*, 1989) is of special value for illustrating the nature of delusions, because, by virtue of his keen intellect, we have access to his own perceptions of his condition, in addition to detailed accounts by his physicians. His first psychotic episode was at the of age 42. He subsequently suffered a more protracted episode in 1893, at the age of 51, when facing a heavy burden of work after appointment as Presiding Judge at the Appeal Court in Dresden. He was discharged from hospital in 1902, but eventually suffered a third episode of illness, after his wife suffered a stroke, and he remained in an uncommunicative, disorganised state until his death.

After obtaining a court order for his discharge from hospital in 1902, he published his memoirs in a volume that includes his own account of his beliefs, and also the report prepared by the asylum director, Dr Weber, opposing his discharge. Schreber believed that he had a mission to redeem the world and restore mankind to its lost state of bliss. His system of delusions included the belief that he was being transformed into a voluptuous female partner of God. Dr Weber reported that, in 1902, Schreber continued to maintain his delusional beliefs in a manner that would accept no contrary argument, although he exhibited a lively interest in his social environment and had a well informed mind and sound judgement. Schreber himself agreed that his beliefs were unchangeable. He considered that they belonged to a domain that was exempt from normal logic. "I could even say with Jesus Christ: My kingdom is not of this world; my so-called delusions are concerned solely with God and the beyond."

In many instances, the delusions of schizophrenia appear to arise from an altered experience of self or of external reality. The phenomena identified by the German psychiatrist Kurt Schneider (1959) as the 'first-rank' symptoms of schizophrenia (discussed in greater detail in Chapter 11) include several symptoms that entail an aberrant experience of ownership of one's own thought, will, action, emotion or bodily function, which the patient attributes to alien influence.

The experience of alien control of action in schizophrenia can be remarkably similar to the experience reported by individuals who have suffered an injury to the supplementary motor area located on the medial surface of the brain anterior to the primary motor area. For example, Mellor (1970, p. 18) describes a schizophrenic patient who reported: "my fingers pick up the pen but I don't control them ... I sit there watching them move but they are quite independent. What they do has nothing to do with me." Compare this with an account of a patient with a lesion of the supplementary motor area: "at one point it was noted that the patient had picked up a pencil and begun scribbling with the right hand. She then indicated that she had not herself initiated the original action. She experienced a feeling of dissociation from the actions of the right arm, stating on several occasions that 'it will not do what I want it to do'" (Goldberg *et al*, 1981, pp. 684–685).

It appears that in both the psychotic individual and in the patient with an injury to the supplementary motor area there is a disruption of the neural circuitry responsible for identifying oneself as the source of one's own actions. However, whereas the patient with traumatic injury to the supplementary motor area can usually recognise that he/she is suffering an abnormal, albeit compelling, experience that has arisen from an injury, the psychotic patient not only suffers the abnormal experience of alien influence, but also has an impaired ability to identify the source of that experience, and does not subject it to a test of its veracity.

Although studies employing factor analysis to delineate the relationships between schizophrenic symptoms demonstrate that delusions and hallucinations have some factor in common, there is also substantial evidence that particular subgroups of delusions and hallucinations can be distinguished on factor analytic grounds. In particular, within the range of reality distortion symptoms that are prevalent in schizophrenia, two major subgroups load on distinguishable factors (Liddle, 1987a). One factor has high loadings on Schneiderian first-rank symptoms, such as delusions of control, auditory hallucinations in the third person, as well as bizarre delusions. Most of the items loading on this factor are related to the issue of autonomy, and are fairly specific to schizophrenia. The second factor has high loadings on persecutory delusions, grandiose delusions and second-person hallucinations. The phenomena associated with this second factor are concerned with the relationship between self and others, and are relatively common in other psychotic illnesses. The two factors are moderately correlated with each other.

Thus examination of the relationships between reality distortion symptoms in schizophrenia supports the proposal that there is a pathological feature common to all manifestations of reality distortion, but, in addition, a distinct factor, possibly associated with disorders of the experience of autonomy, contributes to a subgroup of symptoms that is relatively specific for schizophrenia.

## Affective psychosis

As mentioned previously, the delusions and hallucinations of affective psychosis tend to be mood congruent. In depression, delusions focus on themes of low self-worth, guilt or pessimism, while auditory hallucinations tend to be critical. Conversely, during manic episodes, delusions of grandiose identity or ability are common. The content of hallucinations often serves to confirm the exaggerated self-esteem characteristic of mania.

While the existence of mood-incongruent delusions might give grounds for questioning a diagnosis of affective psychosis, the occurrence of psychotic illness dominated by mood disturbance but including mood-incongruent delusions and/ or hallucinations undoubtedly occurs. Persecutory delusions are relatively common. Schneiderian first-rank symptoms occur in about 10–20% of cases (O'Grady, 1990), compared with a prevalence of about 60% in schizophrenia (Mellor, 1970). According to the DSM–IV criteria, a diagnosis of mood disorder with psychotic features is made when delusions and/or hallucinations occur during an illness dominated by a major mood disorder, irrespective of whether or not the content is mood congruent, unless there is a period of at least two weeks when delusions or hallucinations are present in the absence of major mood disturbance.

It is important to note that reality distortion in affective psychosis does not appear merely to be an inevitable consequence of severe mood disturbance, although the bias in thinking associated with the mood disturbance can shape its character. Many patients suffer repeated episodes of severe unipolar depression, perhaps with gross psychomotor retardation or with marked agitation, yet do not develop delusions or hallucinations. The mood disorder and reality distortion are distinguishable dimensions of psychopathology that none the less interact.

## Alzheimer's disease

Various hallucinations and delusions are encountered in a substantial minority of cases of Alzheimer's disease. In a thorough study of 56 patients who were assessed clinically in life and received a definitive diagnosis of Alzheimer's disease at post-mortem examination, Forstl et al (1994) found the most common form of psychotic symptom was delusional misidentification, which occurred in 25% of their cases. Visual hallucinations occurred in 18%, paranoid delusions in 16% and auditory hallucinations in 13%.

The category of delusional misinterpretation embraced several similar types of phenomena, of which the most common was the misidentification of other people. It is likely that it reflects a disorder of the circuitry specialised for the recognition of familiar faces. Only 29% of the cases exhibiting delusional misidentification exhibited paranoid delusions, which indicates a relatively low degree of overlap in the pathophysiology of delusional misidentification and paranoid delusions. On the other hand, among those with auditory hallucinations, 57% had visual hallucinations and 57% had paranoid delusions, which shows that there is a tendency for hallucinations in one modality to be associated with hallucinations in a different modality and also with paranoid delusions.

Thus, in Alzheimer's disease as in schizophrenia, a diverse range of psychotic phenomena occur, although they are somewhat less prevalent in Alzheimer's disease. Some phenomena, such as paranoid delusions and auditory hallucinations, are common in other psychotic illnesses; others, especially delusional mis-identification, are common in Alzheimer's disease and relatively rare in other conditions. It is of interest to note that the neuropathology of Alzheimer's disease, like that of schizophrenia, appears to affect widespread areas of the cerebral cortex, with the most severe tissue loss in the medial temporal regions, particularly in the parahippocampal gyrus (Hubbard & Anderson, 1981). However, in contrast to schizophrenia, where the pathology is quite subtle and possibly involves loss of neuropil rather than cell bodies (Chapter 11), Alzheimer's disease is character-ised by progressive degeneration of both cell bodies and neuropil.

## Overt brain injury and epilepsy

There is a great deal of overlap between the phenomena of schizophrenia and psychosis arising from overt brain damage or degeneration, although at least some studies indicate that visual hallucinations are more prevalent in psychosis arising from overt cerebral damage than they are in schizophrenia (Goodwin *et al*, 1971). The possibility of identifying the relationship between form and/or content of reality distortion and the site of cerebral damage in cases of focal brain injury has prompted many clinical reports. In a comprehensive review of such reports, Davison & Bagley (1969) concluded that lesions of the temporal lobe and diencephalon are particularly significant in the genesis of psychosis.

Temporal lobe epilepsy, a condition characterised by aberrant neural activity rather than a deficit in neural activity, is associated with a schizophrenia-like psychosis characterised by delusions and hallucinations, including Schneiderian first-rank symptoms, but with less of the disorganisation and psychomotor poverty seen in schizophrenia. Of the 69 patients with psychosis associated with temporal lobe epilepsy studied by Slater *et al* (1963), 67 had delusions in clear consciousness and 52 suffered hallucinations in clear consciousness, but only 31 exhibited formal thought disorder and 28 exhibited loss of affective responses.

## Conclusions from clinical observations

The pattern of occurrence of delusions and hallucinations in various conditions supports the proposal that these core features of psychosis share a cardinal aspect of their pathophysiology. The similarities between delusions and hallucinations occurring in diverse disorders, and the fact that antipsychotic medication can be effective in treating these symptoms irrespective of diagnosis, implies that the shared cardinal pathophysiological feature can occur in several different disorders. None the less, the differences in the frequency of specific types of delusions and hallucinations in various conditions suggest that there are aspects of their pathophysiology that are more strongly associated with the specific pathological processes causing particular illnesses.

In general, the evidence suggests that psychotic reality distortion involves at least two stages. The first is the generation of a specific aberrant mental event. The neuronal system involved in this stage would be that specialised for processing the relevant type of information. The second stage, which is specific to psychotic illness, appears to be a failure of the mechanism that evaluates mental events as they enter consciousness. Such a failure might entail malfunction of a neural system specialised for the evaluation of mental events, or result from a miscommunication between the neural system in which the aberrant mental event was generated and the neural system mediating conscious awareness.

With regard to specific brain loci in the network, the temporal lobe is implicated not only by the specific association of these symptoms with overt temporal lobe lesions and temporal lobe epilepsy, but also because the temporal lobe is heavily involved in the neuropathology of schizophrenia (see Chapter 11) and Alzheimer's disease (Hubbard & Anderson, 1981), two conditions in which a diverse range of reality distortion phenomena occur.

# Neuropsychological correlates of reality distortion

In many individuals exhibiting psychotic reality distortion, there is a marked contrast between the dramatic mental aberration generating the delusional idea or hallucinatory experience and the patient's ability to perceive and think in an apparently normal manner in other domains. Furthermore, various studies have shown that deluded schizophrenic patients do not differ significantly from normal individuals in their ability to make rational deductions (e.g. Williams, 1964). Thus the cardinal abnormality is unlikely to be a generalised failure of reasoning.

Although it appears that impaired deductive reasoning is not relevant, various investigators have proposed that delusions are associated with a deficit in the ability to make judgements based on probabilistic evidence. In a study designed to test this hypothesis, Huq et al (1988) presented deluded schizophrenic patients with beads drawn one at a time from a jar containing unequal numbers of beads of two colours, and asked them to predict the colour of the majority of the beads in the jar. The schizophrenic subjects tended to reach their conclusion after being shown fewer beads but made no more errors than healthy controls. On average, the schizophrenic patients made their choice when they had enough information to give a 95% probability of being correct, a level equal to the probability threshold conventionally accepted by statisticians, whereas healthy controls waited until the probability of error was less. Thus, this study indicates that deluded schizophrenic subjects are competent at judgements based on probabilistic evidence, but tend to be less conservative in reaching decisions than healthy control subjects. Unfortunately, the design of the study did not rule out the possibility that this difference was due to greater impulsiveness, unrelated to delusional thinking, in the patients.

A variety of deficits or biases in the processing of information have been reported to be associated with features of reality distortion, and these are discussed under separate headings below.

## Peripheral sensory processes

Clinical observation suggests an association between deafness and paranoid psychosis in the elderly. Formal testing of auditory acuity reveals an association between subtle hearing impairment and auditory hallucinations in patients with severe persistent schizophrenia (Matthew *et al*, 1993). However, most psychotic patients are not deaf, and this is unlikely to be the principal factor leading to the generation of hallucinations.

## Attributional style and biased processing of information

In a series of studies of the attributional style of patients suffering from paranoid psychosis, Bentall (1994) has found evidence that patients with persecutory delusions tend to attribute negative outcomes to causes external to themselves. This bias appears to reflect selective processing of information, as revealed by types of error on memory and attentional tasks.

## Disturbance of figure–ground perception

Several studies have found an association of moderate strength between reality distortion and an impaired ability to distinguish a line drawing of a figure from a distracting background (Robertson & Taylor, 1985; Liddle, 1987b). Evidence from studies of animals indicates that the hippocampus plays an important role in distinguishing figure from ground (Gray, 1982).

## Monitoring of self-generated mental activity

Heilbrun (1980) found that patients with auditory hallucinations have an impaired ability to recognise the origin of thoughts that they themselves have generated. Collicut & Hemsley (1981) proposed that hallucinations arise from a bias in the attribution of the origin of mental events such that unexpected, internally generated experiences are attributed to external events. In a study designed to test the hypothesis that hallucinations are associated with a tendency to judge internally generated stimuli as arising from external sources, Bentall & Slade (1985) compared schizophrenic subjects suffering from hallucinations with non-hallucinating schizophrenic subjects in their ability to distinguish auditory stimuli consisting of a voice plus noise from stimuli containing noise alone. The two groups of patients achieved a similar level of correct identifications, but the patients with hallucinations were more likely to report stimuli as voices than as noise alone. The authors interpreted this finding as evidence that patients with hallucinations are more likely to report imaginary events as real.

Implicit in the hypothesis that hallucinations arise when internally generated mental events are attributed to an external source is the assumption that there is a mechanism for monitoring internally generated mental activity. Frith & Done

(1989) devised a task designed to test the ability to monitor self-generated action. The task was a computer game in which the subject was required to correct the trajectory of a hidden projectile travelling across the screen of a visual display unit, so as to hit a moving target. Success depended on correctly remembering the previously selected trajectory without the benefit of visual feedback. They found that schizophrenic patients with delusions of alien control performed poorly in the task, compared with control subjects. They interpreted this deficit as evidence that delusions of alien control are associated with defective internal monitoring of self-generated mental activity. In a similar study, Mlakar *et al* (1994) also demonstrated that patients suffering from delusions of control have an impaired ability to monitor self-generated plans for action. More recently, Morrison & Haddock (1997) confirmed that patients with auditory hallucinations have an impaired ability to recognise the source of mental activity.

## Conclusions from the neuropsychological evidence

Examination of the neuropsychological correlates of delusions and hallucinations supports the clinical evidence that diverse elements of mental processing contribute to reality distortion. In particular, several different lines of evidence indicate bias in the processing of information. Perhaps most salient are the studies that have indicated that there is a defect in the monitoring of internally generated mental acts, particularly in recognising that such mental activity was in fact generated internally.

As discussed in Chapter 1, human mental activity is relatively free from constraint by the dictates of concurrent external circumstances. This allows for great flexibility in responding to changing circumstances by manipulating information derived from memories of the past to produce hypothetical constructions of the future. However, it makes it important to have a well developed mechanism for labelling the origin of mental representations of reality. It is essential to be able to distinguish mental representations triggered by current external circumstances from representations of past situations and representations of hypothetical situations. The evidence suggests that at the heart of reality distortion lies a disruption of the mechanisms for making this distinction.

# Regional cerebral activity associated with reality distortion

Several early studies employing SPET reported that patients with hallucinations had overactivity within the temporal lobes (Musalek *et al*, 1989; Suzuki *et al*, 1993). In a PET study of schizophrenic patients with stable persistent symptoms, Liddle *et al* (1992) found that reality distortion was associated with an aberrant pattern of cerebral activity that involved overactivity in the left parahippocampal gyrus and hippocampus. Furthermore, the area of parahippocampal activity coincided with an area that is activated in normal individuals during the performance of a novel eye movement task designed to place heavy demands on the need for internal monitoring of self-generated movements (Frith *et al*, 1992). Liddle *et al* (1992) also found evidence for aberrant activity at several other cerebral sites. In particular, they found overactivity in the ventral striatum and left ventrolateral prefrontal cortex, together with underactivity in the left lateral temporal/parietal cortex and posterior cingulate.

In a subsequent SPET study of acutely ill schizophrenic patients, Ebmeier *et al* (1993) confirmed the observation that reality distortion is associated with underactivity in the left lateral temporal cortex, but they did not find evidence of overactivity in the hippocampus. This may be because SPET is less sensitive than PET, especially for activity in structures deep in the brain, although it is also possible that the discrepancies between studies reflect differences in study design, which we shall consider later.

In a SPET study of patients with auditory hallucinations, imaged during the experience of hallucinations and then in the absence of hallucinations, McGuire *et al* (1993) found that the presence of auditory hallucinations was associated with significantly increased activity in Broca's area (the left ventrolateral frontal cortex), consistent with the hypothesis that the genesis of auditory hallucinations involves the aberrant production of internal speech. Furthermore, the increased activity in Broca's area was part of a pattern of activity in a distributed network of cerebral areas, including the left medial temporal lobe and the anterior cingulate cortex. The magnitude of the increase in rCBF in the medial temporal lobe was actually greater than that in Broca's area, but owing to the noisiness of this region of the images this increase did not by itself achieve statistical significance.

In a PET study of hallucinating schizophrenic subjects, Silbersweig *et al* (1995) found that the occurrence of auditory hallucinations was correlated with increased rCBF in the hippocampus and parahippocampal gyrus, and also in the cingulate gyrus, thalamus and ventral striatum.

## Conclusions from functional imaging

The most consistently reported abnormality associated with reality distortion is overactivity in the medial temporal lobe, especially in the parahippocampal gyrus and hippocampus (Musalek *et al*, 1989; Liddle *et al*, 1992; McGuire *et al*, 1993; Silbersweig *et al*, 1995). Other replicated findings include overactivity in the ventral striatum (Liddle *et al*, 1992; Silbersweig *et al*, 1995); overactivity in the left ventrolateral frontal lobe (Liddle *et al*, 1992; McGuire *et al*, 1993); and underactivity in the left superior temporal gyrus (Liddle *et al*, 1992; Ebmeier *et al*, 1993).

The observation of overactivity in the medial temporal lobe is likely to be of special relevance, because it is engaged during several aspects of mental processing that were implicated in reality distortion by the neuropsychological evidence we considered above. In particular, the hippocampus is involved in memory for context (Chun & Phelps, 1999). In addition, the site of aberrant parahippocampal activity which Liddle *et al* (1992) found to be associated with reality distortion coincided with the site that Frith *et al* (1992) found to be active during a task designed to place heavy demands on internal monitoring of the source of intended action.

Other sites at which overactivity has been reported include loci that might be expected to be involved in the generation of the specific mental acts that form the content of the delusions or hallucinations. In particular, some of the evidence indicates that Broca's area, which is specialised for the production of speech, is activated in patients with auditory hallucinations. Furthermore, areas related to the selection of mental activity, including the anterior cingulate and medial prefrontal cortex, are also implicated. As will be discussed in Chapter 7, these areas are also implicated in the disorganisation syndrome, perhaps accounting for the moderate overlap between the occurrence of reality distortion and disorganisation reported in some studies (Liddle & Barnes, 1990).

The finding that reality distortion is associated with overactivity in the ventral striatum is potentially of particular significance for understanding the mechanism of antipsychotic treatment. Studies of the induction of immediate early genes by various pharmacological agents in the brains of animals indicate that all known antipsychotic agents, both typical and atypical, act on the ventral striatum (Robertson & Fibiger, 1992). Immediate early genes, such as *c-fos*, are expressed rapidly after the pharmacological stimulation of a cell. The functional significance of the expression of these genes is not known.

Despite the substantial level of agreement between the various studies of regional cerebral activity associated with reality distortion, not all studies have observed the same abnormalities. One possible explanation is that, due to differences in study design, some studies might be expected to detect the abnormalities associated with the actual occurrence of reality distortion, while others might be more sensitive to the trait abnormalities that predispose to reality distortion. For example, the studies by Susuki *et al* (1993), McGuire *et al* (1993) and Silbersweig *et al* (1995) were all longitudinal studies that compared cerebral activity during the occurrence of hallucinations with that in the same patients when hallucinations were absent. Therefore, these studies would be expected to identify features associated with the occurrence of hallucinations. All of these studies reported cerebral overactivity, but not sites of cerebral under-activity.

The study of Ebmeier *et al* (1993) was a cross-sectional one that determined the correlation between severity of reality distortion and rCBF, across subjects. Such a study would be more sensitive to the trait that determines the propensity to suffer reality distortion. Ebmeier *et al* observed underactivity in the lateral temporal cortex. The study by Liddle *et al* (1992) was also cross-sectional but it included only patients with persistent symptoms, so that it is likely that the patients were experiencing symptoms during scanning. Thus this study would be expected to reveal sites associated with both the predisposing trait and the actual experience of reality distortion. Liddle *et al* observed underactivity in the lateral temporal lobe, as observed by Ebmeier *et al*, but also overactivity at the diverse sites found to be overactive in the studies of McGuire *et al* (1993) and Silbersweig *et al* (1995). Thus it is plausible that sites of cerebral underactivity reflect the propensity to suffer reality distortion, whereas the sites of cerebral overactivity reflect the actual occurrence of reality distortion.

# Neurochemistry and pharmacology of reality distortion

The success of antipsychotic drugs that block dopamine $D_2$ receptors in alleviating delusions and hallucinations provides strong circumstantial evidence implicating dopamine in the pathophysiology of reality distortion. Indirect dopamine agonists such as amphetamine tend to exacerbate delusions and hallucinations in schizophrenic patients. Furthermore, in a study using SPET with the specific $D_2$ ligand iodobenzamide (IBZM), Laruelle et al (1996) obtained evidence indicating that the exacerbation of psychotic symptoms induced in schizophrenic patients by the administration of amphetamine is associated with increased levels of intrasynaptic dopamine. When amphetamine is administered, endogenous dopamine displaces IBZM from receptors in the basal ganglia. Laruelle et al observed that the amount of displacement of IBZM was greater in schizophrenic subjects than in healthy subjects. Furthermore, in the patients, the amount of IBZM displaced following the administration of amphetamine was correlated strongly with the magnitude of the transient exacerbation of psychotic symptoms (lasting for a few hours after the procedure).

However, not all psychotic patients respond to treatment with $D_2$-blocking medication. For example, in a study of first-episode schizophrenic patients, only 83% achieved remission after one year of treatment with antipsychotic medication (Lieberman et al, 1993). Of those who did not achieve remission, many had persisting delusions or hallucinations. Among patients experiencing their second or subsequent episode, the proportion achieving a satisfactory remission is even lower. A substantial minority of patients who do not respond to typical antipsychotic medication respond to clozapine. Clozapine is effective against the entire spectrum of schizophrenic psychopathology, including reality distortion (Meltzer, 1992). As clozapine blocks a variety of types of receptor, it is uncertain which aspect of its complex pharmacological action is responsible for its enhanced therapeutic effect. Comparison with other atypical antipsychotic drugs suggests that blockade of 5-HT$_2$ receptors may play a part (Meltzer et al, 1989).

The fact that antipsychotic drugs induce the expression of the gene *c-fos* in those neurons with which they interact provides a tool for identifying the likely sites of their action. In rats, typical antipsychotics such as haloperidol induce *c-fos* in both the dorsal and ventral striatum. The induction of *c-fos* in the dorsal striatum is consistent with the widely accepted view that haloperidol generates parkinsonism by blocking dopamine receptors there. Atypical antipsychotics such as clozapine do not induce *c-fos* in the dorsal striatum, consistent with the lack of parkinsonian side-effects of these drugs, but they do induce *c-fos* in the ventral striatum and prefrontal cortex (Robertson & Fibiger, 1992). Thus

**97**

circumstantial evidence indicates that the ventral striatum is the most likely site for the therapeutic actions shared by typical and atypical antipsychotic drugs. It also suggests that the enhanced therapeutic effects of clozapine might arise through action in the prefrontal cortex. It is of interest to note that the pharmacological destruction of dopamine neurons abolishes the induction of *c-fos* by typical and atypical antipsychotics in the ventral striatum, but does not abolish its induction by clozapine in the prefrontal cortex, implying that the effect in the prefrontal cortex does not involve dopaminergic neurons. As discussed above, the circumstantial evidence provided by the observation of *c-fos* induction in the ventral striatum and prefrontal cortex is consistent with the evidence from PET studies (Liddle *et al*, 1992; Silbersweig *et al*, 1995) implicating these areas in the experience of reality distortion.

While dopamine is the neurotransmitter most heavily implicated in reality distortion, other neurotransmitters are also implicated. Agents that interact with serotonin receptors, such as the hallucinogenic drug lysergic acid diethylamide (LSD), which is a serotonin 5-HT$_2$ receptor agonist, have a hallucinogenic effect. LSD stimulates autoregulatory presynaptic 5-HT$_2$ receptors in the raphe nucleus, thereby inhibiting neuronal firing. The net effect is decreased cerebral serotonergic transmission. It is noteworthy that serotonin inhibits dopamine release in some brain areas, by acting at presynaptic heteroreceptors located on dopaminergic neurons (see Chapter 5). Thus reduced serotonergic transmission might promote dopaminergic release. However, it is not certain that diminished serotonergic transmission due to reduced firing in the raphe nucleus is responsible for the hallucinogenic effect of LSD. Direct stimulation of cortical 5-HT$_2$ receptors might also play a role.

Drugs that block glutamatergic receptors, such as the psychotogenic anaesthetic agent ketamine, can produce symptoms of reality distortion, together with other symptoms typical of schizophrenia. Carlsson & Carlsson (1990) have argued that blockade of glutamatergic input to the indirect cortico-striato-thalamo-cortical feedback loop would promote psychosis. The indirect loop provides negative feedback to the cortex (see Chapter 4), and reduction in transmission through this loop would lead to disinhibition of input to the cortex from the thalamus. Since dopamine acts to inhibit transmission through the indirect loop, glutamate and dopamine have potentially opposing effects on transmission in this pathway. Thus, according to the hypothesis proposed by Carlsson and Carlsson, psychosis arises from a shift in the balance between glutamatergic and dopaminergic activity in the indirect pathway, in favour of excess dopaminergic activity.

# Synthesis and hypothesis

Examination of the clinical characteristics and neuropsychological correlates of delusions and hallucinations indicates that the mechanism of reality distortion is likely to involve the failure to label internally generated mental events correctly.

A delusion is an internally generated idea that is labelled as if it were an externally validated fact, and therefore exempt from logical analysis. A hallucination is an internally generated perception that is labelled as if it had been derived via the external senses. The content of the delusions and hallucinations is likely to be determined by the cerebral area in which the relevant mental event arises. For example, it is probable that overactivity in the left ventrolateral frontal cortex is associated with the generation of verbal hallucinations (McGuire *et al*, 1993). The primary mental events might in themselves be either pathological, as in the case of ideas that are distorted by depressed mood, or normal, as in the case of a new untested idea, or normal inner speech. The essential feature of reality distortion appears to be a failure to label such an event appropriately.

In this section we shall draw upon our understanding of the role of the hippocampus in memory for contextual information (see Chapter 3) and the role of the cortico-striato-thalamo-cortical feedback loops (see Chapter 4) to propose a mechanism for the generation of delusions and hallucinations, and for the action of antipsychotic medication.

## The relevance of context for the evaluation of ideas and perceptions

Memories for items of information ('declarative memories') are either episodic or semantic. Episodic memories are memories of specific events experienced by the subject. Their credibility is usually determined by contextual information. Semantic memories are memories for facts whose validity transcends the context within which they were learned. For example, an individual might know that Paris is the capital city of France without remembering the specific circumstances in which he first learned this fact. Novel ideas are initially evaluated in relation to the context in which they arose. Eventually an idea may be sufficiently consolidated (perhaps by cross-reference to other accepted information) that it is accepted without reference to the context of its origin. At that point it becomes an accepted item in semantic memory. This implies that the cerebral representation of a novel idea is normally linked to the representation of the context of its origin.

## The role of the hippocampus in the processing of context

The observation that bilateral damage to the hippocampus abolishes recent episodic memory (Milner, 1966) without damaging semantic memory suggests that the hippocampus may play a role in the linking of an idea to its original context. This hypothesis is strengthened by the subsequent observation that hippocampal damage impairs the ability to employ previously presented contextual information to locate a target in a visual search task (Chun & Phelps, 1999). As discussed in Chapter 3, Rolls (1989) has proposed a model based on the connections of the hippocampus, according to which the CA3 region of the hippocampus acts as an auto-association memory device. An auto-association memory device is a neural network in which memories are stored by strengthening the connections within the network in such a manner that re-exposure of the network to part of a previously presented pattern of inputs reactivates the entire pattern of activity evoked by the previous pattern of inputs. Since inputs from many areas of the neocortex converge on pyramidal neurons in the CA3 region of the hippocampus, these neurons would be expected to fire whenever a previously encountered pattern of distributed cortical activity occurs.

Hippocampal neurons project via glutamatergic fibres to the corpus striatum, where they synapse on GABA-ergic spiny interneurons, which are components of the cortico-striato-thalamo-cortical feedback loops that regulate frontal cortical activity (see Chapter 4). As demonstrated by Grace et al (1998), input from the hippocampus to the striatum facilitates feedback via these loops. Thus the connections and architecture of the hippocampus provide it with the capacity to identify and reinforce specific patterns of cerebral activity.

When the pattern of cerebral activity associated with a particular mental event coincides with a pattern of cerebral activity that represents its appropriate context, hippocampal firing would tend to reinforce that pattern of mental activity. Thus, under normal circumstances, hippocampal firing may act to reinforce mental events that are contextually appropriate. If the pattern of cerebral activity represented an incidental mental event – one occurring without any supporting context – it would be less likely that the pattern of cerebral activity would be adequately reinforced. On the other hand, once an idea has been repeatedly reinforced, its cerebral representation might be reinvoked without reference to context.

What might happen in pathological conditions in which aberrant hippocampal firing occurred? One possibility is that concurrent mental activity would be experienced as if it had occurred before. This is the phenomenon of déjà vu, which occurs in temporal lobe epilepsy. However, less massive aberrant firing of hippocampal neurons might produce more subtle effects. Patterns of neural activity representing incidental thoughts might be reinforced irrespective of context. Thus reality might become distorted in one of several ways.

One possibility would be that an incidental idea would become firmly linked with concurrent perceptual processing. By such a means, delusional perceptions might arise. A delusional perception is the misinterpretation of a normal perception as proof of an unrelated idea. For example, in a case reported by Mellor (1970), a young Irishman at breakfast in a lodging house correctly perceived his companion pushing the salt cellar towards him, and interpreted this as evidence that he should return home since the Pope was about to visit his family because one of the young man's sisters was about to give birth to the Christ child.

In situations where a thought related to concurrent mental activity was reinforced inappropriately, such as excessive reinforcement of ideas of unworthiness during an episode of depression, the reinforced idea might achieve delusional intensity. In other circumstances, the fleeting idea that a situation contained a threat to one's safety might be reinforced so as to become a delusion of persecution. Hallucinations might arise if aberrant hippocampal firing occurred during the production of subliminal internal speech. For example, if aberrant hippocampal firing occurred during the formation of an internally directed utterance such as 'You fool!', the pattern of cerebral activity corresponding to that utterance might be reinforced without reinforcement of the preceding mental events. Thus the utterance might enter consciousness without any awareness of its internal origin.

These speculations imply that the cardinal event leading to the genesis of delusions and hallucinations is aberrant hippocampal activity. However, the tendency to reality distortion might be greatly enhanced if the aberrant hippo-campal activity occurred in association with dopaminergic hyperactivity, which tends to promote positive feedback via the cortico-striato-thalamo-cortical loops (Alexander & Crutcher, 1990a). As discussed in Chapters 7 and 8, dopaminergic overactivity would also be expected to promote other symptoms, such as disorganisation and psychomotor excitation. Individuals prone to dopaminergic overactivity at times of stress (see Chapter 5) would be expected to be prone to acute psychotic episodes in which reality distortion occurred in association with psychomotor excitation and disorganisation.

## The action of antipsychotic drugs

For typical antipsychotics, the level of dopamine $D_2$ receptor occupancy in the basal ganglia is correlated with the therapeutic effect (Nordstrom *et al*, 1993). Dopamine blockade would be expected to diminish the excessive positive feedback via cortico-striato-thalamo-cortical circuits that is presumed to underlie not only delusions and hallucinations, but also symptoms of disorganisation and psychomotor excitation. However, in some cases, psychotic symptoms persist despite a high level of $D_2$ receptor blockade (Wolkin *et al*, 1989). Our hypothesis implies that full remission of reality distortion in acute psychosis will occur only if dopamine blockade is accompanied by suppression of aberrant hippocampal firing (possibly mediated by a decrease in activity in the abundant glutamatergic projections from the frontal cortex to the hippocampus). In individuals in whom aberrant hippocampal firing persisted despite dopaminergic blockade, delusions and hallucinations would be resistant to treatment with typical antipsychotics.

Even in individuals in whom aberrant hippocampal firing was alleviated by antipsychotic treatment, the patterns of cerebral activity representing mental events that had previously been inappropriately reinforced might still be maintained via normal hippocampal activity, but would be amenable to rational scrutiny and would be expected to fade with time. However, in cases with a prolonged duration of psychosis before treatment, it would be anticipated that delusions would be firmly entrenched and, therefore, more resistant to treatment.

The dorsal striatum is principally involved in feedback to the premotor cortex, while the ventral striatum is more strongly involved in feedback to the prefrontal cortex, which is involved in higher mental functions (Alexander *et al*, 1986). Therefore, it would be expected that dopaminergic modulation of the ventral striatum rather than the dorsal striatum would be relevant to the relief of psychotic symptoms. This expectation is supported by the observation by Robertson & Fibiger (1992) that both typical and atypical antipsychotics induce the immediate early gene *c-fos* in the ventral striatum in rats, whereas only typical antipsychotics, which are prone to produce movement disorders as side-effects, induce *c-fos* in the dorsal striatum.

## Summary

The principal postulates of the proposed mechanism for the generation of delusions and hallucinations are:

(1)  Under normal circumstances, hippocampal firing acts to reinforce mental events that are contextually appropriate.
(2)  Aberrant firing of hippocampal neurons leads to reinforcement of mental events irrespective of context, thereby leading to delusions or hallucinations.
(3)  Dopaminergic overactivity will increase the propensity to delusions and hallucinations by virtue of promoting positive feedback via the cortico-striato-thalamo-cortical loops. Therefore, delusions and hallucinations are most likely to arise during periods of acute dopaminergic overactivity.
(4)  Antipsychotic drugs decrease the severity of a psychotic episode by diminishing excessive positive feedback to the frontal cortex via the cortico-striato-thalamo-cortical loops, but the cardinal requisite for alleviation of delusions and hallucinations is the abolition of aberrant hippocampal firing.

Thus it might be predicted that, during the treatment of acute psychosis, there would be a reduction in neural activity in the cortico-striato-thalamo-cortical loops, and also in the hippocampus. Furthermore, the degree of reduction of hippocampal activity would predict the degree of resolution of reality distortion. To test these hypotheses, my colleagues and I performed a study using PET to measure changes in regional cerebral metabolism during treatment with the antipsychotic risperidone in first-episode schizophrenic patients (Liddle *et al*, 2000). We performed PET scans before the start of treatment, 90 minutes after the administration of the first dose of risperidone and again after six weeks of treatment. Reduced activity in the frontal cortex, ventral striatum and thalamus was discernible after the first dose (Plate 15) and became more extensive after six weeks' treatment. This reduction was not preferentially correlated with a reduction in severity of any specific group of symptoms. In addition, we observed that reduction in hippocampal metabolism following the first dose was strongly predictive of the degree of subsequent alleviation of delusions and hallucinations after six weeks' treatment (Plate 16).

These findings provide strong support for the hypothesis that reduction of hippocampal activity is essential for the alleviation of delusions and hallucinations. They provide indirect support for the hypothesis that delusions and hallucinations arise as a consequence of aberrant hippocampal firing, which reinforces concurrent mental activity irrespective of context.

I

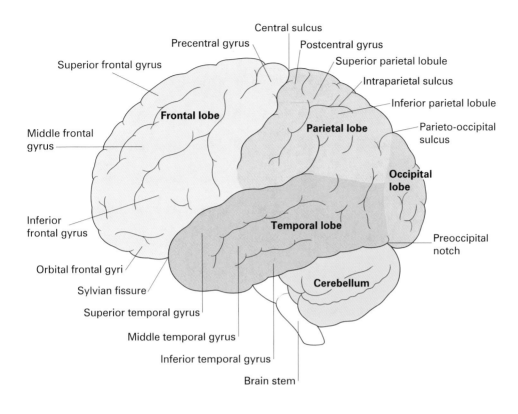

**Plate 1** Lateral aspect of the brain, including the brain stem, left cerebellum and the left cerebral hemisphere, showing lobes, sulci and gyri.

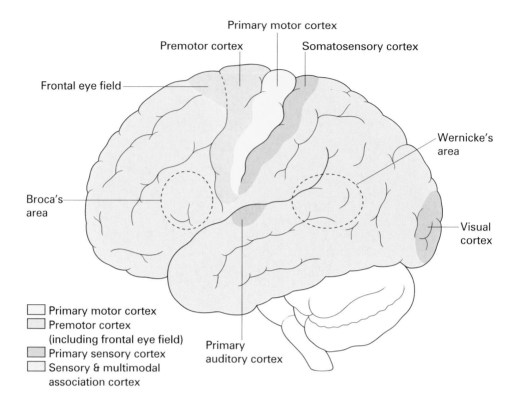

Primary motor cortex

Premotor cortex

Somatosensory cortex

Frontal eye field

Wernicke's area

Broca's area

Visual cortex

☐ Primary motor cortex
☐ Premotor cortex
(including frontal eye field)
☐ Primary sensory cortex
☐ Sensory & multimodal
association cortex

Primary auditory cortex

**Plate 2** Lateral aspect of the left cerebral hemisphere, showing functionally distinct regions.

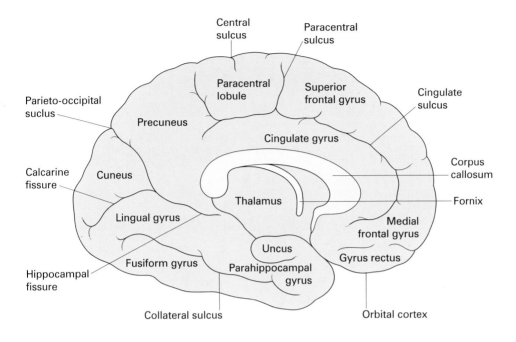

**Plate 3** Medial aspect of the left cerebral hemisphere.

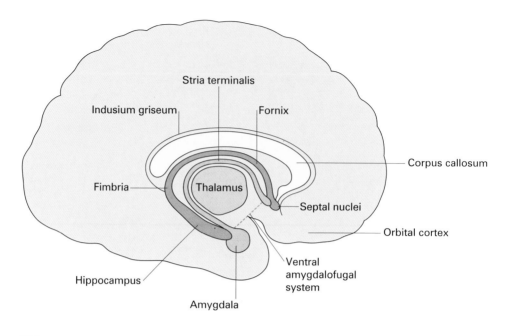

**Plate 4** A schematic illustration of the limbic system, projected onto a parasagittal plane.

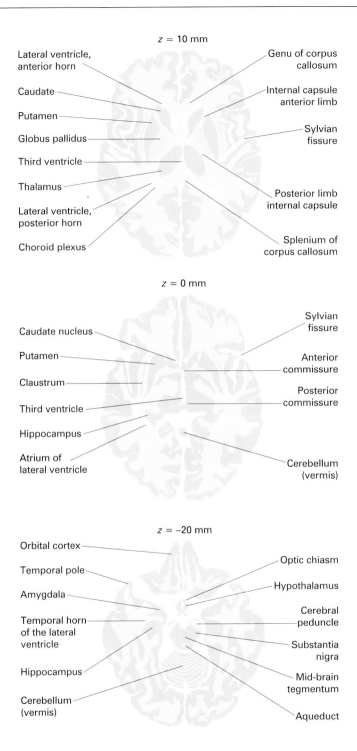

**Plate 5** Axial slices through the brain at 10 mm above, 0 mm above, and 20 mm below the intercommissural plane.

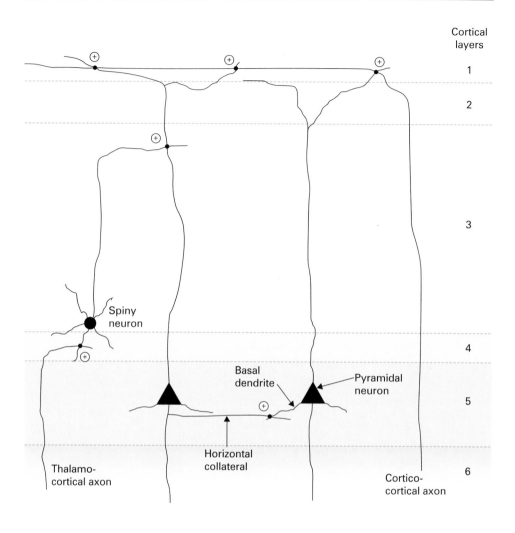

Cortical
layers

1

2

3

Spiny
neuron

4

Basal
dendrite

Pyramidal
neuron

5

Horizontal
collateral

Thalamo-
cortical axon

Cortico-
cortical axon

6

**Plate 6** Schematic illustration of the glutamatergic connections mediating the local spread of excitation in the cerebral cortex. Only one example of each type of connection is illustrated, whereas, in fact, each pyramidal cell receives tens of thousands of synapses, many of which are excitatory. Furthermore, connections that mediate the spatially focused transmission of information, such as feed-forward cortico-cortical fibres terminating in layer IV, are not shown. Although not shown, pyramidal cells are also prevalent in layer 3.

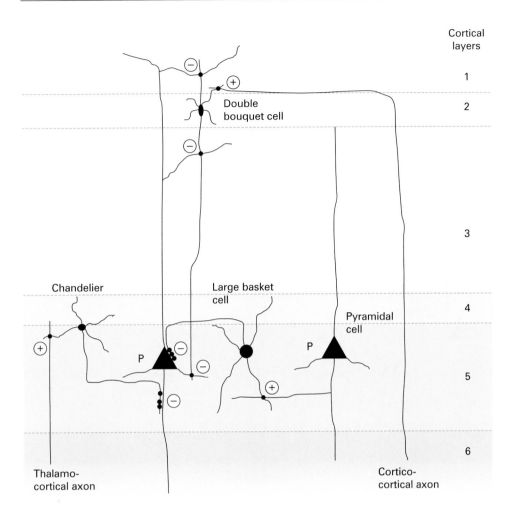

**Plate 7** Local inhibitory circuits in the cerebral cortex. The chandelier cell makes inhibitory synapses with the initial segment of the axon of pyramidal cell P1. The large basket cell makes inhibitory synapses with the pyramidal cell body. The double bouquet cell exerts an inhibitory influence on the dendrites. Each inhibitory cell itself receives multiple inputs. For simplicity, only a single input to each inhibitory cell is shown. Although not shown, pyramidal cells are also prevalent in layer 3.

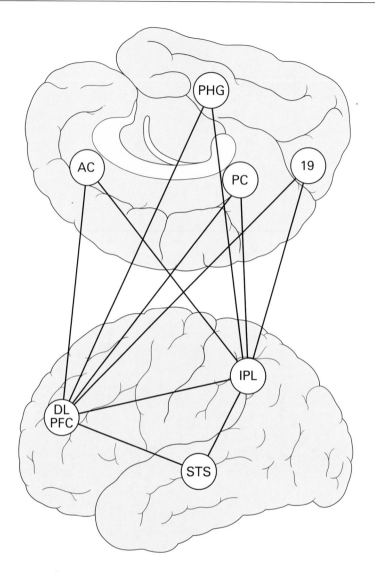

**Plate 8** Diagrammatic representation of the reciprocal connections of both the dorsolateral prefrontal cortex and parietal cortex revealed in anatomical studies of rhesus monkey, superimposed on lateral and medial views of the human cerebral hemispheres, after Goldman-Rakic (1988). The circuit has been proposed to mediate visuo-spatial working memory (Selemon & Goldman-Rakic, 1988). Note that the positions of homologous areas in monkey and human may differ slightly, due to differentiation and expansion of the cortex during evolution. For eamaple, some tissue in the ventral bank of the monkey intraparietal sulcus (and hence in the IPL) may be located in the dorsal bank of the human intraparietal sulcus (and hence in superior parietal lobule). None the less, the basic circiut arrangements can be assumed to be conserved. DL PFC = dorsolateral prefrontal cortex; IPL = inferior parietal lobule; STS = superior temporal sulcus; AC = anterior cingulate; PC = posterior cingulate; PHG = parahippocampal gyrus; 19 = area 19 (extra-striate visual cortex). Reprinted with permission, from the Annual Review of Neuroscience, volume 11 © 1998 by Annual Reviews www.AnnualReviews.org.

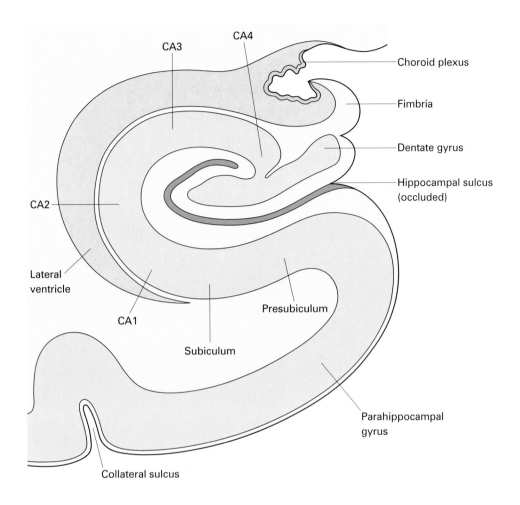

CA4

CA3

Choroid plexus

Fimbria

Dentate gyrus

Hippocampal sulcus
(occluded)

CA2

Lateral
ventricle

Presubiculum

CA1

Subiculum

Parahippocampal
gyrus

Collateral sulcus

**Plate 9** Schematic coronal section through the medial temporal lobe, showing the hippocampal formation.

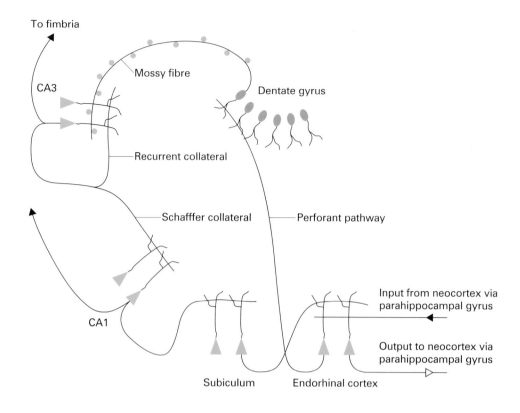

To fimbria

CA3

Mossy fibre

Dentate gyrus

Recurrent collateral

Schafffer collateral

Perforant pathway

CA1

Input from neocortex via parahippocampal gyrus

Output to neocortex via parahippocampal gyrus

Subiculum

Endorhinal cortex

**Plate 10** Schematic representation of connections in the hippocampus. The anterior part of the parahippocampal gyrus is known as the entorhinal cortex, while the posterior part is known as the parahippocampal area; these two regions have different connections. The major input from the cortex enters via the entorhinal cortex. Fibres from the entorhinal cortex project via the perforant pathway to granule cells in the dentate gyrus. These granule cells project via mossy fibres to region CA3, where they synapse with pyramidal neurons. Axons of the CA3 pyramidal cells project to the fimbria and thence via the fornix to the septal area. Collateral fibres (the Schaffer collaterals) project from CA3 to CA1. Fibres from CA1 project to the subiculum and thence back to the entorhinal cortex. Thus the entorhinal cortex acts as the major portal for entry and exit of information from and to the neocortex. It should be noted that the entorhinal cortex is located in the anterior part of the parahippocampal gyrus, so the perforant fibres projecting to posterior regions of the hippocampal formation travel parallel to the long axis before perforating the subiculum. In addition to the illustrated perforant pathway, perforant fibres also project directly to regions CA1, CA2 and CA3.

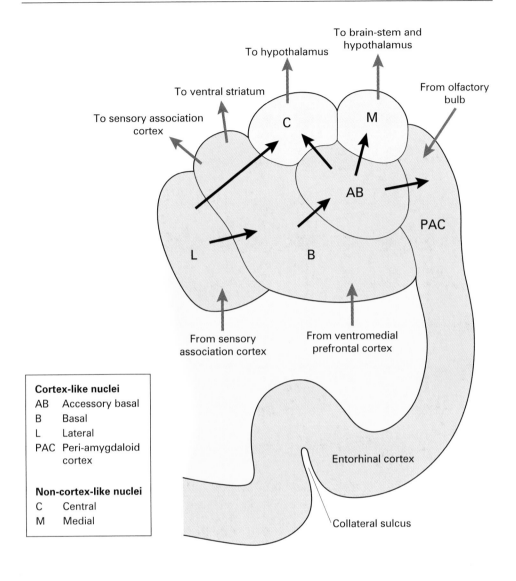

**Plate 11** Diagrammatic coronal section through the anterior medial temporal lobe, showing the amygdala with its principal intrinsic and extrinsic connections.

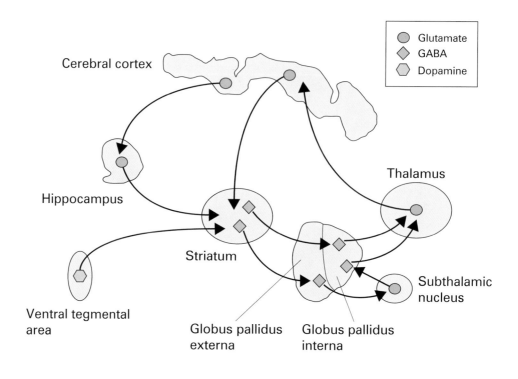

**Plate 12** Cortico-striato-thalamo-cortical circuit. (Reprinted from Liddle *et al*, 2000.)

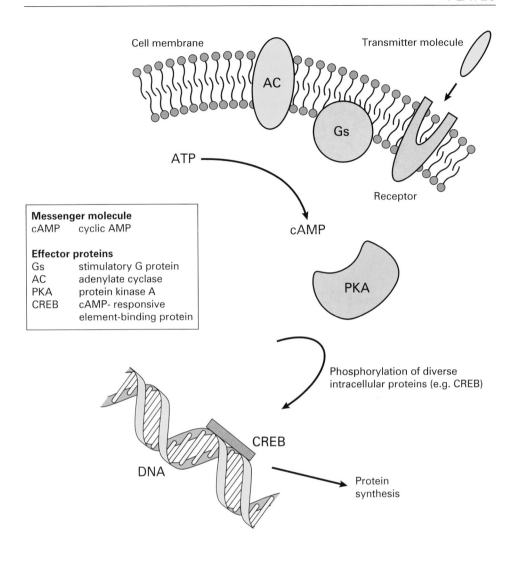

**Plate 13** The cAMP second messenger system. Binding of a transmitter molecule to its receptor activates a G protein, which in turn activates the effector enzyme, adenylate cyclase. Adenylate cyclase acts on ATP to produce cAMP. cAMP activates protein kinase A, which phosphorylates, and thereby activates, diverse types of intracellular effector protein. For example, activation of CREB leads to transcription of DNA and subsequent protein synthesis.

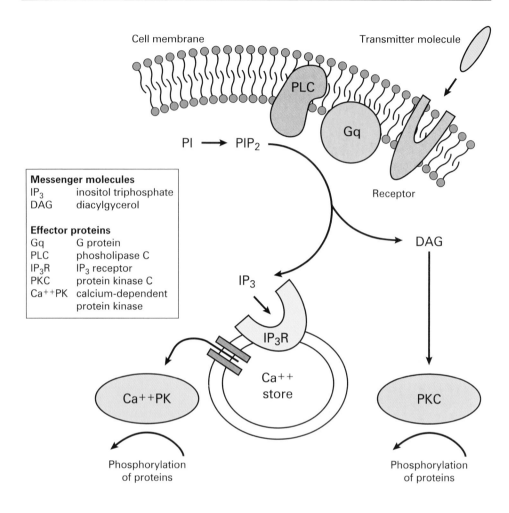

**Plate 14** The phosphatidyl inositol (PI) second messenger system. Membrane-bound PI is initially converted to PI biphosphate (PIP$_2$). Binding of a neurotransmitter molecule activates a G protein (for example, Gq), which in turn activates the enzyme phospholipase C. Phospholipase C hydrolyses PIP$_2$, producing inositol triphosphate (IP$_3$) and diacylglycerol (DAG). IP$_3$ promotes the release of calcium from intracellular stores, initiating a series of calcium-dependent metabolic processes, including protein phosphorylation by calcium-dependent kinases. DAG activates PKC, which regulates a wide range of intracellular processes by phosphorylation of proteins.

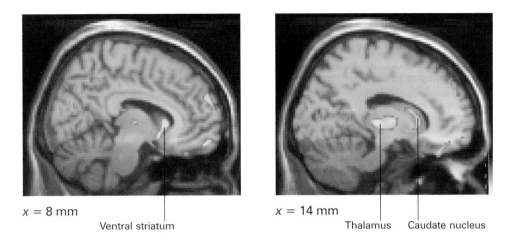

$x = 8$ mm

Ventral striatum

$x = 14$ mm

Thalamus    Caudate nucleus

**Plate 15** Right parasagittal slices at $x = 8$ and 14 mm, showing the sites of significant decrease in cerebral metabolism in schizophrenic patients produced by 2 mg risperidone. (Reprinted from Liddle *et al*, 2000.)

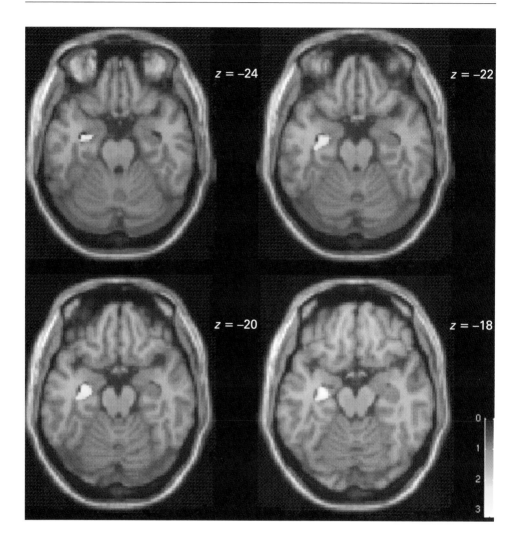

**Plate 16** Decreases in cerebral metabolism in the left hippocampus after the first dose of risperidone predict the subsequent resolution of reality distortion. The warm hues denote voxels in which there is a significant correlation of reduction in immediate metabolism after the first dose with reduction in severity of reality distortion after six weeks of treatment. The colour scale denotes values of the $z$ statistic. Axial slices at 18, 20, 22 and 24 mm below the intercommissural plane are shown. (Reprinted from Liddle *et al*, 2000.)

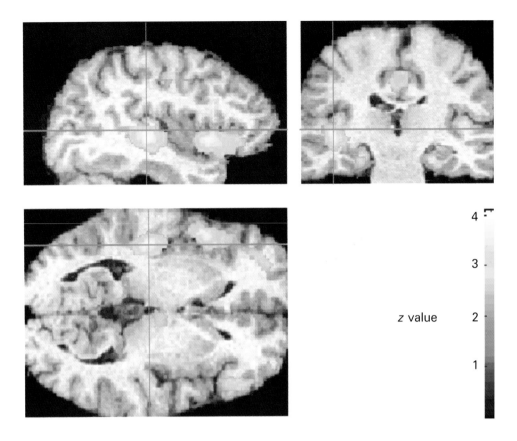

z value

Plate 17 Decreases in rCBF associated with thought form disorder in schizophrenia measured using PET. (Reproduced with permission from McGuire *et al*, 1998.) Shades of red and yellow indicate voxels in which there is a significant negative correlation between rCBF and severity of thought form disorder, assessed as patients describe pictures while in the scanner. Decreases in rCBF with increasing thought disorder are seen in the ventrolateral frontal cortex bilaterally, cingulate gyrus (arrow) and in the left superior temporal gyrus (cross-hairs). Reduced engagement of the superior temporal gyrus would be expected to interfere with word finding, and underactivity of the ventrolateral prefrontal cortex would be expected to promote the intrusion of inappropriate material into current mental processing. The horizontal slice is at the level of the anterior and posterior commissures, the sagittal section is 42 mm left of the midline and the coronal section is 24 mm behind the midpoint of the anterior commissure.

Decreases

Increases

1. Left lateral

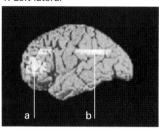

2. Left medial

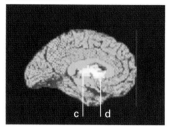

3. Right lateral

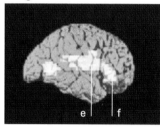

4. Right medial

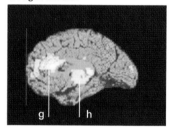

5. Left lateral

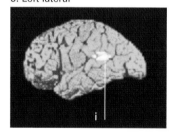

6. Left medial

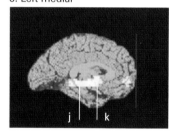

**Plate 18** Patterns of rCBF associated with schizophrenic symptoms (reprinted with permission from Liddle, 2000a). The areas of significant correlation between rCBF and severity of each of three groups of characteristic symptoms are shown rendered onto the cortical surface.
1. Negative correlations of psychomotor poverty with rCBF in the left prefrontal cortex (a) and inferior parietal lobule (b).
2. Positive correlations of psychomotor poverty with rCBF in the thalamus (c) and basal ganglia (d).
3. Negative correlations of disorganisation with rCBF in the right insula rendered on to the overlying temporal cortex (e) and ventrolateral frontal cortex (f).
4. Positive correlations of disorganisation with rCBF in the right anterior cingulate and adjacent medial prefrontal cortex (g) and thalamus (h).
5. Negative correlations of reality distortion with rCBF in the left superior temporal gyrus (i).
6. Positive correlations of reality distortion with rCBF in the left parahippocampal gyrus (j) and ventral striatum (k).
Reprinted by permission of Edward Arnold Ltd.

Range of z
scores

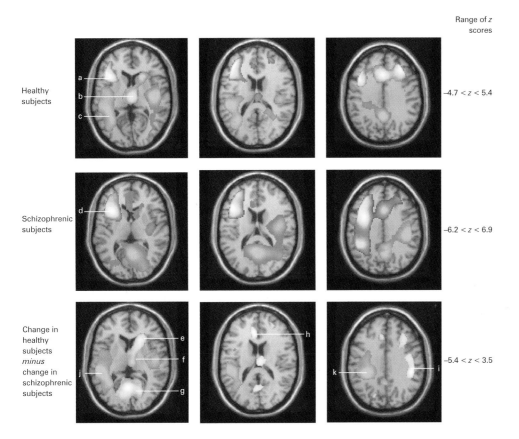

Healthy
subjects

$-4.7 < z < 5.4$

Schizophrenic
subjects

$-6.2 < z < 6.9$

Change in
healthy
subjects
*minus*
change in
schizophrenic
subjects

$-5.4 < z < 3.5$

**Plate 19** Significant changes in rCBF measured with PET during paced word generation in healthy subjects and in schizophrenia. (Reprinted with permission from Liddle, 2000a.) Increases relative to word repetition are shown in red–yellow hues and decreases in blue, in slices at 6 mm (left), 16 mm and 34 mm above the intercommissural plane. In all the clusters of voxels shown in colour, the change is statistically significant at the level $P < 0.05$ after correcting for multiple comparisons. In healthy subjects, rCBF increases in the left lateral frontal cortex (a) and thalamus (b), while it decreases in the temporal cortex bilaterally (c). Schizophrenic subjects exhibit a normal increase in the left lateral frontal cortex (d), but there are abnormalities in many other areas. Relative to healthy subjects, schizophrenic subjects exhibit significantly less increase in rCBF in the right striatum (e), right thalamus (f), lingual gyrus (g), anterior cingulate (h) and right inferior parietal lobule (i), and significantly greater increase in the temporal lobe bilaterally (j) and left inferior parietal lobule (k). Reprinted by permission of Edward Arnold Ltd.

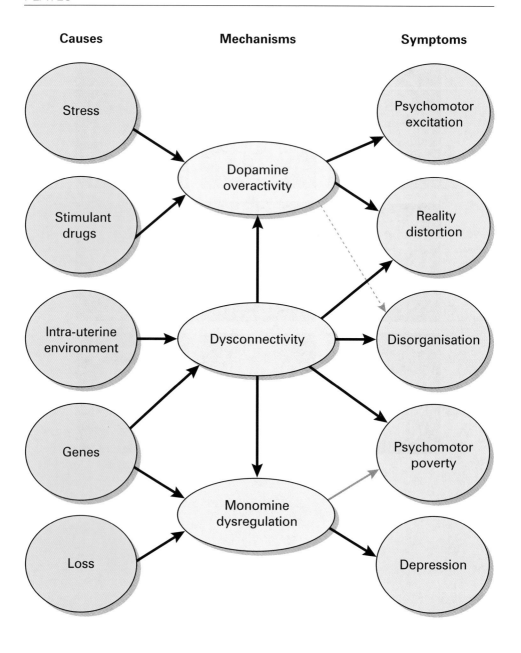

**Plate 20** The developmental dysregulation hypothesis of schizophrenia. The heaviness of the arrows indicates the relative strength of the connections. (Adapted from Liddle, 2000b.)

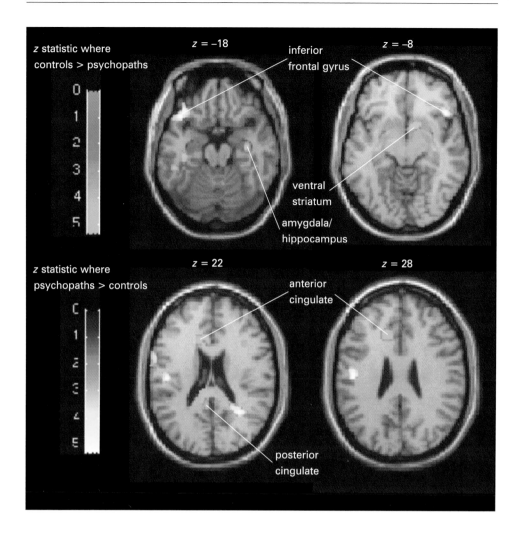

**Plate 21** Differences between psychopaths and healthy subjects in the amount of cerebral activity during the learning, rehearsal and subsequent recognition of lists of emotionally negative words, relative to that during a baseline task in which the subjects were required to learn, rehearse and then recognise similar lists of emotionally neutral words. The blue areas are regions in which the amount of activation during performance of the emotional memory task was greater in healthy subjects than in psychopaths, and the orange areas are regions where the activation was greater in psychopaths. (Data are from the study by Kiehl *et al*, 2000c.)

# Chapter 7

# Disorganisation

## Introduction

The disorganisation syndrome consists of disjointed thought, emotion and behaviour. Its cardinal symptoms are formal thought disorder, inappropriate affect, and bizarre, erratic behaviour. Disorganisation has long been recognised as one of the core features of schizophrenia. Eugen Bleuler, the Swiss psychiatrist who gave the illness its name (Bleuler, 1911), considered that disjointed thought was a fundamental symptom of schizophrenia, insofar as he considered that it is present throughout the illness in all cases; and also a primary symptom, insofar as many of the other symptoms arose from it. He chose the name schizophrenia to reflect the fragmentation of mental activity that was reflected not only in fragmented thinking but also in the split between thought, emotion and behaviour. While the nature of the core feature of schizophrenia is still a subject of debate, the evidence that we shall consider in this chapter provides at least partial support for Bleuler's speculations. In particular, we shall see that subtle disorganisation of mental activity is often an enduring feature of schizophrenia that is strongly associated with poor outcome.

While most characteristic of schizophrenia, disorganisation of thought, emotion and behaviour can follow overt damage to the frontal lobes, especially the orbital frontal cortex. When arising from frontal lobe injury, it is known as the pseudo-psychopathic syndrome, although it should be noted that this group of symptoms does not include the callous disregard for others that is typical of psychopathy (Chapter 14). A modified form of the disorganisation syndrome is also seen in mania, although the presence of euphoric or irritable mood modifies the expression of disjointed emotion. In contrast to the situation in schizophrenia, there is usually a greater coherence between thought and emotion in mania, and the disjointed thought and behaviour characteristic of mania tend to be a transient feature that is present only during the acute phase of the illness.

# Clinical characteristics of disorganisation

## Assessment of disorders of thought form

The disorders of the form of thought that occur in psychotic illness are a heterogeneous collection of phenomena. Most prevalent in schizophrenia is the disruption of connections between ideas that is perhaps most aptly described by Bleuler's term 'looseness of associations'. In his classic description of schizophrenia, he defined this disorder in the following manner: "Of the thousands of associative threads which guide our thinking, this disease seems to interrupt, quite haphazardly, sometimes such single threads, sometimes a whole group, and sometimes even large segments of them. In this way, thinking becomes illogical and often bizarre" (Bleuler, 1911, p. 14).

In practice, abnormalities of the form of thought are inferred from abnormalities of the form of speech. In the case of psychotic illnesses, it is usually assumed that observed abnormalities of the form of speech reflect abnormalities of the form of thought. Some justification for this assumption is provided by the fact that similar anomalies occur in the written output of psychotic patients, thereby demonstrating that the primary abnormality is not at the level of production of vocal output. It is usual to use the term 'disorders of the form of thought', despite the fact that the observable abnormalities are usually abnormalities of speech. More strictly, they should be described as abnormalities of the form of thought and language.

Comparison of the findings of different investigators regarding thought form disorder is difficult because of the differences in the terminology and definitions employed. For the purposes of the present chapter, we shall mainly employ the nomenclature and definitions proposed by Andreasen (1979a) in her scale for the assessment of Thought, Language and Communication (TLC). In recent years, this scale, in either its full or abbreviated form, has been widely used for assessing thought form disorder, although, as we shall see in our subsequent discussion, even this scale has limitations that reflect the difficulty of providing explicit and reliable definitions of some of the subtleties of schizophrenic thought.

The TLC item derailment corresponds most closely to Bleuler's concept of looseness of associations. Derailment is defined as a pattern of speech in which ideas slip off the track onto another one that is either obliquely related or completely unrelated. In addition, loss of goal, tangentiality and incoherence also entail weakening of the links between ideas. Loss of goal is the failure to follow a chain of thought through to its logical conclusion. It often occurs in association with derailment. Tangentiality is defined in the TLC as replying to a question in an oblique, tangential or even irrelevant manner. Incoherence is defined as speech that is essentially incomprehensible because a series of words or phrases seem to be joined together arbitrarily.

Other types of thought form disorder defined in the TLC reflect odd or idiosyncratic use of language. These include neologisms, word approximations and stilted speech. Neologisms are new words invented by the patient. Word approximations are words chosen in an unconventional manner, or words constructed by an unconventional combination of existing words. Andreasen gives the example of a patient who referred to a glove as a hand-shoe. Stilted speech is speech that is inappropriate for the setting. It might be inappropriately pompous, legalistic, philosophical or quaint.

The TLC scale also includes various items concerned with the flow of thought and speech, including poverty of speech and pressure of speech. These phenomena should be regarded as components of the psychomotor poverty and psychomotor excitation syndromes respectively, and will be discussed in Chapter 8. In this chapter we shall deal only with the various abnormalities of the form of thought.

The various published factor analytic studies of TLC items (Andreasen & Grove, 1986; Peralta et al, 1992a) have demonstrated a complex pattern of interrelationships between the different TLC items. Although the findings from these studies differ in detail, the broad outline is similar and demonstrates that two major factors account for the relationships between the disorders of thought form. The first factor might be described as reflecting looseness of associations. Derailment, tangentiality, loss of goal, illogicality and incoherence load on this factor. The second factor is related to the idiosyncratic use of language. Stilted speech, word approximations and neologisms load on the idiosyncratic language factor.

Thought form disorder is most likely to be apparent when a patient is generating thought in a relatively unconstrained way. Because of this, it is difficult to devise a reliable way in which to elicit it. While the TLC definitions provide a fairly comprehensive coverage of the thought form disorders that occur in schizophrenia, the fact that a standardised way of eliciting these phenomena is not specified presents a problem in longitudinal evaluations within subjects, or when making comparisons between subjects. Johnston & Holzman (1979) developed an alternative scale for assessing thought form disorder called the Thought Disorder Index (TDI), which utilises responses made to Rorschach inkblots and also the responses made to the verbal sub-scales of the Wechsler Adult Intelligence Scale, to assign scores for a very comprehensive set of anomalies in thought and language. As we shall see below, the TDI has proved especially useful for delineating the differences between the thought disorders that occur in schizophrenia and in affective psychosis. However, the TDI is too cumbersome for routine use.

In an attempt to combine the merits of the TLC and the TDI, I developed a scale called the Thought and Language Index (TLI) that employs a standardised procedure for eliciting disorders of thought form (Liddle, 1999). The items of the TLI embrace the phenomena from the TLC and the TDI that are most prevalent in schizophrenia. These include:

(1) poverty of speech – decreased number of words per minute;
(2) weakening of goal – vague speech that conveys little information owing to a lack of necessary elaboration or overgeneralisation;
(3) perseveration – unwarranted repetition of ideas;
(4) looseness – derailed or tangential responses;

(5)   idiosyncratic word use – unusual choice of words, neologisms;
(6)   idiosyncratic sentence construction – unusual construction of sentences that hinders understanding;
(7)   idiosyncratic logic – reasoning that does not employ the normal rules of logic;
(8)   distractibility – intrusion of ideas arising from an external stimulus.

Scores are assigned on the basis of responses to pictures from the Thematic Apperception Test or, alternatively, the Rorschach inkblots. The Rorschach stimuli are more ambiguous and usually elicit more abnormal phenomena, but scoring is more difficult because it is less easy to judge whether or not a response is abnormal. This scale has been externally validated by functional imaging studies using both PET and fMRI that demonstrate a consistent pattern of brain activity during the occurrence of these phenomena, irrespective of whether they are elicited using the Thematic Apperception Test pictures or the Rorschach inkblots (McGuire *et al*, 1998; Kircher *et al*, 2000).

## Disorganisation in schizophrenia

Factor analysis of schizophrenic symptoms yields a disorganisation factor whose cardinal components are: thought form disorder; inappropriate affect; and bizarre behaviour (Liddle, 1987a; Mortimer *et al*, 1990; Liddle & Barnes, 1990; Arndt *et al*, 1991; Frith, 1992; Peralta *et al*, 1992b; Malla *et al*, 1993). In several of these studies, there was evidence for some overlap between the features of the disorganisation syndrome and the reality distortion syndrome. For example, Liddle & Barnes (1990) found that thought form disorder loaded heavily on the disorganisation factor (factor loading 0.69) but also on the reality distortion factor (factor loading 0.46). This suggests that there is some aspect of the pathophysiology of these syndromes that is shared. A minority of the studies that have employed factor analysis to examine the relationships between schizophrenic symptoms have failed to identify a discrete disorganisation factor, but have found that the symptoms of disorganisation and reality distortion load on a single positive-symptom factor (Eaton *et al*, 1995).

While the factor analytic studies point to a degree of overlap between disorganisation and reality distortion, the distinct prognostic implications, the associated neuropsychological deficits and the patterns of brain abnormality associated with the disorganisation syndrome, which are considered in detail below, provide strong grounds for regarding disorganisation as a syndrome separate from reality distortion.

There is good agreement between the majority of studies regarding the composition of the disorganisation syndrome, but there are some discrepancies that arise from the definitions of items within the different symptom rating scales that have been used. In particular, several scales, such as the Brief Psychiatric Rating Scale (Overall & Gorham, 1962) and the Positive and Negative Syndrome Scale (Kay, 1991), include inappropriate affect within the blunted affect item. Usually, this item loads on a negative-symptom factor (or psycho-motor poverty factor) rather than on the disorganisation factor. A similar problem arises in studies employing sub-scale scores from the 1982 version of the Scale for the Assessment of Negative Symptoms (SANS; Andreasen, 1982) as this sub-scale included items reflecting both blunted affect and inappropriate affect. The fact that the composition of the disorganisation syndrome can be influenced by the symptom scale employed to measure it should be borne in mind when interpreting the results of studies of the disorganisation syndrome. However, the most prevalent and therefore dominant component of the syndrome is thought form disorder and, consequently, the character of the disorganisation syndrome is dominated by this item, irrespective of which other clinical features are included within the syndrome.

Florid disorganisation is a characteristic feature of acute psychosis, but a more subtle form of disorganisation, characterised by vague, wandering speech, often persists during the stable phase of the illness (Spohn *et al*, 1986). Persistent disorganisation is one of the determinants of poor outcome in schizophrenia. For example, Harrow *et al* (1983) found that thought form disorder in the post-hospital phase of schizophrenia predicted poor outcome. Andreasen & Grove (1986) found that thought form disorder tended to be more persistent in schizophrenic patients than in manic patients, and that persistent thought form disorder predicted poor outcome, although they noted that the strongest predictor of poor outcome was poverty of speech, which is a feature of the psychomotor poverty syndrome rather than the disorganisation syndrome.

Marengo & Harrow (1987) investigated a cohort of young schizophrenic patients early in their illness and compared them with other psychotic and non-psychotic patients. They found that the schizophrenic patients exhibited more thought form disorder than the other diagnostic groups at hospitalisation and, at two and four years after hospital discharge; 37% of the schizophrenic patients exhibited episodic thought disorder, while 40% exhibited persistent thought disorder. Across all diagnostic groups, patients who were more thought-disordered at follow-up showed higher rates of unemployment and greater rates of readmission to hospital. Liddle (1987a) found that severity of disorganisation in chronic schizophrenic patients was correlated with poor performance at work or school, and poor interpersonal relationships. More recently, Norman *et al* (1999) confirmed that severity of disorganisation persisting despite treatment was a strong predictor of poor occupational and social function in the community.

## Disorganisation in affective psychosis

Factor analysis of the correlations between the symptoms of affective psychosis reveals that thought form disorder is associated with a distinct dimension of psychopathology that also includes bizarre behaviour and inappropriate affect (Maziade *et al*, 1995; Peralta *et al*, 1997a). In the study by Maziade *et al*, scores on the various sub-scales of Andreasen's SANS and Scale of the Assessment of Positive Symptoms (SAPS; Andreasen, 1986) were entered into the analysis. The global positive thought disorder item from the SAPS comprises a selection of the most prevalent thought form items from the TLC, including derailment, tangentiality, illogicality, circumstantiality and distractibility. The other symptom loading on the disorganisation factor was bizarre behaviour. Inappropriate affect was not included in the analysis, because in the early versions of the SANS it was represented by one item within the affective flattening sub-scale, and hence was not adequately represented in the sub-scale scores. However, in the study by Peralta *et al*, the SANS and SAPS item scores, including the inappropriate affect item, were entered in the analysis. In that study, inappropriate affect loaded on the disorganisation factor.

Although disorganisation forms a dimension distinguishable from the mood symptoms themselves, it is important to note that, in affective psychosis, the relationships between the various dimensions of the illness are stronger than is the case in schizophrenia. This is because, in mood disorder, symptoms are much more likely to occur in clearly defined acute episodes. In contrast, symptoms often persist in the chronic phase between episodes in schizophrenia, and it is in this phase that the segregation of symptoms is most clearly discernible. In the manic phase of bipolar disorder, elevated mood, psychomotor excitation and reality distortion with grandiose content coexist. In the depressed phase, depressed mood, psychomotor poverty and reality distortion with a depressive content are more likely to coexist. In affective psychosis, disorganisation is virtually confined to the manic phase of the illness. Consequently, the thought form disorder seen in affective psychosis is usually strongly coloured by coexisting pressure of speech.

## Comparison of schizophrenic and manic thought

The distinction between the disorders of the form of thought occurring in schizophrenia and in mania has been controversial. The most prevalent aspect of looseness defined in the TLC scale, derailment, has a similar prevalence in schizophrenia and mania. For example, Andreasen (1979b) found an identical prevalence of 56% for derailment in schizophrenia and in mania, while in a subsequent study Andreasen & Grove (1986) found derailment had a prevalence of 61% in schizophrenia and 80% in mania. The most clear-cut differences between schizophrenic thought and manic thought revealed by the TLC are disorders of flow rather than form. Poverty of speech is common in schizophrenia and pressure of speech is common in mania.

The observation that associative loosening has similar prevalence in schizophrenia and mania is confirmed by the findings of Solovay *et al* (1987), obtained using a quite different assessment instrument, the TDI. The TDI assigns scores for a wide range of aspects of thought on the basis of the subject's responses to ambiguous material such as Rorschach inkblots. These items are grouped into four categories, one of which is associative looseness. Solovay *et al* found that the prevalence of associative looseness in schizophrenia and in mania is very similar.

However, there is also a great deal of evidence that the thinking of schizophrenic patients can be distinguished from that of manic patients. First, despite the evidence that associative looseness occurs in both disorders, severe disruptions of the connections between ideas leading to incomprehensible speech are more prevalent in schizophrenia. For example, Jampala *et al* (1989) defined a disorder called 'drivelling', which is manifest in utterances in which the syntax appears to be intact but the meaning is lost. They found that drivelling had a prevalence of 16.1% in schizophrenia and 0.9% in mania. Similarly, Jampala *et al* found that non sequiturs, defined as utterances that are unconnected in meaning to the preceding question or to the subject's own speech, occurred in 35% of schizophrenic patients but only 14% of manic patients. Solovay *et al* (1987) found that the subgroup of TDI items designated 'disorganisation', which is composed of items such as incoherence, confusion and vagueness, is more prevalent in schizophrenia than in mania.

Second, items that entail idiosyncratic language tend to be more prevalent in schizophrenia than in mania. For example, Jampala *et al* (1989) found neologisms and private use of words were both much more prevalent in schizophrenia. Solovay *et al* (1987) found that a group of TDI items designated 'idiosyncratic verbalisations', which includes phenomena such as peculiar responses, queer responses and neologisms, is much more prevalent in schizophrenia than in mania.

Third, as implied by the observation that pressure of speech is more common in mania than in schizophrenia, manic thought disorder is likely to be coloured by coexisting psychomotor excitation. Many clinicians have used the term 'flight of ideas' to describe the occurrence of associative disturbances that are apparently driven by pressure of speech. Jampala *et al* (1989) found that flight of ideas, defined as associations (usually voluminous) that do not get to the point, and often include multiple recurrent themes, occurred in 72% of manic patients and only in 9.7% of schizophrenic patients. Solovay *et al* (1987) found that the group of disorders designated 'combinatory thinking', which includes incongruous combinations and playful confabulation, were more prevalent in mania than in schizophrenia.

Finally, thought form disorder tends to be more persistent in schizophrenia (Pogue-Geile & Harrow, 1984). For example, chronic thought form disorder, characterised by vague, wandering speech, persists during the chronic phase of illness (Spohn *et al*, 1986).

Several investigators have applied linguistic analysis to attempt to distinguish the speech of schizophrenic subjects from that of patients with affective psychosis. Morice & Ingram (1982) found that the speech of schizophrenic patients was distinguished by a lack of complexity compared with that of manic patients. Hoffman *et al* (1986) deconstructed discourse into its simplest elements and concluded that schizophrenic patients were unable to generate coherent patterns of discourse, whereas manic patients shifted rapidly from one coherent pattern to another.

In conclusion, schizophrenic thought can be distinguished from manic thought by virtue of its exhibiting more severe disruptions of the connections between ideas, greater idiosyncrasy of language, less likelihood of influence from coexisting pressure of speech and greater tendency to chronicity. None the less, associative looseness, the cardinal feature of the disorganisation syndrome, is common to both. This suggests that a similar mental mechanism may play a part in the thought form disorder of both schizophrenia and mania, but it operates in the context of different modifying factors.

## The pseudo-psychopathic syndrome

The classic case illustrating the effects of frontal lobe injury on behaviour is Phineas Gage, the 19th-century American railroad construction foreman who suffered severe damage to his frontal lobes when an explosive charge detonated prematurely, driving the metal tamping rod upwards through his skull, via the orbital surface. He was transformed from a diligent and reliable person into a feckless individual prone to act in an irresponsible manner (Harlow, 1848). More recently, Blumer & Benson (1975) have described a pseudo-psychopathic syndrome that arises following damage to the orbital frontal cortex. This syndrome is characterised by irresponsible behaviour, fatuous affect, garrulous speech and thought form disorder, which Blumer & Benson describe as an inability to maintain specific meanings. For instance, a patient who had suffered a right orbital frontal injury was asked whether the injury had affected his thinking. He replied, "Yeah – it's affected the way I think – it's affected my senses – the only things I can taste are sugar and salt". When the examiner persisted with, "How has it affected the way you think?", he replied, "Yes – I am not as spry on my feet as I was before". These replies would be rated as tangential according to the TLC.

In a study of the language impairments that follow injury to the frontal lobes, Kaczmarek (1987) identified three different patterns. Damage to the left lateral prefrontal cortex produced a pattern dominated by brief replies and lack of elaboration, reminiscent of the poverty of speech in the psychomotor poverty syndrome (see Chapter 8). Damage to the right prefrontal cortex produced distractibility in response to accidental associations, while patients with orbital lesions digressed frequently and did not monitor errors.

## Summary of the clinical observations

The combination of thought form disorder, especially associative looseness, with inappropriate affect and or bizarre behaviour occurs in schizophrenia, mania and traumatic injury to the frontal lobes, especially the orbital cortex. The features of the syndrome differ between the illnesses. In particular, when the disorganisation syndrome occurs in mania, it tends to be strongly coloured by coexisting psychomotor excitation. At least some of the evidence suggests that the thought form disorder of mania results from rapid shifts from one pattern of thought to another. In schizophrenia, there is likely to be more severe disruption of associative links and greater propensity to idiosyncratic use of language. Following trauma to the frontal lobes, behavioural manifestations are the most pronounced abnormalities, but none the less there are abnormalities of language that resemble the associative disorders of schizophrenia. This suggests that a common pathophysiological disruption, probably involving the orbital frontal cortex, is involved in disorganisation in each of the three conditions, but the differential involvement of other neural systems leads to differences in the character of the syndrome in the three conditions.

# Neuropsychological correlates of disorganisation

Decades ago, Broadbent (1958) proposed his seminal 'defective filter' theory of schizophrenia, according to which defects in selective attention played a crucial role in schizophrenic thought disorder. Subsequently, a rich body of evidence has been generated by investigations that have sought to understand schizophrenic thought in neuropsychological terms. In particular, there is evidence for: abnormalities in diverse aspects of attention and working memory (Oltmanns, 1978; Cornblatt et al, 1985; Harvey et al, 1986); failure to use context to form associations (Chapman et al, 1964); failure to inhibit the spreading of semantic and phonological associations (Spitzer et al, 1994); poor discourse planning (Hoffman et al, 1986); inability to take account of the needs of the listener (Cohen et al, 1974); and impaired monitoring of speech output (Harvey et al, 1988). On the other hand, several of the studies that have examined specific aspects of syntactic and semantic processing have not found abnormalities of these processes in thought-disordered schizophrenic patients (e.g. Grove & Andreasen, 1985).

The diversity of neuropsychological abnormalities reported in thought-disordered patients makes it difficult to draw clear conclusions regarding the existence of any cardinal abnormality. None the less, much of the evidence suggests that the core problems involve the executive processes responsible for supervising language and communication, rather than the routine processes employed to interpret or produce speech. The similarities between schizophrenic thought form disorder and the language disorders that Kaczmarek (1987) reported in patients with lesions at various sites in the frontal lobes support the hypothesis that schizophrenic thought form disorder entails impairment at the executive level of language and communication.

While the majority of the studies of the neuropsychological mechanisms of thought form disorder have focused on schizophrenia, a substantial number have examined both schizophrenic and manic patients. These studies have found both similarities and differences in the neuropsychological correlates of thought form disorder in the two conditions. For example, Oltmanns (1978), and also Walker & Harvey (1986), found that thought form disorder is associated with a reduced ability to recall strings of digits, especially in the presence of distraction ('distraction performance'), in both schizophrenia and in mania. Harvey et al (1988) examined the utility of distraction performance to predict subsequent thought form disorder in schizophrenia and in mania. They measured both distraction performance and thought form disorder on two occasions several days

**111**

apart. In both patient groups, poor distraction performance was significantly associated with thought form disorder, at each assessment. However, the impairment of distraction performance at the first assessment predicted severity of thought form disorder at the second assessment only in the schizophrenic patients. Insofar as the temporal relationship between phenomena might indicate causality, these results imply that impaired distraction performance is a part of the mechanism that causes subsequent thought form disorder in schizophrenia. This interpretation is supported by the finding that impairment of digit recall is transient in mania but tends to persist in schizophrenia. For example, Grove & Andreasen (1985) found that in schizophrenic patients digit recall did not improve over a six-month period, whereas in manic patients impairment of digit recall remitted during this period. Thus it is plausible that impaired digit recall is an aspect of a trait that predisposes to thought form disorder in schizophrenia, whereas in mania both impaired digit recall and thought form disorder are aspects of a transient state.

Several studies have reported a specific relationship between disorganisation symptoms and aspects of selective attention. For example, Liddle & Morris (1991) found that severity of disorganisation was correlated with slower performance in the Stroop task (see p. 18), in which correct performance entails suppression of the dominant tendency to respond to the meaning of the word (a colour) instead of the colour of the ink in which it is printed. Subsequently, Baxter & Liddle (1998) and Ngan & Liddle (2000) have replicated the finding that severity of disorganisation is associated with slower Stroop performance. In addition, McGrath (1992) demonstrated that severity of thought form disorder is associated with slower Stroop performance.

Liddle & Morris (1991) also found that severity of disorganisation was correlated with slowed performance in the Trails B task of the Halstead–Reitan neuropsychological battery. In this task a random arrangement of letters and numerals printed on paper is presented and the subject is required to draw a path connecting numerals and letters in the order 1,A,2,B,3,C, and so on. This task entails alternating between the two types of search for the next goal at each step. Additional evidence indicating that disorganisation is associated with impaired response selection is provided by Ngan & Liddle's (2000) finding that disorganisation is correlated with impaired performance in choice reaction time tasks but not in a simple reaction time task.

Disorganisation is also associated with an impaired ability to generate words in a verbal fluency task, which appears to reflect a difficulty in selecting appropriate words. Liddle & Morris (1991) found that severity of disorganisation was associated with reduced verbal fluency, which could not be accounted for by slowness of articulation of words. Allen et al (1993) demonstrated that thought form disorder was correlated with the production of odd or unusual words during a verbal fluency task. Frith et al (1991c) confirmed that both inappropriate affect and thought form disorder were correlated with reduced verbal fluency and with an increased tendency to produce odd or unusual words.

In addition, Frith et al (1991c) found that thought form disorder and inappropriate affect were associated with a tendency to produce errors of commission during a continuous performance task (CPT). In the CPT, a series of stimuli, including a small proportion designated as target stimuli, were presented, and the subject was required to respond only to the target stimuli, while refraining from responding to the non-target stimuli. Errors of commission, in which the subject responds to non-target stimuli, reflect an impaired ability to suppress inappropriate responses.

In summary, many studies have confirmed that disorganisation is associated with slowed performance in tasks that demand selection between competing responses, or with errors of commission in tasks that require suppression of an inappropriate response. These observations suggest that the pathophysiology of disorganisation involves impairment of the neural circuits responsible for response selection and inhibition.

Cohen *et al* (1999) have developed this hypothesis further, in an attempt to clarify the nature of the process by which appropriate responses are selected and inappropriate responses are inhibited. They emphasise the important role of contextual clues in guiding behaviour. They begin by drawing upon the classic studies of Shakow (1962), who was among the first investigators to employ the modern concepts of information processing to explore the mental mechanisms underlying the symptoms of schizophrenia. On the basis of studies of reaction time, Shakow concluded that "we see particularly the various difficulties created by context.... It is as if, in the scanning process that takes place before the response to a stimulus is made, the schizophrenic is unable to select out the material relevant for the response" (p. 4).

In a study using artificial neural networks to model some of the cognitive difficulties that occur in schizophrenia, Cohen & Servan-Schreiber (1992) identified two crucial dimensions of task variation that affect performance. These are the relative strength of competing responses, and the delay between a contextual clue and the response to a query, where the correct response depends on the clue. The design of many of the tasks for which impairment correlates with severity of disorganisation symptoms involves manipulation of one or both of these dimensions. The Stroop task entails manipulation of relative strength of competing responses but, in its usual form, makes minimal demands on keeping contextual clues in mind. In the CPT, in which the subject is required to respond only to designated target stimuli, the strength of the competing responses is manipulated by adjusting the probability of target and non-target stimuli; moreover, the subject needs to hold contextual information in mind, as a delay period is introduced by defining the target stimulus in such a way that it is contingent on previous stimuli (for example by specifying that X is a target only if it follows an A). In the digit recall task employed by Oltmanns (1978) and Harvey *et al* (1986), the subject is required to hold relevant material in mind while ignoring distracting material.

It may seem pertinent to ask whether it is response inhibition and/or the need to keep task-relevant information in mind that is responsible for the observed relationship between impairment in these tasks and severity of disorganisation symptoms. In fact, Cohen *et al* (1999) argue that these two processes are not separate functions. Rather, they propose that a single mental (i.e. neural) process is responsible for maintaining task-relevant information against the interfering and cumulative effects of noise over time. This hypothesis

**113**

is supported by the observation that in the prefrontal cortex of macaque monkeys there are neurons that exhibit sustained, cue-specific activity that persists despite intervening distracters until the appearance of the target stimulus to which the monkey is expected to respond (Miller *et al*, 1996). It appears that these neurons are not merely maintaining the representation of information that may or may not be relevant to later behaviour, but rather maintaining task-relevant information against the interfering effects of noise over time. Consequently, Cohen and colleagues predicted that the ability to maintain relevant information over time and the ability to refrain from inappropriate responses would be correlated in schizophrenic patients and, furthermore, that impairment of both of the processes would be correlated with the severity of disorganisation.

To test their hypothesis, Cohen and colleagues produced modified versions of several tasks, including the Stroop task and the CPT, so as to allow them to manipulate both response inhibition and the period for which it was necessary to sustain relevant information. For example, in their modified Stroop task, the requirement to state either the colour name or the word name was varied randomly from trial to trial. For each trial, the relevant instruction was given either one second or five seconds before the coloured word. In their modified CPT, pairs of letters separated by either one or five seconds were presented. The target stimulus was the letter X following the letter A (AX trials). Eighty per cent of trials were AX trials. The high frequency of AX trials enhanced the probability of false positive responses to the letter X when it was preceded by any other letter (designated BX trials). Five per cent of trials were BX trials, while the remainder were either AY or BY trials, where Y and B denote any letter other than X or A. The short-duration BX trials test the ability to inhibit a prepotent response, while requiring only limited ability to sustain information. The long-duration AX trials test the ability to sustain information while placing little demand on inhibitory mechanisms.

On the basis of their hypothesis that response inhibition and retention of relevant information are performed by the same neural system, they predicted that there would be strong correlations across subjects in the proportion of inhibition failures under the conditions that stressed inhibition and the number of omission errors on target trials under conditions where information had to be retained for a longer period. Their prediction was confirmed, insofar as the correlation between the proportion of inhibition failures and the number of errors of omission in the long-duration trials was stronger than the mutual correlations between other types of errors (such as errors on AY and BY trials) in schizophrenic patients. The correlation between inhibition failures and errors of omission on the long-duration trials was less strong in healthy controls than in schizophrenic patients, which implies that the limiting factor in patients was located in the neural system hypothesised to sustain relevant information over time and to suppress inappropriate responses.

Furthermore, Cohen and colleagues predicted that a composite score reflecting errors in sustaining the relevant information and response inhibition errors would be correlated with severity of the disorganisation syndrome. This hypothesis was also confirmed. These findings have implications regarding the nature of the neural system that might be malfunctioning in the disorganisation syndrome.

# Regional cerebral activity associated with disorganisation

In a study using PET to measure the patterns of cerebral activity associated with persistent symptoms in chronic schizophrenic patients, Liddle *et al* (1992) found that severity of disorganisation was correlated with increased rCBF in the medial frontal cortex, including the anterior cingulate, and also the thalamus and corpus striatum, while it was correlated with decreased rCBF in the insula and contiguous ventral prefrontal cortex, and in the inferior parietal lobule bilaterally.

Using SPET, Ebmeier *et al* (1993) and Yuasa *et al* (1995) both confirmed that disorganisation in schizophrenia is associated with overactivity of the medial frontal cortex, including the anterior cingulate gyrus. In a study of regional glucose metabolism, Kaplan *et al* (1993) failed to find evidence of overactivity of the medial frontal cortex, but did confirm underactivity of the left parietal cortex.

The area of increased activity in the medial frontal cortex observed by Liddle *et al* (1992), Ebmeier *et al* (1993) and Yuasa *et al* (1995) included the site that is maximally activated in healthy individuals during the Stroop task (Pardo *et al*, 1990), which suggests that patients with disorganisation symptoms are continuously engaged in Stroop-like activity, even when not formally engaged in any task. In light of the evidence from studies of monkeys (Mishkin, 1964) that damage to the ventral prefrontal cortex results in an impaired ability to suppress inappropriate responses, it is plausible that, in patients with disorganisation symptoms, underactivity of the ventral frontal cortex allows the intrusion of irrelevant mental activity into the current stream of mental processing, so that the patient is continually faced with the need to select between competing demands for processing resources.

The observation of an association between severity of disorganisation and overactivity in the thalamus and corpus striatum in addition to overactivity in the medial frontal cortex (Liddle *et al*, 1992) suggests that disorganisation is also associated with overactivity in the cortico-striato-thalamo-cortical feedback loops that play a role in regulating frontal cortical activity (see Chapter 4). The association with underactivity in the inferior parietal lobule (Liddle *et al*, 1992; Kaplan *et al*, 1993) suggests that disorganisation is also associated with malfunction in other areas of the association cortex. This observation is consistent with the observation by Shenton *et al* (1992) that severity of thought form disorder is associated with decreased grey matter volume in the left superior temporal lobe and adjacent inferior parietal lobule.

McGuire *et al* (1998) used PET to determine the pattern of cerebral activity

**115**

during the production of thought form disorder in schizophrenic patients. Patients were asked to describe the Thematic Apperception Test pictures that are employed in the TLI to elicit thought form disorder during scanning. The voxels in which there was a statistically significant correlation between rCBF and severity of positive thought form disorder (the sum of scores for looseness, idiosyncratic word use, idiosyncratic sentences and idiosyncratic logic) were identified. Severity of thought form disorder was correlated with reduced activity in the left superior temporal gyrus, bilateral ventrolateral frontal cortex, anterior cingulate and thalamus (see Plate 17). In addition, thought form disorder was correlated with increased activity in the left parahippocampal gyrus and contiguous lingual gyrus.

McGuire *et al*'s finding that thought form disorder is associated with reduced activity in the ventrolateral frontal cortex and left superior temporal gyrus is broadly consistent with the findings of the PET study by Liddle *et al* (1992), in which patients with persistent thought form disorder were found to have underactivity in the right ventrolateral frontal cortex and inferior parietal lobule. At first sight, McGuire *et al*'s finding of decreased activity in anterior cingulate and thalamus during the actual production of thought disorder is contrary to the observation by Liddle *et al* (1992) of overactivity in the anterior cingulate and thalamus in patients with persistent disorganisation. However, the study by Liddle *et al* was designed to measure cerebral activity over a relatively sustained period of time during which the patient experienced disorganisation. This design would be expected to reveal cerebral activity associated with the predisposition to disorganisation, as well as the activity associated with the thought disorder. According to the interpretation presented above, the overactivity of the anterior cingulate in patients with disorganisation reflects the need to deal with the continuous intrusion of inappropriate mental activity, arising as a consequence of defective function of the ventrolateral prefrontal cortex. The actual production of thought disorder would be expected to occur when the anterior cingulate failed to perform this task. Hence it would be predicted that the production of thought form disorder would be associated with a reduction of activity in the anterior cingulate, as was observed by McGuire and colleagues.

More recently, Kircher *et al* (2000) used fMRI to measure cerebral activity in schizophrenic patents while they were describing Rorschach inkblots. As in the study by McGuire *et al*, thought form disorder was evaluated by summing the TLI items for looseness, idiosyncratic word use, idiosyncratic sentences and idiosyncratic logic. Despite employing a different imaging modality and a different set of stimuli to elicit thought disorder, Kircher *et al* replicated the major findings of McGuire *et al*, including the finding of an association between thought form disorder and decreased activity in the left superior temporal gyrus.

In summary, there is converging evidence that disorganisation is associated with underactivity in the ventrolateral frontal cortex, left superior temporal gyrus and adjacent inferior parietal lobule. Furthermore, patients prone to disorganisation have overactivity in the anterior cingulate and thalamus, although the actual production of disorganised thought appears to be associated with a reduction in activity in the anterior cingulate and thalamus. This interpretation should be regarded with caution until further studies provide confirmation.

# Neurochemistry and pharmacology of disorganisation

Disorganisation symptoms observed during acute episodes of psychosis usually respond to treatment with typical antipsychotics, such as flupenthixol, which block dopamine $D_2$ receptors (Johnstone et al, 1978a). However, at least in schizophrenia, a subtle thought disorder characterised by vague wandering speech may persist despite treatment with typical antipsychotics (Spohn et al, 1986), which indicates that there is an underlying pathological process that is not responsive to dopamine $D_2$ blockade. Nonetheless, in patients whose symptoms have not responded to treatment with typical antipsychotics, the atypical antipsychotic clozapine, which blocks several different neurotransmitters in addition to $D_2$ receptors, is often effective in alleviating disorganisation symptoms (Meltzer, 1992). This suggests that neurotransmitters other than dopamine are likely to be involved in the mechanism of disorganisation. In this section, we shall review the evidence for dopaminergic involvement in disorganisation, and also examine the evidence implicating other neurotransmitters.

## Dopamine agonists

Drugs that promote the release of dopamine, or act as agonists at dopamine receptors, can exacerbate thought form disorder in schizophrenic patients. For example, Levy et al (1993) found that methylphenidate, which promotes dopamine release, exacerbates thought form disorder. Zemlan et al (1986) reported that the amount of growth hormone release induced by the dopamine receptor agonist apomorphine (at a dose of 0.75 mg administered subcutaneously) correlated with severity of thought form disorder. In contrast, Levy et al (1993) did not find that apomorphine (0.0075 mg/kg subcutaneously) produced any significant increase in thought form disorder, although it did produce a non-significant increase of approximately 33% in thought disorder score, which raises the possibility that the study was not powerful enough to detect a significant effect.

The effects of dopaminergic agents on cerebral activity are complex. At low oral doses of the indirect dopamine agonist amphetamine, a reduction in cortical blood flow and metabolism is usually observed (Wolkin et al, 1987), although the degree of frontal lobe activation during frontal lobe tasks such as the Wisconsin Card Sorting Test is increased (Daniel et al, 1991). At higher oral doses (above 0.9 mg/kg) amphetamine produces increased metabolism at diverse cerebral sites, with the most significant increases occurring in the anterior cingulate, corpus striatum and thalamus. These metabolic changes are associated with a mania-like syndrome (Vollenweider et al, 1998). Similarly, intravenous amphetamine (at a dose of 0.15 mg/kg) also produces increases in metabolism in the frontal and limbic cortex and in subcortical nuclei, while

**117**

decreasing metabolism in the temporal cortex (Ernst *et al*, 1997). This pattern closely resembles the pattern of cerebral activity associated with disorganisation.

## Glutamatergic antagonists

A growing body of evidence indicates that interference with glutamatergic transmission can also produce disorganised thought and behaviour. The recreational drug PCP and the anaesthetic agent ketamine, which is a derivative of PCP, block the binding of glutamate to NMDA receptors. Both agents can precipitate a psychosis that includes disorganised thought in healthy individuals, and can exacerbate psychosis in schizophrenic patients. The thought disorder produced in healthy subjects is very similar in character to that found in schizophrenia (Adler *et al*, 1999). Adler *et al* (1998) also demonstrated that the degree of ketamine-induced thought disorder in healthy subjects correlates significantly with ketamine-induced decreases in working memory, but does not correlate with ketamine-induced impairments in semantic memory.

In a PET study of the effects of ketamine on rCBF, Tamminga and colleagues demonstrated that ketamine produces an increase in activity in the anterior cingulate in both healthy subjects and in schizophrenic patients (Lahti *et al*, 1997). Using PET to measure regional glucose metabolism, Breier *et al* (1997a) also found that ketamine produced an increase in frontal activity in healthy subjects. Further, the degree of increase in frontal metabolism was correlated with the severity of thought form disorder.

Blockade of glutamatergic neurotransmission tends to enhance dopamine release. In healthy subjects, ketamine infusion promotes the release of dopamine in the corpus striatum, to a similar extent to that achieved by amphetamine (Breier *et al*, 1998). This might suggest that the psychotogenic effects of ketamine are mediated via dopamine release. However, while blockade of dopamine $D_2$ receptors with haloperidol before the infusion of ketamine prevents the adverse effects of ketamine on executive function, it does not block ketamine-induced psychosis (Krystal *et al*, 1999). On the other hand, the atypical antipsychotic clozapine does blunt the psychotogenic effects of ketamine (Malhotra *et al*, 1997). Thus it appears that blockade of NMDA receptors can promote psychosis by a mechanism that does not involve transmission via dopamine $D_2$ receptors, but can none the less be blocked by atypical antipsychotics.

## The effects of antipsychotic treatment

In a study of the effect of the atypical antipsychotic risperidone on regional cerebral activity in schizophrenic patients during the first episode of illness, my colleagues and I found that a single 2 mg dose of risperidone decreased cerebral activity in the frontal cortex and in the cortico-striato-thalamo-cortical circuit (see Plate 15) (Liddle *et al*, 2000). These cortical reductions became more extensive after six weeks of treatment. We interpreted the immediate reduction in cortico-striato-thalamo-cortical circuits as a consequence of the blockade of dopaminergic overactivity, although it should be noted that risperidone blocks both dopamine $D_2$ and serotonin 5-HT$_2$ receptors. The magnitude of this reduction was not correlated with the decrease in any specific group of symptoms. This result is consistent with the interpretation that dopaminergic overactivity creates a predisposition to all the symptoms of acute psychosis, but is not the cardinal process that generates any particular symptom. However, one of the sites of reduction in the frontal cortex coincided with the area where Liddle *et al* (1992) had observed a positive correlation between rCBF and severity of disorganisation. The correlation between reduction in disorganisation severity and reduction in metabolism at this site produced by six weeks of treatment with risperidone was 0.60 ($P = 0.055$) (Lane, 1999). Thus it is likely that this reduction in medial frontal activity was a reflection of the process responsible for the resolution of disorganisation symptoms.

In a further study of the effects of a single 2 mg dose of risperidone on cerebral activity in healthy subjects, we found that it reduced cerebral metabolism in the same medial prefrontal site as had been observed in schizophrenic patients (Lane, 1999). This suggests that the therapeutic effect observed in patients is a consequence of an effect that risperidone produces in the normal brain.

# Synthesis

Disorganisation of thought, emotion and behaviour is a major feature of both schizophrenia and mania. In mania it is usually transient, whereas in schizophrenia a subtle residual disorganisation is often evident during the stable phases of the illness. In both schizophrenia and mania, symptoms of disorganisation are associated with evidence of impaired attention, such as impaired digit recall in the presence of distraction. Extensive studies of the neuropsychological impairments associated with disorganisation in schizophrenia indicate that the primary problem is a difficulty in the selection of mental activity. The precise nature of this abnormality requires further elucidation, but studies by Cohen *et al* (1999) indicate that the defect may lie in a neural system that maintains task-relevant information over time, in the face of distraction.

Functional imaging studies consistently show abnormal function in the ventral prefrontal cortex, left superior temporal gyrus and adjacent inferior parietal lobule, anterior cingulate and thalamus. Underactivity in the ventral prefrontal cortex and left superior temporal gyrus (or inferior parietal lobule) is seen in studies that would be expected to show the patterns of cerebral activity that predispose to disorganisation, as well as in the studies that examine cerebral activity during the production of disorganised speech. The abnormalities reported in the anterior cingulate and thalamus are more complex. The evidence suggests that the predisposition is associated with overactivity in these areas, while the actual occurrence of disorganisation is associated with relative underactivity. While it is necessary to be cautious, the most plausible interpretation of this complex set of observations is that the primary abnormality in disorganisation is a deficit in ventral prefrontal activity. This appears to lead to compensatory overactivity in the anterior cingulate. When the anterior cingulate fails in this task, disorganised thought and behaviour emerge.

The evidence suggests that several different neurotransmitters are involved in the expression of disorganisation. Agents that promote dopaminergic transmission can exacerbate thought form disorder. At least at high doses, the indirect dopamine agonist amphetamine produces effects on regional cerebral activity that resemble the pattern of cerebral activity associated with disorganisation. Dopamine $D_2$ receptor blockers are effective in treating florid disorganisation during acute psychotic episodes, but are ineffective in alleviating the subtle disorganisation that persists in the stable phase of schizophrenia.

Agents that block glutamatergic NMDA receptors, such as ketamine, can also produce disorganised thought and behaviour. These agents produce cognitive impairments similar to those associated with the disorganisation syndrome and also cause an increase in activity in the frontal cortex that is correlated with the severity of the induced disorganisation. The psychotogenic effects of ketamine are not blocked by $D_2$-blocking drugs such as haloperidol, but are blunted by atypical antipsychotics such as clozapine. Clozapine is often effective in treating chronic disorganisation, which is unresponsive to treatment with typical antipsychotics that block dopamine $D_2$ receptors (Meltzer, 1992). Thus the pharmacological evidence indicates that dopamine overactivity can exacerbate disorganisation, possibly by promoting excessive transmission in the cortico-subcortical loops that regulate the frontal cortex, but it is probable that other mechanisms are involved in chronic disorganisation.

The disorganisation of thought, emotion and behaviour that Bleuler considered central to schizophrenia remains enigmatic, but the evidence that we have considered in this chapter provides some understanding of this disabling group of symptoms. They are associated with malfunction at a distributed set of cortical and subcortical cerebral sites, especially the ventral and medial frontal cortex. The evidence suggests that defective function of the ventral frontal cortex allows the intrusion of contextually inappropriate activity in the ongoing stream of mental processing. Furthermore, a similar group of symptoms occurs in other disorders, including frontal lobe injury and mania. Despite some differences, such as the lesser likelihood of chronic disorganisation in mania, the available evidence indicates that similar mechanisms are likely to be involved in the generation of disorganisation in these different conditions.

# Chapter 8

# Psychomotor poverty and psychomotor excitation

## Introduction

The rate at which the mind generates thoughts, feelings and actions fluctuates according to the demands of current circumstances. In a variety of different neuropsychiatric conditions, the mechanism that regulates these fluctuations is disordered, leading either to psychomotor poverty or to psychomotor excitation. Psychomotor poverty is characterised by poverty of speech, flat affect and decreased volitional activity, while psychomotor excitation is characterised by pressure of speech, excited or irritable affect and motor hyperactivity.

Psychomotor poverty occurs in a wide variety of conditions, including schizophrenia, depression, frontal lobe and subcortical dementias, and frontal lobe injury. It can be relatively persistent, as in the chronic phase of schizophrenia and in degenerative conditions such as frontal lobe dementia, or transient, as in depression and in acute schizophrenic episodes. This chapter will address the question of the extent to which there are common pathological processes underlying the psychomotor poverty that occurs in different conditions. Evidence from functional imaging studies and from studies of cerebral biochemistry indicates that the patterns of cerebral activity associated with acute and chronic psychomotor poverty are similar. It is probable that dopaminergic underactivity is a common feature. However, whereas transient psychomotor poverty appears to reflect transient dopaminergic underactivity, much evidence suggests that persistent psychomotor poverty reflects a similar biochemical imbalance associated with more substantial structural brain damage. None the less, even in conditions such as chronic schizophrenia, persistent psychomotor poverty can be at least partially alleviated by psychological or pharmacological stimulation.

Psychomotor excitation occurs in mania and is also quite common in acute schizophrenia. It can also occur in some cases of brain injury. It is usually transient, perhaps because persistent marked psychomotor excitation would be fatally exhausting unless compensating mechanisms were called into play. Although the evidence regarding pathophysiological mechanisms is far from complete, there is substantial evidence that the cardinal biochemical disturbance associated with psychomotor excitation is dopaminergic hyperactivity.

# Clinical characteristics of psychomotor disorders

## Psychomotor poverty in schizophrenia

"Many schizophrenics in the later stages cease to show any affect for years and even decades at a time. They sit about the institutions to which they are confined with expressionless faces, hunched-up, the image of indifference." (Bleuler, 1911, p. 40)

"The patients appear lazy and negligent because they no longer have the urge to do anything, either of their own initiative or at the bidding of another. They can spend years in bed. In mild cases, wishes and desires still exist, they will nevertheless do nothing towards the realization of these wishes." (Bleuler, 1911, p. 70)

In the final two decades of the twentieth century, there was resurgence of interest in the deficits that Bleuler had described so graphically much earlier in the century. Crow (1980) invoked the term 'negative symptoms' to describe these deficits. Negative symptoms reflect the absence or reduction of mental activity that is normally present in healthy individuals. In contrast, 'positive symptoms' are phenomena such as delusions and hallucinations that reflect the presence of mental activity that is not normally present in healthy individuals. However, various studies aiming to determine the nature of negative symptoms, or their responsiveness to treatment, have employed different lists of symptoms. The concept of the psychomotor poverty syndrome developed out of my own attempts to identify the core negative symptoms of schizophrenia.

In the 1970s, using the recently introduced technique of X-ray computed tomography, Crow and his colleagues found that a substantial number of chronic schizophrenic patients had pronounced enlargement of the cerebral ventricles (Johnstone *et al*, 1976). Shortly after, they demonstrated that treatment with a dopamine-blocking antipsychotic drug, flupenthixol, alleviated positive symptoms, but not negative symptoms (Johnstone *et al*, 1978a). These observations led Crow (1980) to formulate the seminal type 1/type 2 classification of schizophrenia. He proposed that there are two pathological processes in schizophrenia: the type 1 process entails biochemical imbalance, most likely dopaminergic overactivity, expressed as positive symptoms that are usually transient; the type 2 process involves structural damage to the brain, resulting in ventricular enlargement, and is expressed as negative symptoms, which tend to be persistent.

Crow regarded poverty of speech and flat affect as the principal negative symptoms. Subsequently he added lack of volition to this cluster of symptoms (Crow, 1985). He regarded delusions, hallucinations and thought form disorder as positive symptoms. Although Crow's choice of the terms type 1 and type 2 schizophrenia to describe the two proposed pathological processes was widely misinterpreted as a classification of schizophrenia into two types of illness, in fact he considered that type 1 and type 2 schizophrenia were two dimensions of a single illness.

Shortly after Crow had presented the type 1/type 2 formulation, Andreasen (1982) developed a scale – the SANS – for assessing negative symptoms that broadened the concept substantially. The SANS included five sub-scales: poverty of speech; flat affect; avolition; anhedonia/asociality; and attentional impairment. The SANS flat affect sub-scale included both flat and inappropriate affect. While the essential concept of avolition was a diminution of drive, the items by which avolition was assessed reflected performance in everyday life. For example, the first item in the avolition sub-scale is decreased performance at work or school. Similarly, the items in the anhedonia/asociality sub-scale largely reflect observable achievement of social relationships. The attentional impairment sub-scale included items covering attention to tasks in daily life and performance on a formal test of attention (serial subtraction of sevens from 100; or spelling 'world' backwards).

Andreasen & Olsen (1982) proposed that the positive/negative distinction might provide a basis for distinguishing two types of schizophrenia: positive schizophrenia, characterised by a predominance of positive symptoms; and negative schizophrenia, characterised by a predominance of negative symptoms. They demonstrated that groups of patients subdivided according to these criteria differed on a number of clinically relevant variables, with the negative schizophrenic patients exhibiting greater ventricular enlargement and greater cognitive impairment. However, they found that approximately one-third of their sample of patients could not be classified satisfactorily into either group, many on account of having a mixture of positive and negative symptoms.

The concepts of type 1/type 2 schizophrenia proposed by Crow and positive/negative schizophrenia proposed by Andreasen & Olsen raised several questions:

(1)   While negative symptoms are usually persistent and positive symptoms usually transient, that is not always the case. Is it symptom type or symptom chronicity that reflects the two pathological processes postulated by Crow?

(2)   Does the positive/negative symptom dichotomy reflect two types of illness or two dimensions within one illness?

(3)   Does the broad range of negative symptoms embraced by Andreasen's SANS reflect a single underlying pathological process? In particular, should inappropriate affect and attentional impairment be included among the negative symptoms? Do the items reflecting performance in everyday life that are included in the avolition and anhedonia/asociality sub-scales reflect the same underlying pathological process as that accounting for the abnormalities of speech, affect and motor behaviour that are included in the affective flattening and poverty of speech subscales?

As a first step in addressing these issues, I examined the relationships between symptoms in a cohort of chronic schizophrenic patients selected on the basis of persistent, stable symptoms. If the distinction between the biochemical imbalance and structural brain damage postulated by Crow led primarily to a difference in symptom chronicity rather than symptom type, the symptoms would not be expected to segregate into separate positive and negative groups. Because the items of Andreasen's SANS, together with her SAPS, provided a good coverage of the phenomena of schizophrenia, I elected to use these scales. To avoid the assumptions implied by the way in which Andreasen had combined these items into sub-scales, I analysed the relationships between items rather than sub-scales. Furthermore, I set aside the items that reflect performance in everyday life from the initial analysis.

The study provided clear answers to all of the questions posed (Liddle, 1984, 1987a). The symptoms in this cohort of patients with persistent symptoms did segregate into discrete groups, supporting the hypothesis that there are several separate pathological processes, each of which is expressed as different types of symptoms. However, instead of merely segregating into positive and negative groups, the pattern of correlations between symptoms clearly indicated that the symptoms segregated into three groups, as shown in Table 8.1. The first group, of six items, which between them represent poverty of speech, flattening of affect and decreased spontaneous activity, reflects a diminution of psychological and motor activity. This group of symptoms corresponds very closely to the concept of negative symptoms proposed by Crow (1980, 1985). Because the meaning of the term 'negative symptoms' had been broadened by Andreasen, I used the descriptive title 'psychomotor poverty syndrome' to designate this group of

**Table 8.1** Factor analysis of the characteristic symptoms of schizophrenia in a sample of 40 patients with persistent, stable symptoms

| Symptoms | Factor 1 | Factor 2 | Factor 3 |
|---|---|---|---|
| *Psychomotor poverty (high loading on factor 1)* | | | |
| Poverty of speech | **0.80** | −0.01 | −0.03 |
| Decreased spontaneous movement | **0.95** | −0.04 | −0.03 |
| Unchanging facial expression[1] | **0.85** | −0.01 | 0.05 |
| Paucity of expressive gestures[1] | **0.97** | 0.02 | −0.04 |
| Affective non-responsivity[1] | **0.82** | 0.02 | −0.00 |
| Lack of vocal inflection[1] | **0.90** | −0.20 | −0.05 |
| | | | |
| *Disorganisation (high loading on factor 2)* | | | |
| Inappropriate affect | 0.19 | **0.84** | 0.09 |
| Poverty of content of speech | −0.08 | **0.57** | 0.01 |
| Tangentiality[2] | −0.05 | **0.94** | 0.03 |
| Derailment[2] | −0.05 | **0.94** | 0.04 |
| Pressure of speech | −0.10 | **0.61** | 0.08 |
| Distractibility | −0.00 | **0.81** | 0.01 |
| | | | |
| *Reality distortion[3] (high loading on factor 3)* | | | |
| Voices speak to the patient | 0.04 | −0.07 | **0.67** |
| Delusions of persecution | −0.19 | 0.06 | **0.51** |
| Delusions of reference | 0.13 | 0.04 | **0.84** |

Factors were extracted by the method of principal factors and subjected to oblique rotation. The correlations between the factors were less than 0.25. Loadings greater than 0.5 are shown in bold.
[1] Aspects of flat affect.
[2] Thought form disorders.
[3] Schneiderian first-rank syndromes were rare and were excluded from this analysis.
(Reproduced from Liddle, 1987a, with permission.)

symptoms. The second and third groups of symptoms, which I designated the 'disorganisation syndrome' and 'reality distortion syndrome' are described in greater detail in Chapters 7 and 6, respectively.

It was clear that the three groups of persistent schizophrenic syndromes did not reflect three separate types of illness, because many patients exhibited evidence of more than one of the syndromes, and a substantial minority exhibited prominent features of all three (Liddle, 1987a).

Inappropriate affect loaded on the disorganisation factor, which indicates that it should not be regarded as a psychomotor poverty symptom. Subsequent studies (e.g. Peralta *et al*, 1992b) have confirmed that inappropriate affect does not belong to the negative or psychomotor poverty dimension. In the revised version of the SANS, encompassed in the Comprehensive Assessment of Symptoms and History (Andreasen, 1986), inappropriate affect is no longer included as a negative symptom.

The situation with regard to poverty of content of speech remains ambiguous. While several of the studies that have examined SANS and SAPS items have confirmed the finding that poverty of content of speech belongs to the disorganisation syndrome rather than to the psychomotor poverty syndrome, one study (Peralta *et al*, 1992b) did find that poverty of content loaded more heavily on the negative (psychomotor poverty) factor than the disorganisation factor. On balance, the evidence indicates that poverty of content as defined in the SANS can reflect either disorganisation or psychomotor poverty.

Finally, my study of the relationships between persistent symptoms revealed that, in the chronic phase of the illness, both the psychomotor poverty and the disorganisation syndromes are correlated with poor occupational and social function, as assessed by the items in the avolition and anhedonia/asociality subscales of the SANS (Liddle, 1987a). In that cohort of patients, the items 'poor grooming and hygiene', 'impersistence at work', 'inability for intimacy' and 'social inattentiveness' were more strongly correlated with severity of disorganisation than with severity of psychomotor poverty. On the other hand, 'relationships with friends and peers' and 'physical anergia' were more strongly correlated with psychomotor poverty.

In several subsequent studies, my colleagues and I have replicated the finding that poverty of speech, flat affect and decreased spontaneous movement constitute a cluster of symptoms that tend to occur together within schizophrenia (Liddle & Barnes, 1990; Liddle *et al*, 1992). Furthermore, studies by other investigators of samples of schizophrenic patients who are more heterogeneous in chronicity using either SANS/SAPS items (Malla *et al*, 1993) or a variety of different symptom rating scales (Kay & Sevy, 1990; Frith, 1992; Thompson & Meltzer, 1993; Bell *et al*, 1994) have identified a negative factor composed principally of items that reflect flattened affect, poverty of speech and decreased voluntary motor activity.

On the other hand, studies using SANS and SAPS sub-scale scores have consistently identified a somewhat broader negative syndrome, including affective flattening; alogia (a sub-scale whose cardinal item is poverty of speech); avolition; and anhedonia/asociality (Kulhara *et al*, 1986; Arndt *et al*, 1991; Peralta *et al*, 1992b). Attentional impairment has been less consistently associated with the negative syndrome (see Peralta *et al*, 1992b). Should avolition and anhedonia/ asociality be regarded as components of psychomotor poverty? My finding that persistent disorganisation is associated with aspects of poor occupational and social function that are assessed in the avolition and anhedonia/asociality sub- scale of the SANS indicates that the scores on these scales embrace a range of phenomena extending beyond psychomotor poverty symptoms, at least in patients with persistent symptoms. The finding that persistent disorganisation is associated with poor functional outcome was confirmed by Norman *et al* (1999). However, these findings do not preclude the possibility that avolition and anhedonia/asociality, evaluated directly rather than via assessment of function, are core features of psychomotor poverty.

Studies that have employed different symptom rating scales support the hypothesis that avolition and anhedonia/asociality are core negative symptoms. In a study that examined the relationships between items from several different symptom scales designed to assess negative symptoms, my colleagues and I (Kibel *et al*, 1993) found that a cluster of five types of phenomena characterised the negative syndrome in schizophrenia:

(1)  poverty of thought and speech;
(2)  blunted affect;
(3)  decreased motor activity;
(4)  apathy and avolition;
(5)  diminished interpersonal interaction.

Overall, the evidence indicates that avolition and anhedonia/asociality are related to the core negative features that comprise the psychomotor poverty syndrome. However, there is no established rating scale that assesses diminished volition in a reliable way. In addition, social interaction is a complex phenomenon that is prone to disruption by causes other than psychomotor poverty. Hence, for the purposes of identifying the brain abnormalities associated with psychomotor poverty, we shall place the greatest reliance on data obtained in studies that examine the correlates of affective flattening, poverty of speech and decreased spontaneous movement.

### The prevalence of psychomotor poverty in schizophrenia

Substantial psychomotor poverty occurs in approximately 50% of patients with schizophrenia. Flattened affect is the most prevalent feature. In an epidemio- logical survey of all patients discharged from hospital with a diagnosis of schizophrenia in the period 1975–85 in the London borough of Harrow, Johnstone *et al* (1991) found that the prevalence of flattened affect was 51.5%, psychomotor retardation 28.6% and poverty of speech 21.4%.

### The reversibility of psychomotor poverty in schizophrenia

One of the cardinal observations that led Crow to propose that negative symptoms in schizophrenia arise from structural brain damage was the observation that core negative symptoms were unresponsive to treatment. More recently, the conclusion that core negative symptoms are immutable has been questioned, as many studies have reported that negative symptoms are at least partially responsive to antipsychotic treatment, especially to the atypical antipsychotics, such as risperidone and olanzapine. For example, Marder & Meibach (1994) found that risperidone at a dose of 6 mg per day produced a 20% reduction in severity of negative symptoms over six weeks, while Tollefson *et al* (1997) found that olanzapine produced a reduction of 19% over six weeks. In both studies, the antipsychotic produced a significantly greater reduction in negative symptoms than the typical antipsychotic haloperidol. These findings not only have substantial implications for clinical practice but also potentially important implications for our understanding of the nature of the pathological process responsible for negative symptoms. They therefore warrant close scrutiny.

There are several potentially confounding issues. The reduction in negative symptoms produced by the novel antipsychotics could reflect resolution of an akinetic syndrome (an expression of one of the components of parkinsonism) produced by prior treatment (Van Putten *et al*, 1990). Alternatively, it might reflect a change in the severity of transient psychomotor poverty associated with depression. Barnes *et al* (1989) have demonstrated that episodic depression in schizophrenia is associated with both poverty of speech and decreased spontaneous movement.

The investigators responsible for the risperidone and olanzapine trials addressed these issues by the post-hoc application of path analysis. Path analysis is a statistical procedure that employs the observed correlations between variables to take account of the extent to which a change in an outcome variable, such as change in negative symptom severity, might be accounted for by changes in other variables, such as depression or parkinsonism. Path analysis applied to the data from the risperidone study (Moller *et al*, 1995) and from the olanzapine study (Tollefson & Sanger, 1997) indicated that the observed therapeutic effect of neither medication on negative symptoms could be accounted for by changes in either parkinsonism or depression.

An additional issue that is perhaps even more important, regarding the implications of the findings for the reversibility of core negative symptoms, is the fact that the score for negative symptoms employed in most treatment trials is potentially contaminated by disorganisation phenomena. For example, the trial by Marder & Meibach (1994) employed the Positive and Negative Syndrome Scale (PANSS). The PANSS item for flat affect includes inappropriate affect and the PANSS score for disturbed volition includes both diminished and disorganised voluntary activity. It is virtually impossible to determine retrospectively whether or not the change associated with treatment was due to a change in psychomotor poverty or disorganisation.

In this regard, it is informative to examine the study by Dollfus & Petit (1995) of the course of symptoms during resolution of the acute phase of schizophrenia. In that study, in which the patients were treated mainly with typical antipsychotics, the SANS total score decreased by 24%. While SANS total score and SANS sub-scale scores, like the PANSS items, confound features of psychomotor poverty with features of disorganisation, SANS item scores are not confounded in this way. Inspection of the changes in SANS item scores reported by Dollfus & Petit reveal that the most significant changes were in those SANS items that are likely to be influenced by changes in severity of the disorganisation syndrome. For example, there were highly significant changes in the items measuring 'inappropriate affect', 'poverty of content of speech', 'poor grooming and hygiene', 'decreased ability for intimacy' and 'social inattentiveness', all of which have been shown to be correlated with severity of the disorganisation syndrome (Liddle, 1987a). Changes in the core negative symptoms that are the cardinal features of the psychomotor poverty syndrome were less significant. There was no change at all in scores for poverty of speech or decreased spontaneous movement, while affective non-responsivity decreased by 21% (a change significant at the level $P < 0.05$, provided that no correction is made to allow for the fact that multiple comparisons were performed).

Thus the findings by Dollfus & Petit are indeed in close agreement with the original observation by Johnstone et al (1978a) that flupenthixol does not produce substantial reduction in the core negative symptoms. Overall, the question of whether or not treatment with antipsychotics, typical or atypical, produces a substantial reduction in these symptoms remains inadequately answered.

None the less, there is indirect evidence suggesting that the core negative symptoms of schizophrenia are not immutable. First, in the famous Three Hospital study, which compared three large asylums that for administrative reasons had adopted differing policies with regard to the rehabilitation of patients, Wing & Brown (1970) observed that the severity of a cluster of features that they termed 'clinical poverty', and which closely resembled the core negative symptoms that make up the psychomotor poverty syndrome, was associated with poverty of environmental stimulation. Furthermore, clinical poverty decreased when environmental stimulation increased.

Nearly a century ago, Bleuler noted that "even the most demented schizophrenic patient can under proper conditions demonstrate productions of a highly integrated type" (Bleuler, 1911, p. 72). The challenge of creating the proper conditions to promote the reversal of the core deficits of the illness remains. The revolution in the social management of schizophrenia that has occurred since the days of asylum care has done much to reduce the poverty of environmental stimulation that accentuates psychomotor poverty. Despite the caution warranted in evaluating the claim that the atypical antipsychotics also help relieve negative symptoms, there is emerging evidence that pharmacological approaches might also play a role in overcoming these core deficits. We shall return to a more detailed discussion of these pharmacological strategies below.

## Psychomotor poverty following frontal lobe damage

In his comprehensive studies of the consequences of frontal lobe damage, Kleist (1934) identified two principal types of clinical outcome. He observed that damage to the ventral frontal cortex led to a pattern of poorly regulated behaviour, resembling the disorganisation syndrome, while damage to the upper convexity resulted in lack of psychic and motor initiative. Patients with such lesions exhibited impoverished and stereotyped patterns of thinking.

Blumer & Benson (1975) subsequently introduced the term 'pseudo-depression' to describe this lack of psychic and motor initiative in patients with frontal lobe lesions. According to Blumer & Benson, patients suffering from this syndrome appear to have lost all initiative. In test situations, where the initiative is provided by the examiner, they can achieve normal scores, but they are unable to function independently in everyday life. They are slow, indifferent and apathetic. Blumer & Benson describe how one of their patients was able to perform sexual intercourse only as long as his wife told him, step by step, what he had to do. They describe another patient who required amputation of the left frontal pole after sustaining a compound depressed fracture of the frontal bone in a road traffic accident. After the surgery, he recovered motor function, had normal sensation and had an IQ of 118. However, in contrast to his previous lively, energetic, sociable character, he became unable to care for himself because of apathy and lack of concern. He would speak when spoken to but did not make spontaneous conversation. He made no friends.

Blumer & Benson emphasise that the feature that distinguishes pseudo-depression from retarded depression is the fact that the apathy in pseudo-depression reflects empty indifference rather than sadness. The pseudo-depressed syndrome described by Blumer & Benson in patients with lesions of the frontal convexity is remarkably similar to the psychomotor poverty syndrome of schizophrenia.

## Psychomotor disorders in frontal lobe dementia

In a classic paper describing the features of frontal lobe dementia, Neary *et al* (1988) identify two broad types of behavioural pattern. One is characterised by slowness, apathy, inertia and lack of spontaneity. Speech tends to be economical in output, concrete and stereotypic. The other pattern is characterised by restlessness, overactivity, distractibility and disinhibition. In patients exhibiting this picture, speech can be pressured, off the point and involve play on words. These two patterns sometimes coexist, although the majority of the individual cases described by Neary *et al* fall predominantly into one or other category.

For example, the first case they presented was a 55-year-old woman with mental slowing, apathy and neglect of personal hygiene, in whom occasional incontinence of urine led to no distress. She did not volunteer conversation and her answers to questions were economical and unelaborated. Her full-scale IQ was 81. On the other hand, their second case was a 61-year-old woman who spent her days wandering aimlessly. She had outbursts of rage and acted impulsively. She exhibited pressure of speech that was frequently off the point and contained stereotyped phrases and plays on words. Her full-scale IQ was 75. The first case presents a picture that is dominated by the clinical features of the psychomotor poverty syndrome. The second case shows features of psychomotor excitation, such as emotional lability, pressure of speech and motor restlessness, but also prominent features of the disorganisation syndrome described in Chapter 7.

## Psychomotor disorders in basal ganglion degeneration

There is a group of degenerative disorders in which the degeneration has its major impact on the basal ganglia. Patients with these disorders present primarily with motor symptoms, but also have a high prevalence of psychomotor and mood symptoms. The disorders include Parkinson's disease, multiple system atrophy (MSA), progressive supranuclear palsy (PSP), corticobasal degeneration (CBD) and Huntington's disease. Symptoms such as apathy, mental slowing (brady-phrenia) and depression can occur in all of these disorders; and excitation or euphoria in some of them. However, the prevalence of these psychomotor and mood symptoms differs substantially between the different disorders. Thus a comparison of these disorders has the potential to help delineate the differing neuropathological processes that are responsible for these symptoms.

### Parkinson's disease

The cardinal pathological process in Parkinson's disease is degeneration of the dopaminergic projections from the substantia nigra to the basal ganglia. The characteristic symptoms are rigidity, akinesia and tremor, but mental symptoms are also common. Therefore, the question of whether or not the akinesia of Parkinson's disease is accompanied by flattened affect and poverty of speech is an important one in our quest to understand the psychomotor poverty syndrome. An epidemiological study of psychiatric symptoms in Parkinson's disease in Norway found at least one psychiatric symptom in 61% (Aarsland et al, 1999). The commonest emotional symptom was depression, which occurred in 38% of cases. Anxiety and apathy were also relatively common. Thus this study suggests that depression is more prominent than blunted affect in Parkinson's disease, although it is possible that the reported apathy reflects blunting of affect.

Starkstein et al (1992a) examined a consecutive series of 50 patients for the presence of apathy, depression, anxiety and neuropsychological deficits. Of these patients, 12% showed apathy as their primary mental symptom, and 30% were both apathetic and depressed. Patients with apathy (with or without depression) showed significantly more deficits in both tasks of verbal memory and time-dependent tasks. The impairments in time-dependent tasks imply bradyphrenia. These findings demonstrate that a form of psychomotor poverty, manifest as apathy, bradyphrenia and other cognitive impairments, does occur in Parkinson's disease.

### Multiple system atrophy

In MSA there is substantial neuronal loss in the caudate and ventral striatum. It produces motor symptoms, including akinesia, similar to those seen in Parkinson's disease. However, MSA differs markedly from Parkinson's disease in the prevalence of depression and blunted affect. For example, Fetoni et al (1999) found that patients with Parkinson's disease were more depressed and anxious than patients with MSA, who, by contrast, showed blunted affect. After treatment with the dopamine precursor L-dopa, the depression and anxiety of patients with

Parkinson's disease improved significantly, whereas the affective blunting of patients with MSA did not change. Thus, in contrast to patients with Parkinson's disease, patients with MSA commonly exhibit a psychomotor poverty syndrome resembling that seen in schizophrenia.

## Progressive supranuclear palsy

Progressive supranuclear palsy is a rapidly progressive recessive genetic condition dominated by motor symptoms similar to those seen in Parkinson's disease. In particular, slowness is a major feature. In a survey of neuropsychiatric aspects of the disorder, Litvan *et al* (1996) found that PSP patients exhibited apathy (91%), disinhibition (36%), dysphoria (18%) and anxiety (18%), but rarely irritability or agitation. Thus, PSP resembles MSA rather than Parkinson's disease, insofar as apathy is more prevalent than depression.

## Corticobasal degeneration

Corticobasal degeneration is a rapidly progressive degenerative disorder whose clinical hallmarks are parkinsonism unresponsive to L-dopa and limb ideomotor apraxia. Its microscopic pathology is very similar to that of PSP. In both disorders, filamentous tau protein inclusions are found in neurons and glia. Both PSP and CBD have similar biochemical alterations in the tau protein, with the abnormal tau protein containing predominantly four-repeat tau. However, in PSP, the degeneration is mainly in the basal ganglia, whereas in CBD degeneration occurs in the cortex and basal ganglia.

In a study comparing the neuropsychiatric symptoms of CBD with those of PSP, Litvan *et al* (1998a) reported that patients with CBD exhibited depression (73%), apathy (40%), irritability (20%) and agitation (20%). CBD patients were more likely than patients with PSP to exhibit depression and irritability. Conversely, patients with PSP exhibited significantly more apathy than patients with CBD. Thus, as in Parkinson's disease, depression predominates over classic psychomotor poverty in CBD.

## Huntington's disease

In Huntington's disease, which is associated predominantly with hyperkinetic motor symptoms, psychiatric symptoms are often prominent in the early stages. In the later stages, dementia supervenes. It is a dominant genetic condition, arising from multiple repetitions of the trinucleotide sequence CAG on chromosome 4. It leads to severe degeneration of the basal ganglia, although the molecular mechanism of the disease is unknown. The predominance of hyperkinetic motor disorders is thought to be due to a preferential failure of the indirect cortico-striato-thalamo-cortical feedback loop (see Chapter 4), in contrast to the situation in predominantly hypokinetic conditions such as PSP, in which the principal failure is more likely to be in the direct feedback pathway.

In a comparison of the neuropsychiatric symptoms of Huntington's disease with those of PSP, Litvan *et al* (1998b) reported that patients with Huntington's disease exhibited significantly more agitation (45%), irritability (38%) and anxiety (34%), whereas patients with PSP exhibited more apathy (82%). Euphoria was present only in patients with Huntington's disease. While Litvan *et al* found that apathy and depression were relatively rare in Huntington's disease, both symptoms none the less do occur.

### Summary of neuropsychiatric symptoms in diseases of the basal ganglia

This brief review of the various neuropsychiatric symptoms occurring in degenerative diseases of the basal ganglia demonstrates that in some disorders, such as Parkinson's disease and CBD, depression is the predominant mental symptom, although apathy can be associated with the depression and, in a minority of cases, apathy is the primary symptom. In other conditions, such as MSA and PSP, blunted affect and apathy are more prevalent than depression. In yet other conditions, such as Huntington's disease, agitation and irritability are common, and even euphoria can occur, but apathy is relatively rare.

These observations strongly suggest that the mechanism of psychomotor poverty (including apathy) is distinct from that of depression. This conclusion is confirmed by the results of a study by Levy *et al* (1998), in which they compared neuropsychiatric symptoms in 30 patients with Alzheimer's disease, 28 with frontotemporal dementia, 40 with Parkinson's disease, 34 with Huntington's disease and 22 with PSP. Apathy did not correlate with depression in the combined sample. Apathy correlated with lower cognitive function as measured by the Mini-Mental State Examination ($r = -0.40$, $P < 0.0001$), but depression did not show such a correlation.

While apathy is more strongly associated with cognitive malfunction than is depression, the contrast between CBD, which is associated with predominant depression, and PSP, which is associated with blunted affect or apathy, indicates that it is not merely a propensity to more extensive neuronal degeneration that leads to more marked blunting or apathy. The microscopic pathology is similar in CBD and PSP, but it tends to be more widely distributed in CBD. It is more likely that the difference is due to differences in the neural pathways that are most affected. It is possible that the differences arise from differential involvement of the various feedback loops serving different regions of the frontal cortex. The association of apathy with greater cognitive impairment suggests a greater involvement of the cortico-subcortical loop providing feedback to the dorsolateral prefrontal cortex, since malfunction of the dorsolateral aspect of the frontal cortex is more likely to produce extensive cognitive impairment than damage to any other part of the prefrontal cortex. In Huntington's disease, the greater propensity to hyperactivity and irritability might reflect greater involvement of indirect rather than direct pathways.

## Subcortical dementia

The evidence we have examined regarding the mental symptoms associated with basal ganglion degeneration indicates that apathy should be distinguished from depression and, furthermore, that apathy is associated with evidence of mental slowing and other cognitive impairments. This constellation of clinical features is sometimes designated subcortical dementia. In a review of the concept of subcortical dementia, Cummings & Benson (1984) described it as a cluster of clinical features including slowness of mental processing, forgetfulness, lack of ability to manipulate acquired knowledge, apathy and depression, which occurs in a variety of conditions that involve degeneration of subcortical structures such as the basal ganglia, thalamus and related brain-stem nuclei.

While Cummings & Benson included depression among the features, the evidence considered above, especially the findings of the study by Levy et al (1998), clearly demonstrates that depression is not a central component, although it can coexist with subcortical dementia. The affective feature most characteristic of subcortical dementia is emotional indifference. This is illustrated by a report by Laplane et al (1984). They described three patients who exhibited psychic akinesia after toxic encephalopathy that produced bilateral lesions of the basal ganglia. Despite only mild motor disorders, they exhibited marked underactivity, impoverished imagination, poverty of speech and a tendency to indifference towards emotional issues. Laplane et al noted that the akinesia was reversible when the patients were stimulated, which indicates that the problem was a loss of ability to take the initiative. The clinical syndrome of subcortical dementia is very similar to the psychomotor poverty syndrome that occurs in schizophrenia.

## Psychomotor disorders in major depression

Over a century ago, when the natural history of depression was less modified by pharmacological treatment than it is nowadays, psychomotor symptoms played an important part in descriptions of the illness. For example, in the first edition of his famous textbook of psychiatry, Kraepelin (1883) defined three types of melancholia: melancholia simplex, which was depression without marked psychomotor features; melancholia activa, which included prominent anxiety and agitation; and melancholia attonica, characterised by slowness, poverty of speech and emotional withdrawal. In its severe form, melancholia attonica was depressive stupor. In a later textbook, he provided the following description of depressive stupor: "The patients lie mute in bed, give no answer of any sort, at most withdraw themselves timidly from approaches.... They sit helpless before their food.... Now and then periods of excitement may be interpolated" (Kraepelin, 1921, p. 80).

A noteworthy feature of this description is the observation that the motility disorder in depression exhibits bipolarity, with the possibility of an abrupt switch into a state of excitement. This can occur without an associated switch from depressed to euphoric mood. In other words, there is a bipolarity of motility disturbances in depression that is distinct from the bipolarity of mood that characterises bipolar mood disorder.

The clinical relevance of recognising that the mechanism of psychomotor slowing is distinct from the mechanism of depression is confirmed by the fact that the presence of psychomotor slowing predicts aspects of the response to

**133**

treatment. In two of the major randomised controlled trials of electroconvulsive therapy, the Northwick Park trial and the Leicester trial, the presence of psychomotor retardation was a major determinant of response to treatment (Buchan et al, 1992).

## Psychomotor excitation in mania

Although symptoms of elation, disorganisation and reality distortion are all common in manic episodes, the predominant symptoms of mania are exaggerated mood, motor hyperactivity and pressure of speech. These psychomotor symptoms are present throughout the episode, but are especially predominant in the early stage. In their classic description of the stages of mania, Carlson & Goodwin (1973) list the following symptoms as characteristic of the first stage:

(1)  Mood: labile affect, euphoria or irritability.
(2)  Thought: racing thoughts, grandiosity and expansivity.
(3)  Behaviour: increased initiation and rate of speech, increased psychomotor activity, increased spending and telephone use.

## Catatonia

Kahlbaum (1874) introduced the term 'catatonia' to describe a brain disease with a cyclic course, characterised by episodes of melancholy, mania, stupor, confusion and eventually dementia. He also recognised that it did not always end in dementia. Because of the tendency towards dementia, Kraepelin (1919) included catatonia within schizophrenia. In current practice (American Psychiatric Association, 1994), catatonia is regarded a set of motor symptoms that can occur in schizophrenia or affective illness, or that can arise as a result of any one of many different overt brain disorders. Catatonic symptoms fall into three groups: diminished voluntary motor activity, excessive voluntary motor activity, and peculiar movements.

Isolated catatonic symptoms are quite common. Late in the nineteenth century, Maudsley (1873) found that motor symptoms were present in nearly all cases of severe mental illness. A century later, neurological examination of 100 patients hospitalised with persistent mental illness (including 86 with schizophrenia) revealed abnormalities of purposive movement in 97% (Rogers, 1985). Further-more, such abnormalities had been recorded in the case notes before the start of antipsychotic treatment in 87% of cases. Sudden transient changes in the level of psychomotor activity were common. In a recent study, approximately 10% of hospital admissions for psychosis satisfied Kalhbaum's classical description of catatonia (Peralta et al, 1997b). Furthermore, the majority of these cases were not typical of either schizophrenia or bipolar affective disorder, which implies that separate 'motility psychoses' may exist. Overall, there is strong evidence that bipolar disturbances of voluntary motor function are a relatively common feature of psychotic illness.

## Summary of the clinical evidence

A specific triad of symptoms – flat affect, poverty of speech and decreased spontaneous movement – occurs in a range of illnesses, including schizophrenia, basal ganglia degeneration, frontal lobe injury, frontal lobe dementia and depression. In schizophrenia, this psychomotor poverty syndrome tends to be persistent, whereas in depression it is transient. Furthermore, there is evidence indicating that psychomotor poverty can be a component of a bipolar syndrome, with a cluster of symptoms characterised by agitation and motor hyperactivity at the opposite pole. In particular, catatonia, a condition that can occur in affective illness, schizophrenia or as a consequence of a general medical condition, is characteristically a bipolar psychomotor disorder.

# Neuropsychological correlates
# of psychomotor poverty

Psychomotor poverty has been reported to be associated with impairment in a wide variety of tasks, including tests of memory, abstraction and concentration. However, the most frequently replicated finding is an association with impaired performance in tasks that entail the initiation of activity or the formation of a plan for action. For example, psychomotor poverty in schizophrenia is associated with a decreased rate of production of words in verbal fluency tasks, which demand the production of words within a given category or beginning with a particular letter (Liddle & Morris, 1991; Frith et al, 1991c; Allen et al, 1993; Norman et al, 1997). It is also associated with slower response in a two-choice guessing task, in which the choice of response is determined only by the patient (Baxter & Liddle, 1998) and in both simple reaction time and choice reaction time (Ngan & Liddle, 2000).

It is of interest to note that the association between psychomotor poverty and slow initiation of responses is stronger in patients with persistent illness than in patients with remitting illness, even after matching for current severity of symptoms (Baxter & Liddle, 1998; Ngan & Liddle, 2000). One interpretation is that the level of cognitive impairment is associated with an underlying trait that determines the likelihood of persistent psychomotor poverty symptoms.

Fewer studies have attempted to identify the cognitive impairments specifically correlated with psychomotor poverty in disorders other than schizophrenia. There have been attempts to identify the cognitive impairments that distinguish subcortical dementia associated with degeneration of the basal ganglia from other dementias. As discussed above, subcortical dementia is very similar to psychomotor poverty. Unfortunately, the research strategy in these studies usually entails comparison of different diagnostic groups rather than groups that differ in a specific symptom profile. None the less, a review of such studies led Cummings & Benson (1984) to identify poor problem solving due to slowness and impaired planning as the cognitive hallmark of subcortical dementia. They also concluded that subcortical dementia is associated with difficulty retrieving learned material (forgetfulness) whereas cortical dementia is associated with difficulty learning new material (amnesia). Overall, there is a striking similarity between the cognitive profile characteristic of subcortical dementia and that associated with psychomotor poverty in schizophrenia.

# Regional cerebral activity associated with psychomotor poverty

In a study of the patterns of rCBF associated with psychomotor poverty in patients with persistent schizophrenia, Liddle *et al* (1992) found a negative correlation between severity of psychomotor poverty and rCBF in the frontal cortex bilaterally and in the left inferior parietal lobule. The frontal underactivity was more extensive in the left hemisphere and extended from the dorsolateral cortex via the frontal pole to the medial frontal cortex. There was also a positive correlation between psychomotor poverty and rCBF in the basal ganglia bilaterally. Furthermore, an examination of the patterns of underactivity associated with specific psychomotor poverty symptoms revealed that poverty of speech was associated with left lateral frontal underactivity, while decreased spontaneous movement was associated with medial frontal underactivity (unpublished data).

Ebmeier *et al* (1993) subsequently confirmed the association between psychomotor poverty and decreased rCBF in the left frontal cortex in a sample of schizophrenic patients that included predominantly acute cases. Wolkin *et al* (1992) found that negative symptoms, assessed in a manner that placed the main emphasis on blunted affect, was associated with decreased glucose metabolism in the right frontal cortex. Yuasa *et al* (1995) confirmed that psychomotor poverty is associated with decreased frontal rCBF and with increased rCBF in the basal ganglia and the thalamus.

Several studies have found that more broadly defined negative symptoms of schizophrenia are associated with decreased activation of the frontal cortex during tasks that normally engage that area. For example, Andreasen *et al* (1992) found that, in schizophrenic patients, severity of negative symptoms was associated with reduced activation of the medial frontal cortex during the Tower of London task, which is a test of planning ability.

The available evidence indicates that psychomotor poverty in conditions other than schizophrenia is associated with a similar pattern of cortical underactivity. For example, Dolan *et al* (1993) demonstrated that poverty of speech is associated with reduced rCBF at sites in the left lateral frontal cortex and the inferior parietal lobule that are virtually identical in major depression and in schizophrenia. Craig *et al* (1996) found that apathy in Alzheimer's disease is associated with reduced rCBF in the frontal and temporal lobes.

Overall, the evidence indicates that, in a variety of disorders, psychomotor poverty symptoms are associated with decreased rCBF in the frontal and parietal cortex. There is some evidence suggesting that different frontal regions are more strongly associated with specific aspects of psychomotor poverty. Poverty of speech is specifically associated with left lateral prefrontal underactivity, motor underactivity more with medial frontal underactivity, and flat affect possibly more with right frontal underactivity.

# Brain structure and psychomotor poverty

According to Crow's type 1/type 2 hypothesis, the core negative symptoms of schizophrenia, which correspond to the symptoms of psychomotor poverty, arise from structural brain abnormality, such as might be reflected in ventricular enlargement (Crow, 1980). In a review of studies using X-ray computed tomography, Lewis (1990) found that five of the 18 studies addressing the issue reported a significant association between negative symptom severity and ventricular enlargement. This indicates that there is probably a real relationship, but that the size of the effect is small and prone to be obscured by noise. Unfortunately, most of the studies used broad definitions of negative symptoms, and made no attempt to distinguish persistent negative symptoms from transient ones.

The only study that has explicitly focused on brain structure associated with persistent psychomotor poverty symptoms is a small one by Chua *et al* (1997) that employed a novel, voxel-based technique for assessing brain structure from $T_1$-weighted MRI images. They employed a voxel-based technique to avoid the need to specify regions of interest in advance, because the specification of regions in the cerebral cortex is largely arbitrary, owing to the paucity of consistent structural landmarks. They found that the severity of psychomotor poverty in a group of chronic patients with persistent symptoms was associated with reduced grey matter in an extensive area of the frontal cortex, bilaterally. The region of diminished grey matter extended from the dorsolateral cortex via the frontal pole to the medial surface. While the findings of this study support the hypothesis that persistent psychomotor poverty in schizophrenia is associated with diminished grey matter in the frontal cortex, the findings must be regarded with caution because of the small sample size and also on account of the novel technique employed to assess the volume of grey matter.

# Neurochemistry and pharmacology of psychomotor poverty

In primates, including humans, the administration of dopamine-depleting agents, such as alpha-methyl-para-tyrosine, leads to marked slowing of physical and mental activity; this suggests that dopaminergic underactivity could play a cardinal role in psychomotor poverty. In accord with this prediction, there is strong evidence that dopaminergic underactivity is associated with psychomotor retardation in depression. Homovanillic acid (HVA), which is produced by the metabolism of dopamine, accumulates at only half the rate in the cerebrospinal fluid of depressed patients with psychomotor retardation than in depressed patients without psychomotor retardation (van Praag & Korf, 1971). Similar findings were reported by Papeschi & McClure (1971) and Banki *et al* (1981). Furthermore, van Praag & Korf (1975) demonstrated that, in depression, L-dopa, administered with a peripheral decarboxylase inhibitor to prevent its rapid removal from the body by peripheral metabolism, improves motor activity and the level of initiative, and normalises the HVA level, but has no influence on the depressed mood itself.

Although stimulants, which promote dopaminergic activity, are used in the treatment of depression, there is only equivocal support for their efficacy as antidepressants. Nonetheless, there is evidence that they alleviate apathy. For example, in a series of cases of treatment-resistant depression, Masand *et al* (1998) found that, in every case, augmentation of the prior antidepressant therapy with stimulants produced significant improvement, mainly through a reduction in apathy. Marin *et al* (1995) reported that, in a range of diseases, including frontal lobe dementia, cerebral infarction, intracranial haemorrhage and traumatic brain injury, pharmaceuticals that promote dopaminergic activity, such as amphetamine, bromocriptine, bupropion and methylphenidate, are effective in alleviating apathy.

Furthermore, there is evidence that low HVA in a variety of illnesses is associated with the type of cognitive impairments seen with psychomotor poverty. Wolfe *et al* (1990) demonstrated that in major depression, Alzheimer's disease and Parkinson's disease, patients with low levels of HVA in the cerebrospinal fluid are slower in processing timed information, and showed greater benefit from semantic structure during a verbal fluency test (i.e. the patients were more impaired in finding words beginning with a specified letter than in finding words belonging to a semantic category).

In schizophrenia, the relationship between psychomotor poverty and indicators of dopaminergic underactivity is less consistent. Low levels of HVA in the cerebrospinal fluid have been reported to be associated with lassitude and slowness of movement (Lindstrom, 1985). Unfortunately, the evidence in schizophrenia is clouded by many factors, including the effects of concurrent treatment with dopamine-blocking antipsychotics, failure to distinguish between acute and chronic symptoms and the use of broad definitions of negative symptoms. There is strong evidence that typical antipsychotics (such as haloperidol), which block dopamine $D_2$ receptors, can worsen some features of psychomotor poverty in schizophrenia, at least in the short term. For example, Van Putten *et al* (1990) described a neuroleptic-induced akinetic syndrome characterised by motor underactivity, apathy and poverty of speech, which developed in a dose-dependent manner during the first few weeks of treatment with haloperidol. On the other hand, Dollfus & Petit (1995) found that, over a somewhat longer period, negative symptoms improved during treatment with typical antipsychotics. However, as discussed above, most of this improvement was due to the alleviation of symptoms of disorganisation rather than of psychomotor poverty. Blunted affect was the only feature of psychomotor poverty to exhibit improvement.

Studies in animals indicate that serotonin 5-HT$_2$ blockade may promote dopaminergic activity in the frontal cortex (Kapur & Remington, 1996), which raises the possibility that the combination of 5-HT$_2$ blockade with D$_2$ blockade might alleviate psychomotor poverty symptoms while also achieving an anti-psychotic effect. Duinkerke et al (1993) demonstrated that augmentation of concurrent typical antipsychotic medication with the 5-HT$_2$ receptor blocker ritanserin produced a significant reduction in total negative symptom score, measured using the SANS, in schizophrenia. The individual SANS items contributing the largest amount to the reduction, in order of the magnitude of their contribution, were: decreased facial expression; physical anergia; inappropriate affect (a feature of disorganisation); impaired relationships with friends; decreased social attention (a non-specific negative symptom); and decreased affective response. Thus the majority of the items that made a large contribution to the therapeutic effect were aspects of psychomotor poverty.

As mentioned above, Marder & Meibach (1994) found that the atypical antipsychotic risperidone, which blocks 5-HT$_2$ receptors and D$_2$ receptors, produced a small reduction in negative symptoms assessed using the PANSS, relative to that produced by a moderately high dose (20 mg) of haloperidol. There are many reasons for serious concern about the interpretation of this study, including a much higher drop-out rate in the haloperidol group, and the ambiguity that arises from the fact that the features of disorganisation are included in individual negative symptom items in the PANSS. Nonetheless, on balance, the evidence indicates that combining blockade of 5-HT$_2$ receptors with blockade of D$_2$ receptors has a small beneficial effect on psychomotor poverty.

Overall, there is compelling evidence that psychomotor poverty symptoms are associated with dopaminergic underactivity and can be alleviated by drugs that promote dopaminergic transmission in episodic conditions such as depression. On the other hand, in schizophrenia, where psychomotor poverty has an intrinsic tendency to persist, the effect of drugs that modify dopaminergic neuro-transmission is much more complex, which implies that additional factors play a major role in the pathophysiology of these symptoms.

It is probable that other neurotransmitters also play an important role in psychomotor poverty. In particular, the observation that benzodiazepines, which modify GABA transmission, produce at least temporary alleviation of both catatonia and psychomotor retardation in schizophrenia suggests that GABA may play a role (Schmider et al, 1999). In a SPET study using iodomazenil to measure GABA$_A$ receptor density in 10 akinetic catatonic patients, Northoff et al (1999) found decreased GABA$_A$ receptor density in the left sensorimotor cortex, compared with healthy controls. The degree of reduction was correlated with the severity of catatonia. Furthermore, in the same patients, the degree of catatonia was correlated with decreased rCBF in the right lateral frontal cortex and right parietal cortex, which suggests a relationship between the reduction of GABA$_A$ receptors in the sensorimotor cortex and decreased rCBF in the frontal and parietal cortex. In this regard it is of interest that Liddle (1994) reported a case of hypokinetic catatonia with reduced rCBF in the left lateral frontal cortex and parietal cortex.

# Neurochemistry and pharmacology of psychomotor excitation

A strong case can be made for the hypothesis that dopaminergic hyperactivity plays a major role in psychomotor excitation. The evidence supporting this hypothesis includes the following.

(1)  Drugs that promote dopaminergic neurotransmission cause psychomotor excitation in healthy subjects. For example, in a study by Jacobs & Silverstone (1986), in which a single 20 mg dose of amphetamine was administered to healthy subjects, the major changes in mental state were increases in arousal, including increased energy, restlessness and racing thoughts. Mood changes were less pronounced but included increased euphoria and irritability, suggestive of affective lability.
(2)  The dopaminergic precursor L-dopa reliably precipitates mild manic features in bipolar patients (Murphy *et al*, 1971).
(3)  Dopamine-blocking medication alleviates psychomotor excitation, irrespective of diagnosis. In particular, it is effective in reducing psychomotor excitation in mania and in schizophrenia.

While it is probable that impaired function in other neurotransmitter pathways plays an important role in the predisposition to mania, and also that other neurotransmitters are involved in the expression of a manic episode (see Chapter 12), the evidence indicates that dopamine overactivity is a major factor in the mechanism of psychomotor excitation symptoms.

# Synthesis

A psychomotor poverty syndrome comprising poverty of speech, decreased spontaneous movement and either apathy or affective blunting can be discerned in a variety of different conditions, including schizophrenia, depression, frontal lobe trauma, frontal dementia and degeneration of the basal ganglia. These clinical features are associated with impaired performance on tasks that require the initiation of mental and motor acts. In all of these conditions, the syndrome is associated with malfunction of the frontal lobes and/or of components of the cortico-subcortical feedback loops that help regulate frontal lobe function. Some of the evidence indicates that specific aspects of the psychomotor poverty syndrome are associated with malfunction in specific frontal areas. In particular, there is evidence supporting the hypothesis that the left dorsolateral cortex is more strongly associated with poverty of speech, the medial frontal cortex with decreased spontaneous movement, and the right dorsolateral frontal cortex with blunted affect. Other cortical areas, such as the left inferior parietal lobule, which have strong reciprocal connections with the prefrontal cortex, are also involved.

The evidence indicates that psychomotor poverty is associated with dopaminergic underactivity. In those conditions in which psychomotor poverty is usually transient, such as major depressive illness, treatment that enhances dopaminergic transmission tends to alleviate psychomotor poverty symptoms. In those conditions in which psychomotor poverty tends to be more persistent, such as schizophrenia, existing pharmacological treatments have only modest effects on psychomotor poverty symptoms. There is preliminary evidence indicating that structural damage to the frontal cortex plays a role in severe persistent psychomotor poverty in schizophrenia. None the less, there is also a substantial body of evidence, including the beneficial effects of a stimulating environment and of atypical antipsychotics, that suggests that psychomotor poverty in schizophrenia can be at least partially reversible.

A syndrome of psychomotor excitation comprising motor overactivity, pressure of speech and affective lability also occurs in several conditions, most notably in mania, but also in schizophrenia. This syndrome is usually transient. A compelling body of evidence indicates that it is associated with dopaminergic hyperactivity. The evidence for dopaminergic overactivity in psychomotor excitation and dopaminergic underactivity in psychomotor poverty suggests that, in some respects, psychomotor excitation and psychomotor poverty are bipolar opposites. However, they are not symmetrical opposites, insofar as psychomotor excitation is usually a transient condition whereas psychomotor poverty is commonly persistent. Furthermore, there is much more evidence linking cognitive impairment to psychomotor poverty than to psychomotor excitation.

It is probable that psychomotor poverty is more directly associated with structural damage to the brain. None the less, the observation that some patients with frontal lobe dementia exhibit excitation (Neary et al, 1988) suggests that frontal lobe damage can predispose to psychomotor excitation. Furthermore, diminished frontal lobe volume is related to a propensity to excessive dopaminergic transmission at times of stress in schizophrenia (Breier et al, 1993).

Overall, the evidence indicates that damage to the frontal lobes or basal ganglia can produce dysregulation of dopaminergic neurotransmission, leading to either dopaminergic underactivity and psychomotor poverty, or dopaminergic overactivity and psychomotor excitation. In those cases where dorsal frontal damage is relatively pronounced, there is likely to be substantial persistent psychomotor poverty, accompanied by cognitive impairment.

# Chapter 9

# Depression and elation

## Introduction

A lowering of mood in response to loss or other adverse circumstances is an almost universal human experience. Conversely, the achievement of success or the satisfaction of needs usually elevates the spirits. Mood might be described as a modulator of behaviour, especially social behaviour and communication. Mood states tend to be sustained beyond the duration of the circumstances from which they arose, which suggests that elevated mood plays a role in maintaining motivation in the absence of stimuli that provide immediate feedback. The mood evoked by a situation can be stored as a part of the memory of that situation, and can be experienced again when the memory is reactivated. Consequently, current behaviour can be modulated in a subtle way by the mood evoked when similar circumstances were experienced previously. Mood, by virtue of its sensitivity to subtle aspects of a situation that may defy verbal delineation, is especially important in the domain of social interaction. Mood plays a part in establishing attachment to other people, to things and even to abstract concepts.

## Clinical characteristics of mood disorders

### Depression

When lowering of mood is disproportionate to the circumstances, and is accompanied by other symptoms, the individual may be described as suffering from clinical depression. Typically, disproportionate lowering of mood is accompanied by a characteristic cluster of cognitive distortions, together with certain characteristic somatic symptoms.

The cardinal symptom of the depressive syndrome is depressed mood itself. Depressed mood is a subjective experience that can be described as feeling sad, miserable or empty. However, it is more than a subjective feeling. It is an attribute of the mental state that shapes virtually the entire range of non-verbal social communication, including facial expression, vocal inflection and bodily posture and, in addition, interacts reciprocally with thinking. In the depressive syndrome, depressed mood is often associated with anhedonia: the loss of the capacity to experience pleasure. Hedonic response, like mood, appears to be an important part of the mechanism for sustaining motivation. However, it is more related to immediate feedback from concurrent activity or circumstances. In severe depression, anhedonia results in the absence of any response to stimuli that would normally give pleasure.

The cognitive distortions occurring in the depressive syndrome involve a negative bias in the evaluation of self, one's situation and the future. Self-esteem falls and the patient tends to blame him/herself unreasonably and to lose hope for the future. The combination of low self-esteem, guilt and hopelessness can lead to suicidal ideation and, in severe cases, to completed suicide. A major problem with cognition in depression is a bias in the selection of ideas. In addition, when the depression is accompanied by psychomotor retardation there is also a reduction in the amount of thought. Perceptions often become distorted. There is enhanced awareness of bodily dysfunction and of pain. As with depressive cognitions, the main problem with perception appears to be a bias in the selection of the material entering into conscious awareness.

The most prominent somatic disturbance is usually disrupted sleep, which in some cases appears part of a disorder of diurnal rhythm, resulting in early waking. In such cases mood is usually worst in the morning. Other somatic symptoms include poor appetite and weight loss, anergia, fatigue and loss of libido.

The depressive syndrome is frequently accompanied by other clusters of symptoms. Three noteworthy groups of associated symptoms each impart their own distinctive character to a depressive episode:

(1)   Depression is frequently associated with psychomotor disturbances. Sometimes it is associated with psychomotor retardation but, conversely, it can be associated with agitation. As discussed in Chapter 8, Kraepelin (1883) subdivided melancholia into melancholia simplex (simple depression), melancholia activa (agitated depression) and melancholia attonica (retarded depression). Because depression is so often accompanied by an altered level of psychomotor activity, it is probable that the neural pathways involved in simple depression are closely related to those involved in psychomotor abnormalities. However, the fact that these clusters of symptoms can be segregated on clinical grounds suggests that they reflect abnormalities in distinguishable neural pathways.

(2)   Anxiety and related disorders, such as agoraphobia, OCD and panic attacks, occur commonly in association with depression. Not only is there a tendency for anxiety symptoms to coexist with the depressive syndrome, but there is also an increased lifetime risk of depression in those with anxiety disorders. For example, in a population-based study of the prevalence of mental disorders, Andrade et al (1994) found that patients with panic attacks are 11 times more likely to suffer depression than would be expected by chance, which suggests that there are predisposing factors common to both conditions.

(3)   In a minority of severe cases, the depressive syndrome is accompanied by reality distortion, characterised by delusions, with depressive themes such as nihilism, and hallucinations, which are usually judgmental.

## Elation

Mood can vary along a bipolar continuum. The polar opposite of the simple depression syndrome does not have a widely accepted name but might best be called clinical elation. This syndrome is characterised by euphoria, elevated self-esteem and decreased need for sleep. Clinical elation occurs in the manic phase of bipolar affective disorder, although it is not the most consistent feature of manic episodes. As will be discussed in Chapter 12, the most consistent feature of mania is psychomotor excitation. Clinical elation can also occur as a consequence of a variety of endocrine conditions; and as a reaction to drugs, especially stimulants such as cocaine and amphetamine. Marked pathological elation rarely occurs in the absence of psychomotor excitation. Conversely, while excitation is often accompanied by elation, this is not always the case, and so it is appropriate to distinguish between clinical elation and psychomotor excitation.

# Disorders involving mood symptoms

## Major depressive disorder

Major depressive disorder is characterised by one or more episodes of markedly depressed mood and associated symptoms that cannot be attributed to some other identifiable psychiatric or general medical condition. In other words, it is depression that cannot be attributed to bipolar disorder, schizophrenia or other psychiatric disorder; nor is it a consequence of the direct physiological effects of overt brain damage, systemic medical illness or drugs. Thus major depressive disorder is defined as much by what it is not as by what it is.

The word 'major' in the name of the disorder implies substantial disruption of mental functioning. The DSM–IV diagnostic criteria of the American Psychiatric Association (1994) for a major depressive episode require the presence of at least five from a list of characteristic symptoms present during a two-week period. Furthermore, the definition of an episode includes the requirement of change from previous functioning. The criteria distinguish major depressive episodes from dysthymia, a persistent condition manifest as a sustained, mild form of the depressive syndrome that lasts for at least two years. The degree to which there is overlap in the pathophysiology of dysthymia and major depression remains uncertain. Individuals with dysthymia frequently suffer major depressive episodes superimposed upon the persistent background of relatively mild depressive features. Also, there is an elevated risk of dysthymia among the close relatives of patients with major depression, which suggests that the conditions are related.

Major depression occurs in 15–20% of the population and approximately half of those affected suffer recurrent episodes. A variety of aetiological factors appear to contribute to major depression, including genes, previous traumatic experiences and recent psychological stresses (Kendler *et al*, 1993). In each case, several of these factors seem to contribute in concert. Attempts to subdivide the illness into discrete reactive and endogenous subtypes on the basis of the presence or absence of precipitating stressors have been largely unsuccessful. Stressors play a role in the precipitation of most episodes, but the severity and nature of the disturbance usually go far beyond an understandable reaction to the particular stress.

## Mood disturbances in bipolar affective disorder

Bipolar affective disorder is discussed in detail in Chapter 12. In this section we shall consider some aspects of bipolar disorder that might illuminate the relationship between the mechanisms of the depressive and manic syndromes.

Bipolar disorder is characterised by the occurrence of one or more episodes of manic, hypomanic or mixed affective features that cannot be accounted for by a general medical condition, drug toxicity, schizophrenia or other psychotic illness. In most cases of bipolar disorder, major depressive episodes also occur. Cases with manic episodes only are regarded as bipolar. Cases of pure mania tend to occur in the families of people with manic and depressive episodes. In contrast, the majority of patients in whom depressive episodes occur without mania or hypomania do not have close relatives with bipolar disorder, which suggests that unipolar depression has relatively little genetic overlap with bipolar disorder.

The clinical features of a depressive episode occurring in bipolar disorder are similar to those of a depressive episode occurring in major depressive disorder. The depressive syndrome itself is virtually indistinguishable, although the relative frequency of the associated symptoms tends to differ, with both psychomotor retardation and reality distortion being more common in the depressive episodes of bipolar disorder than in unipolar major depression.

Within bipolar disorder, episodes of mania and depression do not usually exhibit mirror-image symmetry. In many cases, depressive episodes are more protracted. Quite commonly, a florid manic episode is followed by a prolonged depressive episode. It is also common for a manic episode to emerge if a depressive episode is treated with antidepressant medication. These temporal relationships imply that at least some aspects of the neuronal mechanisms of mania and depression are antithetical. However, the occurrence of mixed episodes, characterised by coexisting manic and depressive features, suggests that other aspects of the neuronal malfunction in these disorders are shared. This speculation is consistent with the observation that mood-stabilising drugs, such as lithium, carbamazepine and valproic acid, are effective in treating both manic and depressive episodes.

## Mood disorder associated with brain injury or degeneration

Overt damage to the brain can result in a depressive syndrome that consists of similar affective, cognitive and somatic disorders to those occurring in major depression. There are three main brain areas in which injury is associated with an increased risk of depression: the frontal cortex, the basal ganglia and the thalamus.

Several studies of the incidence of depression following stroke have shown a strong negative correlation between the likelihood of depression and distance of the site of the stroke from the frontal pole. For example, Robinson & Szetela (1981) found a correlation of $-0.78$ between severity of depression and distance of the stroke site from the frontal pole (as a percentage of total brain length), but only in the left hemisphere. Fedoroff *et al* (1992) found a similar relationship between likelihood of depression and distance of the lesion from the frontal pole in cases of focal trauma. However, in the case of focal traumatic injury, Jorge *et al* (1993) demonstrated that the relationship applies only to depression within a few months of the injury.

The depression associated with frontal lobe injury should be distinguished from the syndrome of pseudo-depression, comprising apathy, motor slowness and poverty of speech, which Blumer & Benson (1975) attributed to damage to the frontal convexity. In particular, Blumer & Benson noted that the characteristic affective disturbance in this syndrome is apathy, which reflects empty indifference, rather than depression.

Depression is also relatively common in disorders that predominantly affect the basal ganglia, especially Parkinson's disease (Starkstein *et al*, 1992a; Aarsland *et al*, 1999; see also Chapter 8).

Because of the prominent role in the regulation of cortical function played by loops projecting from the frontal cortex via the basal ganglia and thalamus back to the cortex (Chapter 4), destructive lesions affecting these regulatory loops have a high propensity to produce symptoms similar to those produced by frontal lobe damage.

Focal brain lesions that give rise to elation are much less common. Orbital frontal lesions can be associated with a shallow jocularity. However, this symptom is often overshadowed by features of the disorganisation syndrome (Chapter 7).

## Mood disorder associated with general medical conditions

Episodes of depression occur frequently in association with systemic illness. The prevalence of depression among hospital patients admitted on account of physical illness is typically reported to be in the range 20–40%. However, before assuming a specific relationship mediated by a direct physiological influence of the systemic disease on the function of the brain, it is important to take account of the high prevalence of depression in any circumstances that entail the experience of severe loss. For example, in women who have an abortion on account of foetal malformation, the incidence of depression in the following year is high (Iles, 1989). The loss of a wanted baby, which entails a bereavement without the social and cultural rituals that help to ameliorate the loss, might well have special potential for generating depression, but many serious illnesses also entail devastating loss. Therefore, it is likely that many cases of depression associated with physical illness are mediated by loss rather than by the specific patho-physiology of the physical condition.

None the less, there are some illnesses where the relationship does not appear to be mediated by the severity of the loss or other psychological trauma, but involves a direct physiological influence of the systemic disease on the brain. In particular, hormonal disorders are associated with depression. Relatively mild degrees of hypothyroidism can be accompanied by depression, and correcting the thyroid imbalance alleviates the depression (Lishman, 1987). There is also strong evidence for a specific association between Cushing's syndrome and depression. In particular, there is an association between the elevation of plasma cortisol and depressed mood, and correction of the cortisol abnormality by treatment of the primary disease results in alleviation of the depression (Kelly *et al*, 1983).

General medical conditions give rise to the elation syndrome less commonly than to depression. The classic clinical picture associated with the late stages of cerebral syphilis includes grandiosity and disinhibition. Disorders associated with increased levels of cortisol, such as Cushing's syndrome, can also be associated with pathological elation, although depression is equally common (Lishman, 1987).

## Drug-induced mood disorders

A diversity of medications and other drugs have been reported to produce depression. The drugs implicated most consistently are:

(1) drugs that deplete monoamine levels, such as reserpine;
(2) corticosteroids;
(3) drugs that promote the inhibitory neurotransmitter GABA, such as benzo-diazepines, some anticonvulsants and alcohol.

In a study of epileptic patients who developed a major depressive episode while taking the anticonvulsant vigabatrin, which enhances the effect of GABA by inhibiting GABA transaminase, Ring *et al* (1993) found a strong temporal relationship between start of treatment or recent increase in dose and the onset of depression.

Several different classes of drugs are prone to produce elation. These include stimulant drugs such as cocaine and amphetamine; and other addictive drugs such as opiates and cannabinoids. These drugs produce a diverse range of consequences in addition to elation. The stimulants produce substantial increases in psychomotor activity (Jacobs & Silverstone, 1986), while the opiates tend to depress central nervous system activity. While most drugs that produce elation are associated with a risk of addiction, addiction itself has several facets. It is possible to distinguish between motivational dependency, which is probably a direct consequence of the tendency for these drugs to produce elation, and a

**147**

craving for the drug after withdrawal, which is more likely to reflect the negative effects of withdrawal. The evidence examined in the neurochemistry and pharmacology section below indicates that the feature common to all the drugs that promote elation is enhancement, either direct or indirect, of dopaminergic neurotransmission in the mesolimbic dopamine system.

## Mood disorder in schizophrenia

Depressed mood is common in all phases of schizophrenia (Hirsch *et al*, 1989). Depressive features occur frequently during the prodrome of psychotic episodes. During the psychotic episode, a full depressive syndrome can often be identified. Depressive episodes are also a well recognised feature of the aftermath of a psychotic episode, giving rise to the proposal that post-psychotic depression is a distinct entity. Depressive episodes also occur during the chronic phase of the illness. In this phase of illness, a depressive episode may be superimposed upon persistent psychomotor poverty, but is clearly distinguishable from the psychomotor poverty itself (Barnes *et al*, 1989).

It is probable that various factors contribute to the aetiology of depression in schizophrenia. For example, in the post-psychotic phase, the emergence of awareness of the potentially devastating effect of schizophrenia may play a part. It is also possible that antipsychotic drugs enhance depression under some circumstances. However, the occurrence of depression in all phases of the illness, and the observation that during acute psychotic episodes depression sometimes follows a time course parallel to that of the psychotic symptoms (Donlon *et al*, 1976), strongly suggest that depression is an integral part of the schizophrenic disease itself.

Although hyperactive episodes occur in schizophrenia, the mood is not usually one of elation. In the words of Eugen Bleuler (1911, p. 210): "Ordinarily the schizophrenic manic is capricious rather than euphoric. The patients delight in all kinds of silly tricks, stupid and bad jokes".

## Summary of the clinical evidence

Simple depression occurs in a very diverse range of conditions. When it arises in association with structural damage to the brain, the damage is commonly to the frontal cortex, basal ganglia or thalamus. However, the observation that frontal lobe injury can produce other syndromes that are distinct from depression, such as the pseudo-depression syndrome, suggests that the location of the injury alone cannot account for the depression. The observation that the relationship between risk of depression and distance from the frontal pole applies only to depression within a few months of the injury implies that it is not merely the lack of brain tissue in a particular region of the frontal cortex that is relevant. Rather, it suggests that depression arises from a dynamic response to the injury. The association of depression with endocrine disorders implicates both cortisol and thyroid hormone in the pathophysiology of simple depression, while the association with Parkinson's disease and with the toxic effects of monoamine-depleting drugs suggests that the monoamine neurotransmitters – dopamine, noradrenaline and serotonin – are involved.

Pathological elation is a rare consequence of overt brain damage, although at least a semblance of elation, in the form of jocularity, is quite commonly associated with orbital frontal lesions. Furthermore, drugs that induce dopaminergic overactivity, especially in the mesolimbic dopamine system, are prone to induce elation.

# Neuropsychological correlates of depression

There is no clear evidence linking neuropsychological deficits with elation, and so this section will deal with depression only.

The neuropsychological deficits associated with depression fall into three categories. First, there is some evidence of a bias in the processing of information such that material with a negative connotation is attended to and recalled preferentially (Gotlib, 1981). However, not all studies have confirmed an abnormal affective bias in memory and attention (Ilsley et al, 1995).

In the second category are well replicated deficits of declarative memory and other abnormalities attributable to temporal lobe malfunction. For example, Ilsley et al (1995) found that depressed patients were impaired in free recall of material (both immediate and delayed). Zakzanis et al (1998) performed a meta-analysis regarding cognitive function in 726 patients with depression and 795 healthy controls. The largest deficits in the depressed subjects were on measures of encoding and retrieval from declarative episodic memory. Intermediate effect sizes were recorded on tests of psychomotor speed and tests that require sustained attention. Minimal effect sizes were found on tests of semantic memory and working memory.

In the light of the susceptibility of the hippocampus to damage by elevated levels of cortisol, it is of interest that Van Londen et al (1998) demonstrated that intellectual functioning was negatively correlated with mean baseline plasma concentrations of cortisol in medication-free patients during a major depressive episode.

Third, depressed patients exhibit impairments of executive function, in particular speed of processing and the ability to plan mental activity. For example, Weingartner et al (1981) found that depressed patients performed as well as controls in remembering words that were clustered into semantically related groups, but performed significantly worse when the material was presented in random order, which implies a deficit in generating a plan for organising material. Degl'Innocenti et al (1998) administered a battery of executive function tests to depressed subjects and to healthy controls. They found that depressed patients were generally slower than the controls, as reflected in longer retrieval times for both words and colours. Furthermore, the depressed patients showed impairment in the ability to alter behaviour in response to feedback.

**149**

In a comprehensive study of neuropsychological function in patients with Parkinson's disease, Starkstein *et al* (1989) found that patients with depression showed more cognitive impairments than those without depression, especially in frontal lobe tasks. Furthermore, in a study of a sample including patients with Alzheimer's disease, Parkinson's disease and major depression, Wolfe *et al* (1990) found that slowed processing of information together with impaired performance on a word generation task was associated with low levels of the dopamine metabolite HVA in the cerebrospinal fluid, which implies that dopaminergic underactivity is associated with mental slowing and impaired executive function, irrespective of the diagnosis. These deficits could be regarded as aspects of the psychomotor poverty syndrome rather than simple depression.

The crucial issue is whether or not the executive impairments that are observed in depression are specifically associated with severity of depressed mood or with features of psychomotor poverty. This issue was addressed by Kuzis *et al* (1999) in a study of cognitive function in patients with Alzheimer's disease, including cases with depression and apathy, cases of depression without apathy, cases with apathy but no depression, and cases with neither depression nor apathy. They found that patients with apathy had significantly lower scores on tests of verbal memory, naming, the ability to shift mental set, and verbal fluency compared with patients without apathy. Patients with depression but no apathy did not show any greater cognitive impairment than those with neither depression nor apathy. Thus, at least in Alzheimer's disease, it appears that the widespread cognitive deficits, including deficits in executive tasks such as set shifting and verbal fluency, are associated specifically with apathy but not depression.

Similarly, in a study of patients with Parkinson's disease, Starkstein *et al* (1992b) found that patients with apathy (with or without depression) showed significantly more deficits in both tasks of verbal memory and time-dependent tasks. They concluded that apathy in Parkinson's disease is significantly associated with specific cognitive impairments, and may have a different mechanism from that of depression.

A study by Pierson *et al* (1996) of ERPs in depressed patients during information processing throws further light on the differences between the cognitive impairments associated with depression and those associated with psychomotor poverty. They found that all depressed patients exhibited slow encoding of stimuli, as reflected in the latency of the P1 component of the ERP, while the P3b component, which is thought to represent decision making, had short latency in anxious/agitated depressed patients, but abnormally long latency in patients with retardation and blunted affect. They concluded that impairments in patients with blunted affect involve effort mechanisms, whereas those in anxious/agitated patients involve perceptual processes.

Overall, the evidence indicates that some of the cognitive deficits reported in depressed patients are associated specifically with depression, while others are associated with accompanying syndromes, especially psychomotor poverty. The deficits most specifically associated with depression itself are impairments of encoding and retrieval from episodic memory. It is probable that the executive deficits in depressed patients are largely attributable to associated psychomotor poverty.

# Brain structure and mood disorders

There is evidence for structural abnormality in various limbic and paralimbic structures in patients with affective disorders. Using MRI, Drevets *et al* (1997) demonstrated reductions in the mean grey matter volume in the subgenual region (i.e. below the genu of the corpus callosum) of the anterior cingulate cortex of 39% in bipolar depressed patients and 48% in unipolar depressed patients. If it is assumed that the observed deficit in grey matter is persistent, the fact that it was observed in 39% of bipolar patients suggests that a deficit in grey matter in the subgenual anterior cingulate can also be associated with mania.

Sheline *et al* (1996) found decreased hippocampal volume in older patients with a long history of depression. Furthermore, they established that this deficit is related to duration of illness, rather than age itself (Sheline *et al*, 1999). In the light of the evidence that episodes of depression are associated with elevation of cortisol levels (Nemeroff, 1996), and that cortisol can damage the hippocampus (Lupien *et al*, 1997), this observation raises the possibility that repeated episodes of depression produce accumulating damage to the hippocampus, which in turn might make the patient more susceptible to further depression.

# Regional cerebral activity in mood disorders

## Depression

There have been many studies of cerebral metabolism or blood flow in depressive illness, although relatively few have examined the cerebral activity associated with the depressive syndrome *per se*. Virtually all the studies of regional cerebral activity that have compared patients suffering from depressive illness with healthy controls have found underactivity of the frontal cortex. In particular, there is underactivity of the lateral prefrontal cortex, especially on the left (Buchsbaum *et al*, 1986; Baxter *et al*, 1985, 1989; Bench *et al*, 1992). Studies that have assessed changes during treatment have reported that this lateral prefrontal underactivity resolves in parallel with recovery from depression (Baxter *et al*, 1989).

Studies have reported underactivity of the medial prefrontal cortex, including the anterior cingulate (Bench *et al*, 1992; Mayberg *et al*, 1994). In PET studies of both familial bipolar depressives and familial unipolar depressives, Drevets *et al* (1997) found an area of abnormally decreased activity in the prefrontal cortex ventral to the genu of the corpus callosum. This paralimbic region, in which they observed reduced rCBF, coincided with the area in which they observed reductions in grey matter volume.

Several functional imaging studies have also found underactivity in the caudate nucleus (Buchsbaum *et al*, 1986; Mayberg *et al*, 1994). Mayberg *et al* (1994) found

**151**

decreased rCBF in the left anterior temporal lobe. Bench *et al* (1993) and Mayberg *et al* (1999) found that depression was associated with underactivity in the left inferior parietal lobule.

## The paralimbic paradox

A substantial body of evidence indicates that depression is associated with underactivity of the medial frontal cortex, including the anterior cingulate. Paradoxically, other studies have reported that depression is associated with overactivity in the medial frontal cortex, especially the ventral paralimbic areas, including the anterior cingulate gyrus inferior to the corpus callosum. In a PET study of patients with pure familial depression, Drevets *et al* (1992) found that the depressed patients exhibited increased rCBF in an area that extended from the left ventrolateral prefrontal cortex onto the medial prefrontal cortical surface. They also found increased rCBF in the amygdala. The increases in rCBF resolved during treatment. In a study of cerebral activity associated with induced low mood in healthy subjects, Pardo *et al* (1993) found that induction of low mood was associated with an increase in orbital frontal rCBF.

In a comprehensive study, Mayberg *et al* (1999) employed PET to measure rCBF in healthy subjects during the induction of transient sadness, and also to measure changes in regional glucose metabolism in depressed patients during recovery from depression. They found that transient sadness in healthy subjects was associated with increases in paralimbic blood flow (subgenual cingulate, anterior insula) and decreases in neocortical regions (right dorsolateral prefrontal, inferior parietal). In patients, recovery from depression was associated with the reverse pattern, in the same regions. As the depression resolved, paralimbic rCBF decreased, while rCBF in neocortical areas increased. A significant inverse correlation between subgenual cingulate and right dorsolateral prefrontal activity was demonstrated in the healthy subjects during transient sadness, and in the depressed patients during recovery.

Studies comparing treatment responders with those who do not respond to treatment provide a clue to the paradoxical observations regarding rCBF in the paralimbic frontal cortex in depression. In a PET study of regional metabolism in patients with unipolar depression, Mayberg *et al* (1997) found that those who subsequently responded to antidepressant treatment had hypermetabolism in the rostral anterior cingulate, while those who did not respond to treatment had hypometabolism in that area, relative to healthy control subjects. Thus, on balance, the evidence indicates that the ventromedial frontal cortex (i.e. paralimbic orbital cortex) is overactive during induced low mood in healthy subjects and in depressed patients who subsequently respond to treatment, whereas there is underactivity in this area in those patients who respond poorly to treatment. One possibility may be that ventromedial frontal overactivity reflects a compensatory response to depression.

An alternative possibility that is consistent with most of the data is that the experience of depression is normally associated with increased neural activity in the paralimbic cortex, but the overactivity can damage the limbic and paralimbic cortex, leading eventually to chronic underactivity in these regions. During subsequent depressive episodes, an increase in limbic and paralimbic activity is superimposed on a lower baseline, creating the apparently paradoxical situation in which recovery from an episode of depression is associated with a decrease to an abnormally low baseline, rather than with return to a normal level of activity.

The results of PET studies of the regional cerebral activity associated with depression in both Parkinson's disease and Huntington's disease reveal that paralimbic frontal areas are underactive in both groups of patients. Ring *et al* (1994) compared rCBF in depressed patients with Parkinson' s disease with that in three control groups: non-depressed patients with Parkinson's disease; healthy controls; and patients suffering from major depressive illness. They found that the depressed Parkinson's disease patients had reduced blood flow in the medial prefrontal cortex (Brodmann's areas 9 and 32), when compared with either non-depressed Parkinson's disease patients or with healthy controls, but there were no significant differences in Brodmann's areas 9 or 32 when the depressed patients with Parkinson's disease were compared with patients suffering from major depressive illness. Mayberg *et al* (1992) compared regional glucose metabolism in depressed with that in non-depressed patients suffering from Huntington's disease, and demonstrated that depression was associated with hypometabolism of the orbital frontal and adjacent inferior prefrontal cortex.

The functional imaging studies that we have considered so far have compared depressed patients with healthy controls, and therefore do not distinguish the pattern of cerebral activity associated with depression itself from the features related to associated symptoms such as psychomotor poverty or anxiety. In a study of rCBF in which patients with depression were scanned twice, once in the morning when depression was more severe, and once in the evening when the severity of depression was less, Ebmeier *et al* (1997) found that the severity of a symptom factor reflecting the essence of depression was correlated with increased rCBF in the anterior cingulate cortex.

Overall, studies of regional cerebral activity in depression strongly implicate paralimbic areas such as the anterior cingulate, but also demonstrate that limbic sites such as the amygdala and also neocortical areas such as the lateral frontal cortex are involved. Under some circumstances, the paralimbic cortex is overactive relative to healthy controls while under other circumstances it is underactive. This could reflect differences between the predisposition to depression and the actual experience of depression. When neocortical areas are involved, underactivity is the rule. It is probable that neocortical underactivity is at least in part a reflection of associated clinical features, such as poverty of speech.

## Elation

No reported functional imaging studies have examined the pattern of regional cerebral activity associated with elation itself. However, several investigators have used SPET or PET to examine regional cerebral activity during manic episodes in patients with bipolar disorder. It should be borne in mind that psychomotor excitation is a consistent feature of mania, and hence it is difficult to distinguish the cerebral activity associated with elation from that associated with psychomotor excitation.

An early PET study (Baxter *et al*, 1985) indicated that global cerebral metabolism increased as patients made the transition from the depressed to manic state. The administration of D-amphetamine, which promotes both elevation of mood and speeded thinking, produces increased cerebral metabolism in limbic and paralimbic areas, in addition to frontal cortical areas involved in cognitive processes (Mattay *et al*, 1996; Ernst *et al*, 1997). Using fMRI, Breiter *et al* (1997) found that, in cocaine abusers, cocaine-induced feelings of 'rush' and 'high' were correlated with increased activation of the VTA, basal forebrain, caudate, cingulate and most regions of the lateral prefrontal cortex. Using SPET, Schlaepfer *et al* (1998) found that euphoria induced by the mu-opioid receptor agonist hydromorphone, in drug addicts, was associated with increased rCBF in the anterior cingulate, amygdala and thalamus.

On the other hand, some studies indicate that mania is associated with decreased paralimbic or limbic rCBF or metabolism. For example, Blumberg *et al* (1999) used PET to compare rCBF in bipolar patients during a manic episode with that in euthymic bipolar patients and in healthy subjects. They found that decreased orbital frontal activity was associated with mania. In a SPET study of the effects of withdrawal of the mood stabiliser lithium in bipolar patients, Goodwin *et al* (1997) observed a decrease in rCBF in the orbital frontal cortex. However, approximately half the subjects developed manic symptoms and in these cases there was a relative increase in activity in the anterior cingulate and orbital frontal cortex. These observations are mostly consistent with the hypothesis that a predisposition to elation (and other features of mania) is associated with underactivity of the paralimbic cortex, while the experience of elation is associated with a relative increase in paralimbic activity. This hypothesis is also consistent with evidence that orbital frontal damage can produce manic features.

# Neurochemistry and pharmacology of mood disorders

## Depression

An extensive, but inconsistent, body of evidence derived from measurements of metabolites in the cerebrospinal fluid or in plasma, or from neuroendocrine challenge, has implicated serotonin, noradrenaline, acetylcholine, dopamine and GABA in the pathophysiology of depression. Much of the inconsistency may arise from the fact that the depressive syndrome occurs in association with various other clusters of symptoms. Some of the reported abnormalities may in fact reflect the presence of associated symptoms that differ in prevalence in different samples of depressed patients, rather than the depression itself. For example, some studies revealed depletion of the level of the serotonin metabolite 5-hydroxy-indole acetic acid (5-HIAA) in depressed patients, but closer scrutiny indicates that this is an abnormality associated with suicide attempts and other manifestations of impulsivity rather than with depression itself (Lidberg *et al*, 1985a).

Perhaps the most consistent pointer towards the nature of the biochemical disturbance in depression is the well established evidence from clinical treatment trials that approximately two-thirds of cases show an improvement during treatment with drugs that enhance monoamine neurotransmission. These drugs delay the removal of serotonin and/or noradrenaline from the intrasynaptic cleft, either by blocking reuptake of one or both of these neurotransmitters into the presynaptic terminal, or by inhibiting the enzyme monoamine oxidase, which is responsible for degradation of these transmitters. The therapeutic efficacy of such drugs suggests that the pathophysiology of depression involves underactivity of serotonergic and/or noradrenergic neurons. This is consistent with the evidence that drugs such as reserpine that deplete the levels of monoamines promote depression. The hypothesis of serotonergic underactivity receives further support from the observation that the acute depletion of tryptophan, the precursor of serotonin, can produce negative mood states in healthy subjects and trigger a relapse in patients whose depression has remitted (Young *et al*, 1985).

However, the clinical response to reuptake inhibitors and to monoamine oxidase inhibitors typically takes two weeks to develop, which suggests that the essential disorder is a neuronal abnormality that can be reversed only by the synthesis of new cellular constituents. Potential candidates are deficits in the numbers of a particular neuroreceptor or deficits in an enzyme responsible for the synthesis of a neurotransmitter. There is fairly consistent evidence for a reduction in serotonin 5-HT$_{1A}$ receptor density in depression. Using PET with a ligand, $^{11}$C-WAY-100635, that binds selectively to 5-HT$_{1A}$ receptors, Drevets *et al* (1999) found decreased binding in the depressed phase of familial mood disorders in multiple brain regions. Of the regions tested, the magnitude of this reduction was largest in the midbrain raphe, where it was 41.5%. There was also a relatively large decrease of 26.8% in the medial temporal cortex.

The prolactin response to stimulation by tryptophan, mediated by 5-HT$_{1A}$ receptors, is blunted in some depressed patients (Price *et al*, 1991). The 5-HT$_{1A}$ receptors are located presynaptically, especially in the raphe nucleus, and also postsynaptically in areas such as the hippocampus. Both pre- and postsynaptic receptors are implicated in the prolactin response. In addition, the hypothermic response to ipsapirone, which is a partial agonist at 5-HT$_{1A}$ receptors, is blunted in depression (Lesch *et al*, 1990). Paradoxically, treatment with antidepressant medication produces further blunting of this response.

There is also evidence that 5-HT$_2$ receptors are abnormal in depression, but the data are complex. Using PET with the 5-HT$_2$ receptor ligand $^{18}$F-setoperone, my colleague Lakshmi Yatham and I found decreased binding of setoperone, implying decreased receptor density, in widespread areas of the cortex, in depressed patients (Yatham *et al*, 2000). Paradoxically, we found that treatment with the tricyclic antidepressant desipramine significantly decreased the binding of setoperone in similarly extensive cortical areas (Yatham *et al*, 1999a). The production of cortisol following the administration of 5-hydroxytryptophan is mediated by 5-HT$_2$ receptors, and therefore provides an indicator of 5-HT$_2$ receptor function. Consistent with our observations using PET with setoperone, the cortisol response to 5-hydroxytryptophan is diminished by treatment with serotonin reuptake inhibitors (Meltzer *et al*, 1984). In summary, there is evidence that the numbers of serotonergic 5-HT$_{1A}$ and 5-HT$_2$ receptors are decreased in depression but, paradoxically, the data indicate that treatment can produce further decreases.

Various strands of evidence implicate noradrenaline in depression. In particular, depressed patients show abnormal reduction of plasma cortisol in response to the alpha$_2$ agonist clonidine (Siever *et al*, 1984), and an augmentation of cortisol release in response to the alpha$_2$ antagonist yohimbine (Price *et al*, 1985). Since alpha$_2$ agonists inhibit noradrenaline release, these observations suggest that depressed patients have tonic hyperactivity of the noradrenergic neurons projecting from the locus coeruleus to the neurons in the PVN of the thalamus that secretes CRF and thereby promotes the production of cortisol. While hyperactivity in this noradrenergic pathway would be consistent with the enhanced responsivity to stress characteristic of depression, it does not fit well with the observation that noradrenaline reuptake inhibitors alleviate depression.

Dopaminergic neurotransmission is also abnormal in depression. There are reports of an increase in dopamine D$_2$ receptors in the basal ganglia (D'heanen & Bossuyt, 1994) and decreased levels of the dopamine metabolite HVA in the cerebrospinal fluid (Brown & Gershon, 1993). As discussed above, the reduction in HVA correlates with the degree of slowing of mental processing (Wolfe *et al*, 1990), which suggests that this decrease might be explained largely by the involvement of dopamine in the psychomotor retardation that can be associated with the depressive syndrome. On the other hand, in an intriguing study, Naranjo *et al* (in press) found that depressed patients exhibit a much larger elevation of mood than healthy subjects following the administration of amphetamine, an indirect dopamine agonist. This supports the hypothesis that there is a deficit in dopaminergic function in depressed patients, and furthermore indicates that this deficit is related specifically to depressed mood.

## Elation

It is probable that the mechanism of the motivational dependency produced by many drugs of addiction, including the stimulants (cocaine, amphetamine and the various derivatives of amphetamine), the opiates, the cannabinoids and alcohol, is euphoria mediated by enhanced dopamine neurotransmission in the basal ganglia, especially the ventral striatum (Wise & Bozarth, 1985).

Laruelle *et al* (1995) used SPET with the dopamine ligand iodobenzamide to quantify endogenous dopamine release in the basal ganglia following the administration of intravenous D-amphetamine to healthy subjects. The amphetamine produced a mean reduction of 15% in dopamine receptor availability, which implies that a proportion of the receptors had been occupied by endogenous dopamine. The intensity of induced euphoria, alertness and restlessness was correlated with the magnitude of the decrease in available dopamine receptors, which suggests that the severity of these symptoms is related to the amount of dopamine released.

Similarly, Schlaepfer *et al* (1997) used PET with the dopamine ligand [11]C-raclopride to quantify the release of endogenous dopamine in the basal ganglia following the administration of cocaine in 11 cocaine users. All 11 reported euphoria in response to cocaine administration. The occupancy of dopamine receptors by raclopride was decreased significantly after cocaine administration, which indicates that the euphoria was associated with increased release of endogenous dopamine.

Although the pharmacological and behavioural effects of the stimulants and opiates differ in many respects, the opiates, such as morphine, activate dopaminergic neurons in the ventral striatum and hence have the potential to increase dopaminergic release there (Wise & Bozarth, 1985). Furthermore, it appears that opiates and stimulants can act synergistically to produce greater enhancement of dopamine release in the ventral striatum than either drug acting alone, which possibly explains the popularity of combinations such as cocaine and heroin ('speedball') among abusers. Hemby *et al* (1999) demonstrated that the self-administration of cocaine/heroin combinations in rats produced synergistic elevations of dopamine in the nucleus accumbens (the rat analogue of the ventral striatum) that were 1000% above baseline, while cocaine alone produced an increase of 400%, and heroin alone did not produce a significant increase above baseline.

It is of interest to note that while both stimulants and opiates produce euphoria, the euphoria produced by stimulants is usually accompanied by psychomotor excitation, whereas opiates tend to produce a slowing of activity. While it is probable that both euphoria and psychomotor excitation reflect dopaminergic overactivity, it is likely that the mechanism by which this overactivity contributes to euphoria is distinct from the mechanism by which it generates psychomotor excitation. Antipsychotics that block dopamine $D_2$ receptors are effective not only as antipsychotics but also in alleviating psychomotor excitation, but they do not block the elation produced by stimulants (Brauer & De Wit, 1997). On the other hand, the $D_1/D_5$ receptor blocker ecopipam is effective in blocking the euphoric effect of cocaine, in a dose-dependent manner (Romach *et al*, 1999). Thus it appears that euphoria is mediated via a pathway that involves $D_1/D_5$ receptors, while psychomotor excitation and reality distortion (see Chapter 6) are mediated via $D_2$ receptors.

In a review of the effects of the cannabinoids, Ameri (1999) concluded that the reinforcing and abuse-inducing properties of marijuana arise from the ability of psychoactive cannabinoids to increase the activity of dopaminergic neurons in the mesolimbic pathway. Thus, cannabinoids share a final common neuronal action with other major drugs of abuse, such as morphine and ethanol, in producing facilitation of the mesolimbic dopamine system.

# Stress, cortisol and mood

One of the major mechanisms by which the body responds to stress is by increasing cortisol output. The hypothalamus plays a key role in mediating this response via the HPA axis. Cortisol production is regulated by negative feedback at several sites in the HPA axis (Chapter 5). Exposure to a high level of corticosteroids, arising either from adrenal disorders such as Cushing's syndrome or from the therapeutic use of high doses of corticosteroids, can lead to depression (Lishman, 1987). Conversely, depression arising from other causes is associated with elevated cortisol (Plotsky *et al*, 1998). Several abnormalities of HPA axis function – including elevation of basal cortisol; diminished sensitivity to dexamethasone-mediated negative feedback; blunted ACTH release in response to CRF; and increased cerebrospinal fluid levels of CRF – are consistently observed during depressive episodes, but mostly resolve on recovery (Plotsky *et al*, 1998).

It is likely that the hippocampus and amygdala are among the primary sites that drive the hypothalamus to promote cortisol release during stress. The hippocampus and amygdala integrate information from the external environment and from memory, to determine the motivational salience of a situation. Furthermore, glucocorticoid receptors in the hippocampus play a role in the negative feedback from glucocorticoids on the HPA axis (Feldman & Weidenfeld, 1999). Not only it is likely that the hippocampus plays a leading role in the normal response to stress, but the hippocampus itself is vulnerable to damage by stress-induced cortisol release. Lupien *et al* (1997) have shown that induction of stress in healthy elderly people leads to significant memory impairments of the type associated with hippocampal damage. Furthermore, those individuals who had the greatest cortisol elevation in response to the stress situation exhibited the greatest impairment of memory. The administration of cortisol (10 mg) to younger subjects has also been shown to produce similar memory deficits: namely impaired declarative memory without impairment of non-declarative memory (Kirschbaum *et al*, 1996).

Furthermore, in animals, there is evidence that stress levels in infancy influence hippocampal structure so as to impair the subsequent regulation of cortisol and lead to behaviours that resemble features of depression. Rats that were more extensively groomed by their mothers in infancy subsequently exhibit reduced corticosterone response to stress and increased hippocampal messenger RNA expression (Liu *et al*, 1997). Monkeys that had suffered stress in infancy due to variable foraging demands on their mothers subsequently exhibited increased CRF levels in the cerebrospinal fluid, which were correlated with elevated serotonin and dopamine metabolite concentrations in adulthood (Coplan *et al*, 1998). Furthermore, in adulthood, these monkeys exhibited low sociability, increased subordinate behaviour and low tolerance to affective demands. Overall, it is likely that abnormalities of HPA axis function not only play a role in mediating somatic symptoms in depression but also are involved in the process whereby early stress promotes subsequent vulnerability to depression.

# Synthesis

The clinical and laboratory evidence regarding the nature of depression and elation leads to the following conclusions:

(1)    The induction of depression by depletion of monoamines implicates mono-aminergic underactivity in the mechanism of depression.

(2)    The delayed therapeutic response to monoamine-enhancing agents suggests that the pathophysiological mechanism of depression entails a neuronal abnormality that can be reversed by synthesis of new cellular constituents.

(3)    Studies of regional cerebral activity in depression indicate that the lateral and medial frontal cortex, caudate nucleus, anterior temporal lobe and inferior parietal lobule are involved. Evidence from the association between degenerative brain disorders and depression implicates the frontal lobes, together with the cortico-subcortical loops, which play a major role in the regulation of frontal lobe function.

(4)    The association between declarative memory deficits and depression implicates hippocampal malfunction in depression.

(5)    Abnormal function of the HPA axis is consistently reported in depression. It is likely that the hippocampus plays a role in driving the HPA response to stress and, furthermore, that the hippocampus is vulnerable to damage by elevated levels of cortisol. Cortisol-induced damage to the hippocampus is potentially a mechanism by which stress in early life, and also concurrent stress, could increase the propensity to depression.

(6)    Elation is associated with overactivity in the mesolimbic dopaminergic system.

Four interconnected neurohumoral systems are implicated by the evidence considered above: the limbic system, the frontal lobes and related cortico-subcortical loops; the monoaminergic nuclei located in the brain-stem that modulate limbic and frontal lobe function; and the HPA axis. In Chapter 3 we examined the evidence that one major role of the limbic system is the processing of the emotional significance of information. Furthermore, the hippocampus probably plays a part in relating the salience of the current situation to past experiences. The hippocampus influences the monoaminergic nuclei in the brain-stem, which in turn modulate neural activity throughout the cortex, especially the frontal cortex. The hippocampus also has the potential to mobilise the HPA axis to produce an increase in cortisol output from the adrenal glands. The increased cortisol output prepares the body to react to stress and also provides feedback to the brain. The precise mechanism by which abnormal function of these neural systems generates depression or elation is not known. None the less, in the following section, we shall examine a hypothesis that attempts to draw together much of the evidence reviewed above.

# Hypothesis

The apparently paradoxical evidence indicating that depression is associated with underactivity of the limbic and paralimbic cortex, while the actual experience of depression is associated with limbic and paralimbic overactivity, suggests that the cardinal feature of mood disorder is a malfunction of the limbic and paralimbic cortex that renders it hyper-responsive to stress. The primary cause of this hyper-reactivity might be damage at one of several sites. For example, damage to the frontal cortex might impair regulation of the limbic system, while stress-induced cortisol release might damage the hippocampus directly.

By virtue of the ability of the hippocampus to activate the HPA axis, and also to mobilise brain-stem monoaminergic neurons, which in turn modulate activity throughout the brain, this putative limbic hyper-reactivity would have widespread somatic and cerebral effects. The nature of these effects would depend on the association between the current circumstances and past experience. As discussed in Chapter 3, it is probable that the hippocampus mediates the re-creation of previously existing patterns of cerebral activity. In instances where the associations reawaken memories of situations that led to avoidance in the past, the net effect on brain-stem monoaminergic neurons would be underactivity. This in turn would suppress neocortical activity. The patient would suffer depression, with a tendency towards psychomotor retardation. Eventual resolution of the depressive episode would entail a reduction of the limbic hyperactivity and a return to a baseline that might, at least in some cases, be abnormally low. During recovery, neocortical activity would increase. One potential consequence of the activation of the HPA axis would be further cortisol-induced damage to the hippocampus, which would account for the observation that depression is often recurrent and that, in many cases, successive episodes are increasingly severe (Post *et al*, 1992).

In circumstances where the limbic hyper-responsivity triggered overactivity of dopaminergic neurons in the VTA of the midbrain, the consequence would be psychomotor excitation, with or without elation, depending on which of the dopaminergic fibres projecting to the ventral striatum were involved. In the event that $D_1/D_5$ dopamine receptors in the ventral striatum were engaged, the patient would experience elation. The overall clinical picture would be one of mania. If there was preferential engagement of $D_2$ receptors, agitation without elation would be expected, and the clinical picture might be one of agitated depression. Furthermore, concurrent aberrant hippocampal firing might produce reality distortion (see Chapter 6).

It should be noted that, according to this hypothesis, both depression and elation are postulated to reflect limbic (and paralimbic) hyperactivity relative to baseline, although this hyperactivity might be superimposed on an abnormally low baseline level of activity. By virtue of the postulated ability of the hippocampus to reactivate any one of a variety of previously experienced mental states (Chapter 3), limbic hyper-responsivity might lead to either depression or elation, depending on current circumstances and past experience. While the clinical features of depression and elation are bipolar opposites, the limbic hyper-responsivity hypothesis postulates that they arise from a common fundamental cause. Furthermore, the proposal that hippocampal firing might recruit any one of many previously existing patterns of cerebral activity would account for the frequent coexistence of mood disorder with a variety of other symptoms.

# Chapter 10

# Anxiety

## Introduction

Anxiety is a syndrome consisting of feelings of unease, fear or dread, together with certain associated mental experiences and somatic symptoms that reflect overactivity of the sympathetic nervous system. It can occur as the central feature of generalised anxiety disorder, in which it pervades and colours all concurrent mental processing. It can present as a sudden storm in panic disorder, in which circumstance the anxiety is so overpowering that all other mental activity is disrupted. It is a cardinal feature of several specific disorders, including phobias, OCD and post-traumatic stress disorder (PTSD). It is a frequent concomitant of the depressive syndrome in major depressive disorder. It can be a significant component of the clinical picture in schizophrenia, traumatic brain injury and various endocrine disorders. It is a quite common side-effect of drugs and medications, especially drugs that enhance the activity of the sympathetic nervous system. It can also be engendered in virtually any human being in circumstances that are sufficiently stressful.

## Anxiety disorders

### Generalised anxiety disorder

In generalised anxiety, sustained unease, worry, restlessness, inner tension, difficulty in concentration, fatigability and sleep disturbance are present much of the time over many months. This disorder can occur as a single episode or in multiple episodes throughout the patient's lifetime. The anxiety has a free-floating character and is not overtly related to specific precipitants.

## Panic disorder

In contrast to the relatively sustained symptoms of generalised anxiety, panic attacks are brief, dramatic episodes that develop over a time scale measured in minutes, in which intense fear or discomfort is associated with marked somatic symptoms. The fear might be of losing control, of going crazy, of choking, of heart attack, or of dying. Cardiovascular symptoms, such as palpitations and tachycardia, are often associated with sweating, shaking, shortness of breath, nausea and dizziness. The sufferer might experience derealisation (feeling the situation is unreal) or depersonalisation (feeling detached from oneself). Panic is a quite common human experience. Over one-third of the population report suffering at least one such attack (von Korff *et al*, 1985). A much smaller proportion of the population, in the range 1–2%, suffer frequent panic attacks, associated with marked morbidity (Weissman, 1990). Panic attacks can be either cued (in the sense that a specific precipitating event can be identified) or uncued. The diagnosis of panic disorder is made when an individual suffers significant disability owing to repeated panic attacks, at least some of which are uncued. Cued panic attacks can be a feature of other anxiety disorders, such as agoraphobia, other phobias, or PTSD.

## Specific phobia

Specific phobia entails anxiety on exposure to a specific object or situation, such as spiders, snakes, thunderstorms or heights, and often results in avoidance of the feared object or situation. Avoidance tends to reinforce the fear. The success of behavioural treatment, in which the fear is extinguished by graded exposure to the feared object, is consistent with the hypothesis that the association between the object and the fear is a conditioned response, acquired by learning.

## Agoraphobia and social phobia

Agoraphobia involves anxiety about being in public places, such as in a supermarket, on a bus or train, or in a crowded restaurant. These are usually perceived as situations from which escape would be difficult or help would not be readily available in the event of a crisis. The dominant problem is fear of panic itself rather than fear of any external threat posed by the situation. The person tends to avoid the feared situations and cannot face the situation without a trusted companion. In severe cases, the sufferer becomes housebound.

In social phobia, the anxiety is provoked by situations that demand social interaction or public performance. As in agoraphobia and specific phobias, there is a tendency to avoid the feared situations.

## Post-traumatic stress disorder

In PTSD, the repeated re-experience of a traumatic event is accompanied by anxiety symptoms and avoidance of stimuli that could act as reminders of that event. According to the criteria defined in DSM–IV (American Psychiatric Association, 1994), the diagnosis should be made only if the person has been exposed to an event involving the threat of death, or severe injury or threat to the physical integrity of self or others; has suffered intense fear, helplessness or horror at the time; and has subsequently suffered persistent re-experience of the event and persistent symptoms of increased arousal; and has engaged in avoidance of stimuli associated with the trauma. In addition, the criteria demand that the symptoms have lasted over one month and that there is substantial distress or disability.

When exposed to cues that symbolise or resemble an aspect of the traumatic event, the person may experience intense psychological distress or physiological reactivity. The avoidance may take the form of deliberate, conscious avoidance of potential reminders of the trauma; apparently unconscious blocking of memories of aspects of the trauma; and/or a numbing of responsiveness to others and to former interests. The association between features indicating hyper-responsivity and features indicating numbing of responses implies that the pathophysiology of PTSD involves an interplay between a primary tendency to overarousal and compensatory protective responses.

## Obsessive–compulsive disorder

In OCD, the person has recurrent obsessions or compulsions that interfere significantly with daily life and/or cause marked distress. The obsessions take the form of persistent, intrusive thoughts, impulses or images. Compulsions are excessive, unreasonable repetitive activities, such as checking, washing or ordering objects, or mental acts such as counting or repeating words silently, which are aimed at minimising a dreaded event or situation. If the individual is prevented from performing the compulsive ritual, the level of anxiety rises. At least at some stage in the disorder, the person recognises that the obsessions or compulsions are unreasonable, although in some chronic cases insight into the unreasonableness is lost.

## Coexistence of anxiety disorders

There is a high degree of overlap between the various anxiety disorders. Eighty to ninety per cent of those suffering from generalised anxiety have a lifetime history of another anxiety disorder. In many instances, several anxiety disorders coexist. In particular, Yonkers *et al* (1996) found that 41% of individuals with generalised anxiety had suffered agoraphobia coexisting with uncued panic attacks, and 41% had suffered agoraphobia without uncued panic attacks. A further 11% suffered panic disorder. Thus generalised anxiety is strongly associated with both

**163**

agoraphobia and panic. Furthermore, 32% of those with generalised anxiety had suffered social phobia, 18% a specific phobia, and 18% OCD. The comorbidity between the various anxiety disorders supports the proposal that they share common pathophysiological factors.

## Coexistence of anxiety disorders with depression

Anxiety and depression frequently coexist. An international task force that examined the major epidemiological studies concluded that panic disorder is the anxiety disorder most frequently associated with depression (Merikangas et al, 1996). Approximately 50% of patients with panic disorder eventually suffer depression. Generalised anxiety disorder is the next most strongly associated with depression. Of the phobic conditions, social phobia is the most likely to be associated with depression. In general, when anxiety is associated with depression, the anxiety disorder precedes the development of depression. Most of the available medications used to treat depression are also effective therapy for panic disorder.

## Anxiety associated with general medical conditions

Castillo et al (1993) found that 73 out of 309 post-stroke patients seen within two to three weeks of the injury had generalised anxiety. Of these, 58 had concomitant depression. Those with left hemisphere cortical lesions tended to suffer depression and anxiety, while those with right hemisphere strokes tended to suffer anxiety without depression. Patients with subcortical lesions were more prone to depression without anxiety.

Anxiety is common in both respiratory and cardiac disease, such as chronic obstructive pulmonary disease and congestive cardiac failure. The high prevalence of anxiety in these disorders is consistent with the hypothesis that a distorted cognitive appraisal of experiences such as shortness of breath and tachycardia is the primary pathological process in panic disorder. Alternatively, it is possible that the response of brain-stem chemoreceptors to blood levels of carbon dioxide or oxygen can play a cardinal role in triggering panic without the need for cognitive mediation. Hypercapnia and hypoxia can apparently act through brain-stem chemoreceptors to regulate the locus coeruleus, from where noradrenergic neurons project to widespread areas of the cerebrum (Elam et al, 1981). Direct stimulation of the locus coeruleus in animals can produce behaviour resembling human panic (Redmond, 1986). Various chemical manipulations that might be expected to alter pH in the vicinity of brain-stem chemoreceptors, including the infusion of sodium lactate or of sodium bicarbonate and an increase in the concentration of carbon dioxide in the blood, can induce panic in individuals prone to panic disorder. In an attempt to explain the panic-inducing capacity of sodium lactate, Carr & Sheehan (1984) argued that in patients with a predisposition to panic, brain-stem chemoreceptors are abnormally sensitive to changes in pH. However, the mechanism by which sodium lactate induces panic has remained a subject of debate (Nutt & Lawson, 1992).

Anxiety is common in endocrine disorders, especially hyperthyroidism. As discussed in relation to respiratory and cardiac disease, it is possible that misinterpretation of somatic symptoms such as tachycardia plays a part in generating anxiety, although it is also possible that direct hormonal influences on cerebral function are responsible.

# Animal models

It is potentially informative to review some of the findings from studies of standardised situations in which animals are subjected to threatening circumstances. It is necessary to bear in mind the likely differences between the human responses to threat and those of animals. In particular, it might be anticipated that human language and cognition would play an important role in human responses. None the less, several observations demonstrate that many elements of the response to threatening circumstances are consistent across species. The features of the 'fight or flight' response are similar in many species, including humans. The processes of the acquisition and extinction of conditioned responses exhibit similarities across species. Pharmacological agents that are effective anxiolytics in humans are similarly effective in animal models of anxiety.

## Conditioned fear

Animals learn that a tone can predict the occurrence of an electric shock through classical Pavlovian conditioning. Rats trained in this way freeze when they hear the conditioned stimulus. Surgical removal of the amygdala abolishes both the ability to acquire this learned fear response and also the expression of previously learned fear responses. In particular, damage to the central nucleus of the amygdala obstructs the acquisition of conditioned fear (Kapp et al, 1984). In contrast, damage to the dorsal part of the medial prefrontal cortex enhances the conditioned fear response, which suggests that this area plays a role in reducing the fear response. Conversely, Garcia et al (1999) demonstrated that a conditioned aversive tone produces a reduction in the spontaneous activity in prefrontal neurons. The reduction is proportional to the degree of fear. Furthermore, the reduction in prefrontal neural firing is related to amygdala activity rather than being directly related to the freezing response itself. This observation suggests that, under some circumstances, abnormal amygdala-induced modulation of prefrontal neuronal activity may play a part in anxiety disorders.

## The separation response

When a young monkey is separated from either its mother or its peers, it tends to exhibit overactivity initially, followed by a period of withdrawal. The initial phase

**165**

has features resembling an anxiety state. The young monkey becomes agitated and exhibits increased spontaneous motor activity and increased vocalisation (Hinde *et al*, 1966; Mineka & Suomi, 1978). There are marked variations in the severity of the separation response between and within species. In particular, the nature of the mother–infant relationship before separation influences severity of the response to maternal separation. Infants who had experienced more maternal rejecting behaviour exhibit a more severe response (Hinde & Spencer-Booth, 1970).

Breeze *et al* (1973) demonstrated that maternal separation increases the activity of the enzymes that synthesise catecholamines in the adrenal medulla. In a study of squirrel monkeys, Vogt & Levine (1980) demonstrated that maternal separation leads to a marked increase in cortisol release. Individual variations in the magnitude of the cortisol response are determined by factors such as the dominance of the mother. The more dominant the mother, the greater is the cortisol response in the infant after separation.

Overall, the separation response in animals demonstrates the existence of an integrated response involving the mechanisms of cerebral arousal, peripheral autonomic activity and activity in the HPA axis, but there are marked differences between individuals in the severity of this response, apparently reflecting both constitutional and developmental factors.

## The acoustic startle reflex

Sudden loud sounds produce a startle reflex in animals and humans. The observation that this reflex is excessive in patients with PTSD indicates that it is relevant to human anxiety disorders. Studies in rats demonstrate that projections from the amygdala to the brain-stem regulate the acoustic startle reflex. Explicit cues (such as lights or tones) activate the central nucleus of the amygdala. On the other hand, less explicit information, such as exposure to a threatening environment or the intraventricular administration of CRH, activate the bed nucleus of the stria terminalis, which also projects to the startle pathway. As discussed in Chapter 3, the bed nucleus of the stria terminalis is a part of the extended amygdala. These observations suggest that the bed nucleus of the stria terminalis may mediate situational anxiety, whereas activation of the central nucleus of the amygdala may mediate stimulus-specific fear (Davis & Shi, 1999).

## Elevated mazes

The elevated plus-maze provides a setting for testing avoidance behaviour in small animals such as rats and guinea pigs. The maze is elevated by 50 cm and has two open arms (exposed to the drop) and two closed arms. Animals normally make fewer entries into the open arms. The strength of the bias against entering the exposed open arms provides a measure of learned fear (also known as inhibitory avoidance). Clinically effective anxiolytic drugs produce a significant increase in the percentage of time spent on the open arms, while anxiogenic agents have the opposite effect (Pellow *et al*, 1985).

The standard elevated plus-maze test does not by itself allow discrimination between different types of anxiety. A modified version, the elevated T-maze, was developed to provide discrimination between inhibitory avoidance (representing learned fear or conditioned fear) and unconditioned (innate) fear. The apparatus consists of three elevated arms, one enclosed and two open. Inhibitory avoidance is measured by recording the time taken to leave the enclosed arm in three consecutive trials. Unconditioned fear (innate fear) is evaluated by recording the time to escape from an open arm. Anxiolytic agents reduce inhibitory avoidance, but do not affect the time taken to escape the open arm (Graeff *et al*, 1998).

Graeff *et al* (1996) have suggested that the ascending serotonin pathway that projects from the dorsal raphe nucleus to the amygdala and frontal cortex facilitates conditioned fear, while the pathway projecting from the dorsal raphe to the peri-aqueductal grey matter inhibits inborn fight or flight reactions to impending danger, pain or asphyxia. To test the involvement of serotonergic projections from the raphe in anxiety, they injected the 5-HT$_{1A}$ agonist 8-OH-DPAT into the dorsal raphe to inhibit serotonin release. This treatment impaired inhibitory avoidance (i.e. decreased conditioned fear) without affecting one-way escape (unconditioned fear). They also employed various treatments to increase serotonin release from the terminals of dorsal raphe neurons. The least anatomically specific of these treatments was intraperitoneal injection of D-fenfluramine, which would be expected to promote widespread release of serotonin. All treatments that increased serotonin release enhanced conditioned avoidance (i.e. increased conditioned fear). In addition, fenfluramine decreased one-way escape time (i.e. increased unconditioned fear). These findings support the hypothesis that different serotonin pathways are involved in different types of fear response, but do not help to localise the neurons that mediate unconditioned fear.

# Normal response to threat

The normal response to threat in humans involves an increase in arousal; an increase in vigilance; the cognitive appraisal of the threat and the planning of a response; increased autonomic activity, which prepares the body for fight or flight; and increased output of cortisol from the adrenal cortex.

As discussed in Chapter 5, the increase in arousal is probably mediated by an increase in modulatory monoaminergic neurotransmission, especially by increased activity of the noradrenergic neurons of the locus coeruleus in the midbrain, which project widely throughout the brain (Redmond, 1986). The preparation for immediate fight or flight is largely mediated by increased tone in the sympathetic nervous system, which involves an increase in the release of adrenaline from the adrenal medulla and also via action of the autonomic neurons innervating the heart, gut and other organs. In addition, increased release of ACTH from the pituitary leads to increase in release of cortisol from the adrenal (Koob & Bloom, 1985). Studies of animals indicate that the amygdala is likely to play a cardinal role in mobilising these various responses (Ledoux, 1995).

In both animals and man, the response to threat also entails learning that modifies the response to subsequent exposure to the same threat. As discussed in Chapter 3, the limbic system is strongly implicated in such learning processes. The role of the amygdala in conditioned fear in animals (Ledoux, 1995; Garcia *et al*, 1999) suggests that it is also likely to play an important role in the acquisition of fear responses in humans, especially when the threat is immediate. However, in circumstances where the threat is perceived on the basis of a cognitive appraisal of the situation, it is plausible that the hippocampus would play a role. In an elaboration of an earlier theory advanced by Gray (1982), McNaughton (1997) has proposed that at least some instances of clinical anxiety could result from hyperactivity of the septohippocampal system, which might strengthen negative associations of stimuli, with a consequential increase in anxiety when the stimuli are subsequently presented.

# Cognition and information processing in anxiety disorders

According to the cognitive theory of emotional disorders, patients prone to anxiety disorders engage in maladaptive patterns of thought that lead them to jump to anxiety-generating conclusions. For example, Clark (1986) proposed that the primary problem in panic is a catastrophic misinterpretation of interoceptive sensations or thoughts. For example, a patient might interpret tachycardia (a perceived sensation) as indicating a catastrophic event such as an impending heart attack; this would evoke a threat response, which in turn might exacerbate the somatic sensations, thus establishing a vicious circle leading to panic.

There is substantial evidence supporting the hypothesis that bodily sensations can play a primary role in anxiety and panic. For example, the anxiogenic effects of hypoglycaemia depend on intact peripheral sensation. In tetraplegic subjects, it produces sedation rather than arousal (Mathias *et al*, 1979). Furthermore, using a standardised technique to explore subjective experiences during recent episodes of anxiety in patients with panic disorder, Zucker *et al* (1989) found that 85% of the patients reported a bodily experience as the initial event reaching conscious awareness. However, the role of conscious thought in mediating the panic is less clear. Zucker and colleagues found that 70% of the patients reported a feeling of anxiety that preceded any worrying thought. Moreover, panic can occur during sleep (Mellman & Uhde, 1989), in the absence of conscious thought.

Some empirical evidence supports the hypothesis that anxiety disorders are associated with specific patterns of maladaptive thought. The style of thinking of patients with different types of anxiety disorder tends to be consistent with the nature of the specific disorder. For example, Breitholtz *et al* (1999) found that patients with generalised anxiety had an excess of thoughts concerned with interpersonal confrontation, competence, acceptance, concern about others and worry over minor matters, while patients with panic disorder had significantly more thoughts about physical catastrophe. Furthermore, those patients with generalised anxiety together with social phobia had more concerns about social embarrassment than patients with generalised anxiety without social phobia.

However, other investigations provide only partial support for the hypothesis. For example, Becker *et al* (1999) performed two studies in which patients with various types of anxiety disorder were requested to learn a list of words that included words with special relevance to specific types of anxiety, pleasant words and neutral words. The patients were subsequently tested to determine whether their memory was biased towards the words with special relevance to the type of anxiety they suffered. In the first study, in which they compared patients with generalised anxiety disorder, social phobia (specifically, anxiety about speaking) and healthy control participants, the patients did not show any evidence of bias towards the anxiety-related words. In a second study, they compared patients with panic disorder and coexisting agoraphobia with healthy controls. In this study, the panic disorder patients exhibited a highly significant bias such that they were much better at recalling threatening words.

Studies using ERP techniques to provide an indirect measure of brain electrical activity during the processing of information confirm that patients with anxiety disorders process information abnormally. A variety of different abnormalities have been reported in different anxiety disorders. For example, Clark *et al* (1996) found that, during a task that required a response to infrequent target tones embedded in a series of lower-pitched tones, patients with panic disorder exhibited a frontal P300 component of the type that healthy individuals exhibit when confronted with novel, task-irrelevant stimuli.

Levy *et al* (1996) recorded early evoked potentials that reflect brain-stem function to test the hypothesis that the transmission of acoustic sensory information through the brain-stem is abnormal in panic disorder. The patients exhibited a reduced latency of the N3 component that indicates activation in the pons. The N3 latency period significantly correlated with severity of anxiety, assessed using the Hamilton Anxiety Scale. In addition, the N3–5 interval was prolonged. This interval reflects the passage of the signal from the pons to the midbrain. The pons is the site of the locus coeruleus, the nucleus from which noradrenergic fibres project widely throughout the cerebral cortex.

Morgan & Grillon (1999) found that women who suffered PTSD following sexual assault exhibited an abnormally large mismatch negativity when presented with odd auditory stimuli embedded in a train of regular stimuli. Mismatch negativity is an ERP that reflects the operation of a preconscious cortical detector of stimulus change. This finding implies increased sensitivity to stimulus changes in PTSD, at a preconscious level.

# Neurochemistry and pharmacology of anxiety

Drugs with a variety of pharmacological mechanisms are effective in the treatment of anxiety disorders. These drugs include:

(1)   minor tranquillisers, such as the benzodiazepines, which promote the action of the inhibitory neurotransmitter GABA;
(2)   antidepressants, including both noradrenaline and serotonin reuptake inhibitors;
(3)   antipsychotics, which block dopamine.

In addition, beta-blockers have an anxiolytic effect, although this could be due, at least in part, to reduction of peripheral signs of anxiety, such as tachycardia.

## Benzodiazepines and the role of GABA

There is a paucity of good evidence establishing whether one class of anti-anxiety drug is preferable to another. None the less, in the last decades of the twentieth century, benzodiazepines were widely used as the first-line treatment for anxiety disorders. In an international study of expert opinion regarding the treatment of anxiety disorders conducted in 1992, the majority recommended a benzo-diazepine anxiolytic as the first-line treatment for panic disorder, generalised anxiety disorder, simple phobia and adjustment disorder. Very similar results were obtained in a repetition of the study in 1997 (Uhlenhuth *et al*, 1999).

Benzodiazepines promote the action of the inhibitory transmitter GABA, by binding to a specific site on the $GABA_A$ receptor. The nature of the naturally occurring endogenous ligand that binds to the benzodiazepine binding site is unknown. In particular, it is unknown whether it is an agonist, which would be expected to promote the action of GABA, or an inverse agonist, which would antagonise the action of GABA.

### Inverse benzodiazepine agonists

The beta-carboline compound FG 7142 is an inverse agonist at the benzodiazepine site, and is a potent anxiogenic agent. Even in healthy individuals, it can produce intense anxiety (Dorow *et al*, 1983). If the endogenous ligand at the benzo-diazepine site were to be an inverse agonist, it might be expected to play a major role in the mechanism of anxiety. One candidate is tribulin, a naturally occurring substance that can act as an inverse agonist at the benzodiazepine site, but it has not been established that it fulfils this role under normal circumstances. Urinary tribulin levels are increased in patients with anxiety (Clow *et al*, 1988). However, the hypothesis that the usual endogenous ligand is an inverse agonist is inconsistent with the preliminary observation that the benzodiazepine receptor blocker flumazenil provokes panic in patients with panic disorder (Nutt *et al*, 1990). Flumazenil is effective in blocking both agonists and inverse agonists. This observation, if confirmed, would make it unlikely that the endogenous ligand is an inverse agonist.

In PTSD, flumazenil does not promote either the specific symptoms of PTSD nor other anxiety symptoms, which implies that PTSD and panic disorder do not share a similar disorder of benzodiazepine/GABA$_A$ function (Randall *et al*, 1995).

### *In vivo* assessment of benzodiazepine receptors

Several investigators using SPET with the ligand [123]I-iomazenil, which is a partial inverse agonist at the benzodiazepine receptor, to assess the binding potential of benzodiazepines in patients with anxiety disorder (mainly panic disorder) have reported widespread decreases in binding potential, especially in the frontal and temporal cortex (Kaschka *et al*, 1995; Tokunaga *et al*, 1997; Uchiyama *et al*, 1997). Tokunaga *et al* (1997) and Uchiyama *et al* (1997) both reported that the decrease in binding in the frontal and temporal lobes was correlated with severity of anxiety, measured on the Hamilton Anxiety Scale.

In a quantitative PET study using the ligand [11]C-flumazenil to assess benzo-diazepine receptor density in a group of patients with panic disorder who had been unmedicated for at least six months, and who had never abused alcohol, Malizia *et al* (1998) found a global reduction in flumazenil binding throughout the brain in patients compared with healthy controls. The decreases were most substantial in the right orbital frontal cortex and right insula. In contrast, using PET with the same ligand, Abadie *et al* (1999) did not find any regional differences in receptor number or binding affinity in 10 unmedicated patients with anxiety disorder, compared with matched healthy controls. It is possible that differences in patient characteristics might account for this discrepancy. None the less, the balance of current evidence indicates that there is widespread reduction in benzodiazepine receptor density in at least some patients with anxiety disorders, especially panic disorder.

## Noradrenergic overactivity

Noradrenergic neurons project from the locus coeruleus, located in the mid-brain pons, throughout the cerebral cortex, including the hippocampus, and also to subcortical nuclei such as the amygdala, thalamus and hypothalamus. As discussed in Chapter 5, the extensive projections of the noradrenergic system allow it to modulate brain activity in response to stressful environmental change. Exposure to stress produces increased firing of noradrenergic neurons in the locus coeruleus. In animals, increased firing of the locus coeruleus is associated with the behavioural manifestations of fear, such as arched back and pilo-erection in the cat.

In healthy humans, the alpha$_2$ adrenoceptor ligand yohimbine produces anxiety and can trigger panic in patients suffering from panic disorder (Charney *et al*, 1984). It enhances noradrenergic activity by blockade of presynaptic auto-receptors. In particular, it increases the firing rate of noradrenergic neurons in the locus coeruleus. It produces increased production of 3-methoxy-4-hydroxy-phenylglycol (MHPG), the principal metabolite of noradrenaline. Yohimbine also produces anxiety and specific PTSD symptoms in patients with PTSD.

Southwick *et al* (1997) compared the effects of yohimbine to that of the serotonergic indirect agonist m-chloro-phenyl-piperazine (m-CPP) in 26 patients with PTSD and 14 healthy subjects. The subjects each received an intravenous infusion of yohimbine hydrochloride (0.4 mg/kg), m-CPP (1.0 mg/kg) or saline solution, under double-blind conditions, on three separate test days, in a randomised balanced order. Both m-CPP and yohimbine induced significantly more severe symptoms of anxiety, panic and PTSD in the patients, compared with the healthy controls. Eleven (42%) of the patients with PTSD experienced yohimbine-induced panic attacks. Eight of the patients (31%) with PTSD experienced m-CPP-induced panic attacks. Neither yohimbine nor m-CPP induced outright panic attacks in the healthy control subjects. The yohimbine-induced panic attacks tended to occur in different patients from the m-CPP-induced panic attacks, which led the investigators to conclude that their data suggest the presence of two subgroups of patients with PTSD, one with a sensitised noradrenergic system and the other with a sensitised serotonergic system.

Studies in animals suggest that the acoustic startle reflex is a useful model to investigate the mechanism of anxiety and fear states. Yohimbine increases the amplitude of this reflex in laboratory animals. Morgan *et al* (1995) demonstrated that intravenous yohimbine also increases the magnitude and probability of the acoustic startle reflex in patients with PTSD, but not in healthy controls.

While it is probable that the induction of panic by yohimbine arises from a direct action in the locus coeruleus, adrenergic agonists that do not cross the blood–brain barrier, such as the beta-agonist isoprenaline, can also produce anxiety (Pyke & Greenberg, 1986). It is probable that the anxiogenic effects of peripherally acting noradrenergic agents are mediated by cognitive misinterpretation of somatic symptoms.

## Alteration of serotonergic function

As discussed above, the serotonin agonist (m-CPP) can provoke anxiety, including panic, in susceptible individuals (Charney *et al*, 1987; Southwick *et al*, 1997). However, not all agents that increase serotonergic activity provoke anxiety. In particular, 5-hydroxytryptophan, the immediate precursor of serotonin, alleviates anxiety in patients with panic disorder. The effects of serotonin reuptake inhibitors, which act to increase the level of serotonin in the synaptic cleft, are enigmatic. Initially, these drugs tend to increase anxiety, at least in some individuals, but after a period of several weeks they exert an anxiolytic effect, perhaps reflecting adaptive changes in serotonin receptors (Westenberg & den Boer, 1988). Furthermore, in patients with panic disorder who have responded to treatment with a selective serotonin reuptake inhibitor, tryptophan depletion can cause a relapse (Nutt *et al*, 1999).

Evidence such as the observation by Southwick *et al* (1997) that some patients with PTSD suffer panic in response to m-CPP while in others panic is generated in response to yohimbine suggests that some patients have a sensitised serotonergic system while in others the noradrenergic system is more sensitised. However, this does not preclude the possibility of interactions between the serotonergic and noradrenergic systems in the genesis of panic. Goddard *et al* (1995) examined the effect of tryptophan depletion on the propensity of healthy subjects to suffer panic in response to an infusion of yohimbine. They found that five of 11 subjects reported marked nervousness in response to an infusion of yohimbine after tryptophan depletion, whereas only one of the subjects exhibited marked nervousness in response to yohimbine after sham tryptophan depletion. Thus it appears that diminishing serotonergic neurotransmission increases the propensity to suffer anxiety in response to increased noradrenergic activity.

## Cholecystokinin

Cholecystokinin (CCK) is a peptide that was originally isolated from the gastrointestinal system and subsequently shown to occur abundantly in the central nervous system. It has a powerful anxiogenic effect in humans and animals. In humans, infusion of the tetra-peptide form of CCK (CCK-4) produces marked symptoms of anxiety within a few minutes. In the majority of instances, the anxiety takes the form of a short-lived panic attack (de Montigny, 1989).

The issue of which neurotransmitter systems are involved in mediating the panic induced by CCK has been a subject of debate. In the original study by de Montigny (1989), pretreatment with lorazepam (a benzodiazepine) prevented subsequent CCK-induced panic. Le Melledo *et al* (1998) demonstrated that the beta-blocker propranolol decreased sensitivity to CCK-4, which suggests that the panicogenic effects of CCK-4 are mediated, in part, through the beta-adrenergic system. In a study of guinea pigs, Rex *et al* (1997) observed that CCK-4 induced 'anxious' behaviour and potentiated the increase of serotonin release on the elevated plus-maze. The $5\text{-HT}_{1A}$ agonist 8-OH-DPAT, which has anti-anxiety effects, reduces basal serotonin levels and also diminishes the increase in serotonin release on the elevated plus-maze. Rex *et al* observed that 8-OH-DPAT given simultaneously with CCK-4 blocked the effects of CCK-4. The results indicate an interaction between CCK-4 and $5\text{-HT}_{1A}$ mechanisms.

## Corticotrophin-releasing factor

Corticotrophin-releasing factor acts as neuromodulator in a system of neural pathways that mediates the autonomic, neuroendocrine and behavioural changes in response to stress (Gray & Bingaman, 1996). These neural pathways embrace the amygdala, locus coeruleus and hypothalamus. In animals, stress leads to increased CRF release in the amygdala and, furthermore, infusion of CRF into the amygdala produces anxiety-like behaviours in animals (Gray & Bingaman, 1996). Thus it is likely that stress-induced CRF release in the amygdala plays an important role in human anxiety. Animal experiments using antisense oligo-deoxynucleotides directed against the mRNA of both the $CRF_1$ and $CRF_2$ subtypes of CRF receptor suggest that the $CRF_1$ receptor is the mediator of the anxiogenic effects of CRF. Mutant mice in which this receptor subtype has been deleted are less anxious than wild-type mice when experimentally stressed (Holsboer, 1999).

The evidence that CRF plays a role in human anxiety is less direct. Strohle *et al* (2000) found that ACTH levels were increased in patients with panic disorder following induction of a panic attack by infusion of CCK-4, which indicates that induced panic is associated with activation of the HPA axis.

As discussed in Chapter 9, studies in animals reveal that stress in early life leads to subsequent hyper-responsivity of the HPA axis and impaired regulation of stress responses. It is possible that cortisol-induced damage to the limbic structures that regulate the HPA axis plays a primary role in this process. In humans, such damage might predispose to subsequent depression and anxiety. Whereas the existing evidence (e.g. Sheline *et al*, 1999) suggests that damage to the hippocampus plays a major role in depression, the amygdala has been more strongly implicated in animal models of anxiety. This is consistent with the fact that the amygdala receives direct input from unimodal sensory areas, whereas the hippocampus receives input from the multimodal association cortex (Gloor, 1997). Hence the connections of the amygdala would support a role in mobilising a rapid response to threatening situations. None the less, it is probable that both the hippocampus and the amygdala are involved in anxiety.

## Dopamine and stress

The dopaminergic neurons projecting from the VTA in the midbrain to the prefrontal cortex are uniquely sensitive to stress. In animals, they exhibit increased firing at low levels of stress that do not produce discernible effects on other ascending catecholaminergic systems (Horger & Roth, 1996). As discussed in Chapter 5, it is probable that prefrontal dopaminergic activity regulates responses to stress. However, when the stress is too great (or when the prefrontal dopaminergic system is impaired) there is an increase in ventral striatal dopamine activity, which produces overt behavioural signs of stress, such as agitation.

# Regional cerebral activity and anxiety

## Provocation of anxiety in healthy subjects

Chua *et al* (1999) used PET to delineate the neural systems engaged in anticipatory anxiety in healthy subjects. They measured rCBF during motor tasks performed while the subjects received electric shocks and compared it with that during performance of the same tasks in the absence of shock. The most significant increase in rCBF during the shock condition, compared with baseline, was in the left insula. There were also increases in rCBF in the right superior temporal sulcus, left fusiform gyrus and left anterior cingulate. Anxiety, assessed using the State–Trait Anxiety Inventory, was significantly correlated with rCBF in the left orbital frontal cortex, left insula and left anterior cingulate cortex.

Kimbrell et al (1999) also used PET, to measure rCBF during transient self-induced anxiety in healthy subjects. They observed increased rCBF in the left inferior frontal lobe, left temporal pole, left anterior cingulate and cuneus, thus confirming the involvement of the left inferior frontal and paralimbic cortex in the experience of anxiety in healthy subjects.

Benkelfat et al (1995) used PET to measure rCBF during panic induced by CCK-4 in healthy individuals. CCK-4, but not placebo, elicited a marked anxiogenic response, indicated by robust increases in subjective anxiety ratings and heart rate. CCK-4-induced anxiety was associated with rCBF increases in the anterior cingulate gyrus, the claustrum–insula–amygdala region and the cerebellar vermis. They also observed robust and bilateral increases in extracerebral blood flow in the region supplied by the superficial temporal artery and suggested that rCBF increases reported in the temporal pole in other studies might in fact be due to misidentification of increases in extracerebral blood flow.

Javanmard et al (1999) used PET to measure rCBF at two different time points in the course of panic induced by CCK-4. In each subject, they performed either a scan during the first minute following the CCK-4 injection, or a scan during the second minute. The early effects of CCK-4 were associated with increases in rCBF in the hypothalamic region, whereas the late scan showed an increase in rCBF in the claustrum–insula region.

## Mixed anxiety disorders

Rauch et al (1997) used PET to measure rCBF during the provocation of anxiety symptoms in a group of patients with anxiety disorders such as OCD, simple phobia and PTSD. They found that in comparison with the baseline condition, the patients exhibited increased activity in the right inferior frontal cortex, right posterior medial orbital frontal cortex, bilateral insular cortex, bilateral basal ganglia and bilateral brain-stem foci. Furthermore, there was a positive correlation between rCBF in the brain-stem and subjective anxiety scores ($r = 0.744$, $P < 0.001$).

## Post-traumatic stress disorder

Rauch et al (1996) used PET to compare rCBF in patients with PTSD during exposure to audiotaped traumatic scripts compared with that during exposure to neutral scripts. They found increases in rCBF during exposure to the traumatic script compared with the neutral script in right-sided limbic, paralimbic and visual areas. They also observed decreases in the left inferior frontal and middle temporal cortex. They concluded that emotions associated with the PTSD symptomatic state are mediated by the limbic and paralimbic systems within the right hemisphere, while activation of the visual cortex might reflect the visual component of PTSD re-experiencing phenomena.

Bremner *et al* (1997) used PET to measure changes in regional cerebral glucose metabolism after the administration of yohimbine. Infusion of yohimbine produced a significant increase in anxiety in patients with PTSD but not in healthy subjects. Yohimbine produced significantly greater increases in metabolism in the prefrontal, temporal, parietal and orbital frontal cortex in the patients compared with the healthy subjects.

## Simple phobia

Rauch *et al* (1995) used PET to measure the change in rCBF in patients with simple phobia provoked by exposure to the relevant object. They observed significant increases in regional blood flow during the symptomatic state compared with the control state in the anterior cingulate cortex, insular cortex, anterior temporal cortex, posterior medial orbital frontal cortex, somatosensory cortex and thalamus. They suggested that the activation in the somatosensory cortex might reflect tactile imagery related to the specific content of the phobia, while the other activations might reflect the experience of anxiety.

While most studies of regional cerebral activity in anxiety disorders have revealed overactivity in the limbic system and/or paralimbic cortex, a series of PET studies, by Fredrikson and colleagues, of rCBF in phobic patients during exposure to pictures of the feared object, revealed that the strongest activations were outside the limbic system, especially in the visual cortex (Wik *et al*, 1993). In contrast to other studies of anxiety, they found a decrease in rCBF in the hippocampus, orbital frontal, prefrontal, temporopolar and posterior cingulate cortex, compared with that observed during neutral visual stimulation. Furthermore, in the case of a healthy volunteer who experienced an unexpected panic attack while participating in a fear conditioning study, Fredrikson and colleagues observed that the panic attack was associated with decreased rCBF in the right orbital frontal cortex, prelimbic cortex (Brodmann area 25), anterior cingulate and anterior temporal cortex (Fischer *et al*, 1998). These observations raise the possibility that anxiety can be associated with a compensatory suppression of limbic activity. An alternative explanation is that pathological anxiety arises from a failure of normal adaptive limbic activity in response to threatening situations. In other words, the limbic underactivity might reflect the causal mechanism rather than a compensatory response.

## Summary

The balance of evidence from the studies reviewed indicates that in a variety of different anxiety disorders, provocation of anxiety produces activation in the frontal, limbic and paralimbic cortex. These sites are also active in healthy individuals during the experience of provoked anxiety. Thus in both healthy subjects and in patients with anxiety disorders, the functional imaging studies demonstrate that anxiety is associated with activity in the circuits implicated in animal models of anxiety. While the majority of evidence indicates that pathological anxiety is associated with overactivity of the limbic system, the findings reported by Fredrikson and colleagues (Wik et al, 1993; Fischer et al, 1998) suggest that pathological anxiety can be associated with limbic underactivity.

# Synthesis

Increased vigilance and enhanced autonomic activity are part of an adaptive response to threat. In otherwise healthy individuals this can become maladaptive when the stress is too great. In various pathological conditions the anxiety response is disproportionate to the stress, either because of a pathological misinterpretation of threat, or because of hyper-responsiveness at any of a variety of points in the complex network of neural pathways that serve the stress response. Functional imaging studies provide evidence that sites embracing the limbic system, paralimbic cortex and frontal cortex are active during the experience of anxiety, in both healthy subjects and patients with anxiety disorder.

The functional imaging studies do not provide any clear indication of the nature of the abnormality that makes this neural system over-responsive in patients with anxiety disorders. It is probable that the causal factors are different in the different disorders, and possibly even within a given disorder. For example, some patients with panic are prone to suffer exacerbation following infusion of the noradrenergic agonist yohimbine, and this suggests an over-sensitive noradrenergic system, while other patients are more prone to suffer panic following infusion of the serotonergic agent m-CPP. The observation that damage to the medial prefrontal cortex in rats enhances the conditioned fear response suggests the possibility that, in some cases, damage to the frontal cortex leads to impaired regulation of the amygdala, creating a propensity for excessive neuronal firing in the amygdala in response to threat.

The evidence for widespread reduction in benzodiazepine receptors in unmedicated patients with panic disorder indicates that GABA-ergic neurotransmission is abnormal in that condition. The interpretation of this finding depends strongly on whether or not the endogenous ligand for the benzodiazepine receptor is an agonist or an inverse agonist. If it is an inverse agonist, whose intrinsic function would tend to promote anxiety, the low density of benzodiazepine receptors might be merely a compensatory response to excessive anxiety. On the other hand, if the endogenous ligand is an agonist, its normal action would result in a reduction of anxiety. In this case, the low benzodiazepine receptor density observed in panic disorder might be an aspect of the causal mechanism.

In view of the frequency with which anxiety and depression coexist, it is noteworthy that panic disorder and depression are associated with similar disturbances in HPA axis function, and in serotonergic neurotransmission.

**177**

Therapeutic agents that are effective in depression are usually also effective in treating panic. It is probable that hyper-responsivity of the stress response mechanism is common to both conditions.

# Part III

# Mental diseases

# Chapter 11

# Schizophrenia

## Clinical features of schizophrenia

Schizophrenia is a disorder in which subtle but wide-ranging disturbances of brain structure and function disrupt many aspects of mental function. These disturbances embrace the domains of perception, cognition, emotion and volition. While the illness has detectable effects in virtually every sphere of mental activity, it is in the realm of higher mental function, including the experience of oneself as the source of one's own mental activity, and in the selection and initiation of activity, that the most striking features of the illness are seen. The deficits in initiating and organising activity often persist for long periods and so lead to enduring occupational and social disabilities.

### Evolution of the concept of schizophrenia

The current concept of schizophrenia arose from Kraepelin's attempt to distinguish the psychotic illness with a tendency towards persistent disability from those illnesses characterised by episodes of transient disturbance with intervening normal function (Kraepelin, 1896). The former group included hebephrenia, catatonia and dementia paranoides. Kraepelin amalgamated these relatively chronic conditions to form the illness that he called dementia praecox and that his contemporary, Eugen Bleuler (1911), subsequently renamed schizophrenia. Those transient psychoses that are dominated by major disturbances of mood and affect, Kraepelin identified as manic–depressive psychosis. It is uncertain how transient psychoses that do not involve major disturbances of mood and affect should be classified in his framework.

Kraepelin's separation of manic–depressive psychosis from schizophrenia continued to be central to the classification of psychotic illnesses throughout the twentieth century. However, it has remained a problematic distinction. In particular, the question of how to classify transient psychoses that do not involve prominent affective disturbance remains a subject of debate. Furthermore, some individuals suffer psychotic illness with prominent affective features during florid psychotic episodes, but between these episodes suffer persistent non-affective symptoms and disability. Such cases might be labelled 'schizoaffective', although it is difficult to discern any natural boundary that demarcates schizoaffective disorder from schizophrenia on the one hand or from affective psychosis on the other. Furthermore, episodes of depression are common in many cases that unequivocally conform to Kraepelin's concept of schizophrenia. It is possible to assemble a strong case for the existence of a continuum of psychotic illnesses extending from bipolar affective disorder to schizophrenia. None the less, despite the lack of a clear boundary distinguishing schizophrenia from other psychoses, the distinction between schizophrenia and affective psychosis has value, even if only to define the two ends of a spectrum.

Kraepelin's term 'dementia praecox' implies two cardinal features: onset in young adult life, and a subsequent deterioration of mental function. A substantial body of evidence has confirmed that early onset is a cardinal feature. While deterioration is not as remorseless as is implied by the term 'dementia', some relatively persistent deterioration of function remains a cardinal feature of the illness as it is identified in current clinical practice. In his early descriptions of dementia praecox, Kraepelin placed some emphasis on the presence of hallucinations in addition to delusions, but also acknowledged that the essential feature was a "peculiar destruction of the internal connections of the psychic personality. The effects of this injury predominate in the emotional and volitional spheres of mental life" (Kraepelin, 1919, p. 3). In a later essay, in which he speculated on the nature of dementia praecox, he proposed that the cardinal features were weakened or disjointed volitional behaviour (Kraepelin, 1920).

In recognition of the evidence that the mental deterioration is not necessarily progressive, Bleuler (1911) renamed the illness. He chose the name 'schizophrenia' to denote the fragmentation of mental activity that lies at the heart of the condition. The integration of thought, emotion and action is disrupted. As we shall see later in this chapter, modern neuroimaging techniques provide evidence that this mental fragmentation reflects a disorder of the coordination of neural activity at distributed cerebral sites.

Among the symptoms of schizophrenia, Bleuler placed emphasis on loosening of associations and flattened affect. By loosening of association, he meant loss of "the thousands of associative threads that guide our thinking" (Bleuler, 1911, p. 14). He considered that this feature was both fundamental, in the sense of being present at all phases of the illness in every case, and primary, in the sense that other symptoms flowed from it. He emphasised flatness of affect as a hallmark of the chronic phase of the illness. He wrote: "It has been known since the early years of modern psychiatry that an acute curable psychosis became chronic when the affects began to disappear" (Bleuler, 1911, p. 40).

Both Kraepelin and Bleuler placed emphasis on the disorganisation and impoverishment of mental activity, which have such a disabling influence on the lives of individuals with schizophrenia. However, such aspects of the illness do not provide a firm foundation for reliable diagnosis, because they exist on a continuum of severity that merges into the range of mental function observed in healthy individuals. In an attempt to identify a set of symptoms that might provide a more reliable basis for diagnosis, Kurt Schneider (1959) focused on a set of features that have come to be known as Schneider's first-rank symptoms of schizophrenia. These are listed in Table 11.1. Schneider proposed that, in the absence of evidence of overt brain injury, these features could be regarded as diagnostic of schizophrenia. However, he noted that schizophrenia "is not a single flaw in an otherwise perfect stone", implying that the illness entails more than the presence of a single symptom.

The diagnostic utility of the Schneiderian criteria is diminished by the observation that these symptoms can occur in transient, affective psychoses. None the less, the available evidence indicates that if the criteria are elaborated somewhat (for example by demanding both the experience of external interference in one's own mental or bodily function, and the delusional attribution of this interference to an alien agency) they will rarely be met by conditions other than schizophrenia (O'Grady, 1990). The content of several of the Schneiderian symptoms suggests that malfunction of the neural mechanism for recognition of oneself as the source of one's own mental activity is a characteristic feature of schizophrenia.

With the introduction in the 1950s of dopamine-blocking antipsychotic drugs, which are usually effective in alleviating delusions, hallucinations and the more florid features of thought form disorder – the 'positive symptoms' of schizophrenia – therapeutic efforts became focused on these. On the other hand, the observation that many patients remained disabled, despite treatment with this first generation of antipsychotics, led to a clearer recognition of the fact that several pathophysiological processes occur in schizophrenia, each of which warranted attention. In the 1980s there was a renewed focus on the persistent impoverishment and disorganisation of activity. Crow (1980) and Andreasen & Olsen (1982) described the negative symptoms, which entail diminution of mental activity, while Bilder *et al* (1985) and Liddle (1987a) drew attention to the cognitive impairment and disability associated with persistent disorganisation of mental activity.

**Table 11.1** First-rank symptoms of schizophrenia (derived from Schneider, 1959)

| Symptom | Description of the perception, experience or attribution |
| --- | --- |
| Thought insertion | The insertion of thoughts into one's mind by an alien source |
| Thought withdrawal | The withdrawal of thoughts from one's mind by an alien agency |
| Thought broadcast | The broadcast of one's thoughts, so that they are accessible to others |
| Made will | The control of one's will by an alien influence |
| Made acts | The execution of the acts of one's own body by an alien agency |
| Made affect | The experience of emotion that is not one's own, attributed to an alien source |
| Somatic passivity | The control of one's bodily function by an alien influence |
| Delusional perception | The attribution of a totally unwarranted meaning to a normal perception |
| Voices commenting | A hallucinatory voice commenting on one's actions in the third person |
| Voices discussing or arguing | Hallucinations of two or more voices discussing or arguing about oneself |
| Audible thought | Hearing one's own thoughts aloud |

In current clinical practice (American Psychiatric Association, 1994; World Health Organization, 1993), the diagnosis of schizophrenia is based not only on the existence of certain characteristic symptoms, but also on deterioration in occupational and/or social function, and a time course that demonstrates at least some tendency towards persistence. The characteristic symptoms on which diagnosis is based include delusions and hallucinations, with special weight attached to bizarre delusions and hallucinations such as Schneiderian first-rank symptoms, but also include features of disorganisation and psychomotor poverty. It is also necessary to establish that the clinical features could not be better accounted for by some other diagnosis, such as an overt general medical condition or a mood disorder.

## Subtypes and dimensions

As might be expected from the fact that what we now call schizophrenia is an amalgamation of conditions previously regarded as separate illnesses, it is heterogeneous in its clinical features. However, attempts to delineate subtypes of schizophrenia on the basis of symptoms have had limited success because cases that show clinical features characteristic of a mixture of subtypes are common. For example, the classical subdivision into paranoid, hebephrenic, catatonic and simple schizophrenia fails because of the frequency of cases with mixed features. Similarly, the attempt to divide schizophrenia into positive and negative subtypes (Andreasen & Olson, 1982) fails because approximately one-third of cases have a mixture of positive and negative features. Furthermore, subtypes based on symptom profile do not breed true, in the sense that two affected members of a family can have quite different symptom profiles (Gottesman & Shields, 1982).

Alternatively, the heterogeneity of symptom profiles can be described in terms of dimensions. In such a description, each dimension of the illness is represented by a cluster of symptoms that tend to coexist, and vary in parallel over time, within an individual and between individuals. At any point in time, an individual patient might exhibit symptoms from several dimensions. Individuals might differ in their propensity to exhibit the various clusters of symptoms. Such a dimensional approach implies that each cluster of symptoms represents one of a set of distinguishable pathophysiological processes, which can all occur within a single disease entity.

Crow's (1980) type 1/type 2 formulation of schizophrenia (see Chapter 8) is essentially a dimensional approach, insofar as type 1 and type 2 refer to two distinct pathological processes (dopamine imbalance and structural brain damage), which may both occur within a single schizophrenic patient. However, there are two major limitations of Crow's hypothesis. First, the two groups of symptoms that Crow attributed to these two pathological processes do not embrace all the symptoms that occur in schizophrenia. (Crow's list of positive symptoms comprised delusions, hallucinations, thought form disorder and inappropriate affect, while his list of negative symptoms comprised flat affect and poverty of speech.) All of the major clusters of psychiatric symptoms –

reality distortion, disorganisation, psychomotor poverty, psychomotor excitation, anxiety and depression – are common in schizophrenia (Liddle, 1995). The first three of these symptom clusters are especially characteristic of schizophrenia.

Second, Crow's hypothesis implies that positive symptoms can be reversed by correcting the biochemical imbalance, while negative symptoms are irreversible. However, positive symptoms persist in some cases despite adequate blockade of dopamine (Wolkin et al, 1989), while negative symptoms can be transient (Chapter 8). As discussed in Part II of this book, the evidence indicates that each cluster of symptoms arises from malfunction of a specific cerebral circuit. The form and content of the symptoms are determined by the normal role of the relevant circuit. The distinction between biochemical imbalance and structural damage specified in Crow's model accounts better for the differences in chronicity of symptoms than for differences in symptom form and content. This is confirmed by the observation that enlargement of the cerebral ventricles is associated with poor response to treatment, irrespective of symptom type (Lewis, 1990), although it should be acknowledged that negative symptoms (i.e. psychomotor poverty symptoms) do have a greater tendency to persist.

The various symptom clusters are described in detail in Part II of this book. In this chapter we shall review some features that characterise these symptom clusters when they occur in schizophrenia.

## Reality distortion

Any type of delusion or hallucination can occur in schizophrenia. Persecutory delusions and delusions of reference are common, but they are not specific to schizophrenia. More characteristic are bizarre delusions and hallucinations with content far removed from the experiences that healthy individuals might readily imagine. These include the Schneiderian first-rank symptoms (Table 11.1), which include experiences such as alien control of thought, action, will and somatic function, and also the experience of hearing a hallucinatory voice commenting on one's actions, or several voices discussing or arguing about oneself.

## Disorganisation

The disorganisation most characteristic of schizophrenia reflects a marked fragmentation of mental activity so that the threads of connection between thoughts are often so weak that the train of thought becomes peculiarly incomprehensible. Similarly, the split between emotion and experience can be so complete that affect is quite incongruous with the circumstances, although in many instances the degree of incongruity is less severe. In schizophrenia, behaviour can be disconcertingly odd and/or devoid of a discernible goal.

In contrast, when disorganisation occurs in other conditions, such as mania or in overt frontal lobe injury, the associations between thoughts are usually more understandable, affect tends to be more often merely fatuous than frankly inappropriate, and even bizarre behaviour appears more goal directed. During

**185**

the chronic phase of schizophrenia, when florid disorganisation has abated, there can be a lingering subtle fragmentation of mental activity that is manifest as vague, wandering speech, awkwardness of manner and disjointing of goal-directed behaviour.

### Psychomotor poverty

The third group of characteristic symptoms, psychomotor poverty, is especially characteristic of the chronic phase of schizophrenia and, in marked cases, appears to express an emptiness of mental content. In contrast to the psychomotor poverty characteristic of retarded depression, where mental activity appears to be slow rather than absent, in the psychomotor poverty of schizophrenia there appears to be a more profound weakening of the drive that propels thought and action. Affect is often shallow and can disappear entirely.

However, one of the enigmas of schizophrenia is the fact that even profound and sustained psychomotor poverty can be reversed, at least temporarily. In the days when institutional care exacerbated the features of psychomotor poverty, a patient who had spent much of the day sitting slumped in an armchair for months or even years might suddenly be aroused by some event to a bout of ill-directed activity lasting for several days (Liddle, 1998, p. 275).

### Other clinical features

In addition to the characteristic symptoms, virtually any affective or anxiety symptom can occur in schizophrenia. Depression is especially noteworthy. It is very common during the prodromal phase that precedes the first overt episode, and occurs quite commonly during acute episodes. Knights & Hirsch (1981) found major depressive features in 65% of a sample of acute schizophrenic patients. In such circumstances, the depression tends to resolve in parallel with the psychotic symptoms (Donlon *et al*, 1976), which would suggest it is an intrinsic feature of the illness. After resolution of an acute episode, an episode of depression that is at least in part an understandable reaction to the losses that the illness entails is not uncommon. In the stable phases of the illness, episodes of depression are less common, with a point prevalence of approximately 10–15% (Barnes *et al*, 1989).

In addition, a diverse array of relatively subtle cognitive and motor disturbances occur. Most pronounced among the cognitive disorders are disturbances of attention, executive function and memory. The motor disorders include impaired motor coordination and, less commonly, the catatonic disorders of the initiation and selection of voluntary motor action.

## Time course

Perhaps one of the most characteristic features of schizophrenia is the age of onset. Overt illness usually becomes manifest at the end of adolescence or early in adult life. None the less, a minority of cases have onset in later adult life, especially among women, in whom onset in middle age is not uncommon. The mean age of onset of the first psychotic symptom is 26.5 years in males and 30.6 years in females (Hafner *et al*, 1994). However, the earliest manifestations of impending illness are often discernible much earlier and can sometimes be traced to infancy. In family video recordings, infants who subsequently develop schizophrenia tend to exhibit evidence of poorer motor coordination than their siblings (Walker & Lewine, 1990).

Two large prospective studies of human development from infancy through childhood into adulthood provide valuable insights into the development of children who subsequently suffer schizophrenia. The first of these studies was the UK National Survey of Health and Development. The intellectual and social development of a cohort of 5362 people born in the week 3–9 March 1946 was assessed on multiple occasions during childhood. The second study was the UK National Childhood Development Study, in which a cohort of individuals born in the third week of March 1958 were assessed in infancy and at the ages of 7, 11 and 15. Subsequently, the individuals who developed schizophrenia were compared with those who did not. Jones *et al* (1994) examined the 1946 birth cohort, while Done *et al* (1994) examined the 1958 cohort. The two studies revealed very similar childhood antecedents. In particular, the pre-schizophrenic children exhibited significant cognitive and social impairments in comparison with their non-schizophrenic peers. These deficits were most marked in the domains of language development, motor coordination, organisation of behaviour and development of social relationships.

For example, Jones *et al* (1994) found that pre-schizophrenic infants were 4.8 times more likely to have failed to develop speech by the age of two. The mean age at which they first walked was delayed by 1.2 months. Speech problems were still evident at age 15. The pre-schizophrenic children were more likely to prefer solitary play at the ages of four and six, and were rated by their teachers as more anxious in social situations at age 15. Done *et al* (1994) found evidence of impaired school performance, especially in language and arithmetic. In the 1958 cohort, the behaviour most characteristic of the pre-schizophrenic children was inconsequential behaviour, recorded by schoolteachers.

It should be emphasised that disturbances during childhood are not sufficiently specific to allow a diagnosis at this stage. Despite the statistically robust evidence for cognitive impairment discernible in group comparisons, a substantial number of pre-schizophrenic children perform within the normal range on cognitive tests. It is not clear whether the childhood precursors occur in only a proportion of cases, or whether virtually all cases exhibit at least a minor degree of impairment compared with their potential if they had not had a predisposition to schizophrenia.

The onset of overt psychosis can either be acute or emerge gradually from a prodromal phase characterised by features such as increasing social isolation, depressed mood, sleep disturbances, attentional impairment, perplexity, agitation and erratic behaviour. Once overt psychosis has emerged, the illness tends to follow a course characterised by acute episodes of florid illness superimposed upon relatively stable periods in which there is at least some degree of persisting disability.

The florid phase is dominated by symptoms of reality distortion and disorganisation. Transient psychomotor excitation is common, although symptoms of psychomotor poverty and of depression are also seen in many cases. After the initiation of treatment, psychomotor excitation usually resolves rapidly and the severity of delusions and hallucinations abates over a time scale of several weeks (Johnstone *et al*, 1978a). None the less, in a substantial minority of cases, delusions and hallucinations persist. When depression accompanies an acute episode, it tends to follow a similar time course to the florid psychotic symptoms (Donlon *et al*, 1976). Psychomotor poverty symptoms also diminish in severity as the psychotic episode wanes (Dollfus & Petit, 1995), although these symptoms are the most prone to persist.

In the first episode, 83% of cases achieve at least partial remission during the first year of treatment (Lieberman *et al*, 1993). In 50% of cases, remission is achieved within 11 weeks. Within five years of the first episode, 82% of those who had achieved remission experience at least one relapse (Robinson *et al*, 1999). Typically the illness continues with episodes of florid psychosis super-imposed on intervening periods of disability that varies greatly in severity between cases. There is a tendency for episodes to become more severe and for the speed and extent of recovery to be less after each successive episode in the first few years. However, after several decades, the illness tends to wane, and by late middle age over 50% of cases have made a substantial recovery, insofar as they have, at most, minimal symptoms and achieve satisfactory social relationships and occupation (Harding *et al*, 1992).

# Epidemiological evidence regarding the aetiology of schizophrenia

The lifetime risk for schizophrenia is approximately 1% and the prevalence of schizophrenia is remarkably similar world-wide (Jablensky, 1995). However, there are several notable instances of variation with time and place, and these potentially provide clues to aetiology. There is an approximately twofold greater risk for those born in cities compared with those born in rural areas (Mortensen *et al*, 1999). Furthermore, a small excess of winter/spring births is a robust finding, world-wide. This finding suggests that exposure to seasonally varying environmental factors increases the risk. A possible candidate is pre- or perinatal exposure to a viral illness such as influenza. Several studies carried out in the 1980s and '90s reported an increased rate of schizophrenia among individuals who had been in the mid-trimester of intra-uterine development during an influenza pandemic (e.g. Adams *et al*, 1993). However, because more recent studies (Cannon *et al*, 1996; Selten *et al*, 1999) have not confirmed this finding, any effect of prenatal exposure to influenza on the risk of schizophrenia is likely to be small.

There is evidence that prenatal malnutrition increases the risk. In the winter of 1944/45, the population of western Holland suffered severe famine during the occupation by Nazi troops. Individuals who had been *in utero* during the Dutch hunger winter had an approximately twofold increase in their risk of schizophrenia (Susser *et al*, 1996). The evidence also indicates that not only severe physical stress on the pregnant mother but also severe emotional stress experienced by a pregnant woman increases the risk that her child will subsequently suffer schizophrenia. In a study of Finnish children whose fathers died between their conception and birth, Huttunen & Niskanen (1973) found that the rate of subsequent diagnosis of schizophrenia was substantially increased, in comparison to that in a control group whose fathers had died during the children's first year of post-natal life. There was no increase in the rate of obstretric complications among those whose fathers died before their birth. Similarly, individuals who had been *in utero* at the time of the invasion of the Netherlands by the German army in May 1940 had an increased risk of subsequently developing schizophrenia, compared with those from other birth cohorts in the period 1938–43 (Van Os & Selton, 1998). Thus a number of environmental factors acting during development in the womb increase the risk of schizophrenia.

Many studies have indicated that obstetric complications are associated with an increased risk of schizophrenia. In a comprehensive meta-analysis of 20 case-control studies and two cohort studies that have examined the issue, Geddes & Lawrie (1995) found that exposure to obstetric complications increased the child's odds of subsequent schizophrenia by a factor of 2 (with 95% a confidence interval extending from 1.6 to 2.4). However, inspection of the funnel plot illustrating the relationship between the odds ratio reported for each study and study size revealed a paucity of small studies reporting a low odds ratio, which suggests a bias against the publication of small, negative studies. Therefore, the pooled estimate of the odds ratio might be an overestimate.

While much of the evidence for environmental factors implicates pre- or perinatal events that might disrupt early development of the brain, there is also some evidence indicating that factors acting in young adulthood can act as precipitants. Studies of the psychiatric sequelae of head injury indicate that injury in young adult life is more likely to be followed by a schizophrenia-like psychosis, whereas injury later in life is more likely to be followed by an affective illness (Achte *et al*, 1991). Abuse of drugs, including psychostimulants such as cocaine or amphetamine and cannabis (D'Souza *et al*, 2000), can precipitate schizophrenic symptoms. Furthermore, a substantial body of evidence indicates that stressful events or circumstances can precipitate relapse in schizophrenia (Bebbington *et al*, 1995).

# Genetics of schizophrenia

The concordance for schizophrenia in monozygotic twins is 45% while that in dizygotic twins is only 12%; this shows that genes play a substantial role in the aetiology of schizophrenia (Gottesman & Shields, 1982). However, the observation that discordance among monozygotic twins is slightly more common than concordance suggests that non-genetic factors also play a role. The conclusion that genes play a major role is confirmed by adoption studies. These demonstrate that a major part of the risk in adopted children is determined by the biological parents. The patterns of inheritance within families suggest that multiple genes play a role. Studies, including several that have scanned the entire genome to identify genes linked to schizophrenia, have identified many weak linkages. Some of the findings, including linkages to sites on chromosomes 1, 6, 8, 10, 13 and 22, have been replicated in several studies (Brzustowicz *et al*, 1999, 2000; Pulver, 2000). The most plausible interpretation of the findings from linkage studies is that there is no single gene of major effect, but rather that many genes, each with a small effect, contribute to the risk of schizophrenia.

# Cognitive deficits in schizophrenia

There is abundant evidence that schizophrenia is associated with a wide range of cognitive deficits, especially in the domains of executive function, attention and memory (Green, 1998). However, there are substantial differences between individuals in the profile of impairments (Shallice *et al*, 1991). Cognitive impairments are strongly associated with poor occupational and social outcome (Green, 1998).

The impairments are detectable before the first psychotic episode (Done *et al*, 1994; Jones *et al*, 1994; Byrne *et al*, 1999). However, the pattern of variation over time is complex. The cognitive deficits tend to be relatively persistent, despite resolution of symptoms (Goldberg *et al*, 1993). However, at least some of the cognitive impairments are exacerbated during florid psychotic episodes and resolve at least partially during remission. For example, memory deficits become more pronounced at the onset of psychosis (Byrne *et al*, 2000) and can improve after resolution of the first psychotic episode (Albus *et al*, 2000). The picture is made more complex by evidence indicating differential effects of different types of antipsychotic treatment on cognitive performance. There is good evidence that, in comparison with the typical antipsychotics, which block dopamine $D_2$ receptors, second-generation antipsychotics, which block various receptors including $5\text{-HT}_2$ and $D_2$ receptors, produce a relatively greater improvement in several aspects of cognition (Keefe *et al*, 1999). These aspects include working memory (Green *et al*, 1997) and verbal fluency (Meltzer & McGurk, 1999). In the long term, a minority of cases go on to develop profound cognitive impairment comparable to that seen in moderately severe dementia of the Alzheimer type (Johnstone *et al*, 1978b; Liddle & Crow, 1984).

Relatives of patients also exhibit impairments, particularly in the domain of executive function. For example, Byrne *et al* (1999) found that in unaffected young adults with one of more family members suffering from schizophrenia, impairment in the Haylings sentence completion test (B version) was strongly correlated with the degree of genetic loading. In the Haylings B test, the participant is required to complete an incomplete sentence with a word that is not congruent with the context established by the given part of the sentence.

This task places demands upon the mechanism for suppressing pre-potent responses.

Despite the occurrence of impairments that are correlated with genetic loading, studies of discordant monozygotic twins reveal that the twin with schizophrenia is usually the more impaired across a range of aspects of cognition (Goldberg *et al*, 1990). Overall, the evidence indicates that cognitive impairment, especially impaired executive function, is associated with genetic risk for schizophrenia, but factors that determine the occurrence of overt illness can also produce further deterioration in cognitive function. The deterioration is at least partially reversible, although in a minority of cases progressive deterioration occurs.

# Event-related potentials

Perhaps the most robust indices of brain malfunction in schizophrenia are provided by measurement of ERPs. Many studies have demonstrated that schizophrenic patients exhibit reduced amplitude of the P300 component elicited by 'oddball' stimuli. These are rare (sparsely distributed) target auditory stimuli embedded in a series of regular non-target stimuli (McCarley *et al*, 1991). This abnormality is discernible at onset of the illness and can also be detected in first-degree relatives of patients. As discussed in Chapter 2, fMRI studies demonstrate that the detection of rare target stimuli is associated with activation of a large set of sites in the association cortex in healthy individuals, but these activations are greatly reduced in schizophrenia (Kiehl & Liddle, 2001).

Another consistent abnormality of ERPs is reduced amplitude of mismatch negativity (Shelley *et al*, 1991). The intrusion of a long-duration tone within a series of equal-duration tones, presented while the participant is engaged in some other attention-demanding task, leads to a pronounced negative ERP component. The difference between the response to the long-duration tone and that to the regular tones is called the mismatch negativity. The reduction in the amplitude of mismatch negativity tends to persist, largely independent of clinical state. It is also observed in relatives.

When two closely spaced auditory stimuli are presented, the very early positive component that occurs approximately 50 ms after the second stimulus (P50) is reduced in amplitude compared with the corresponding component elicited by the first stimulus in healthy subjects. This reduction of P50 represents the habituation of the early phases of sensory processing that occur in the superior temporal gyrus. The reduction in amplitude arises as a consequence of modulatory influences of acetylcholinergic neurotransmission. The magnitude of the attenuation of P50 is reduced in some schizophrenic patients and also in some family members. The reduction has been reported to be linked to the occurrence of an abnormal gene for the alpha$_7$ nicotinic acetylcholine receptor (Freedman *et al*, 1997). This observation represents the first report linking an abnormality of brain function in schizophrenia to a specific gene. However, the finding should be viewed with caution because measurement of the attenuation of P50 is influenced by factors such as cigarette smoking and sleep deprivation, so the measurements are prone to substantial variation between subjects.

Other abnormal ERP components that have been reported in schizophrenia include reduced amplitude of the N400 component elicited by a semantically incongruous word embedded in a sentence (Niznikiewicz *et al*, 1997); reduced amplitude of the frontocentral negativity that occurs approximately 400 ms after presentation of a 'no go' trial during a 'go/no go' task (Kiehl *et al*, 2000b); and reduced amplitude of the error-related negativity that occurs when a subject makes an erroneous response to a stimulus (Ford, 1999). Overall, the evidence of abnormalities in many different ERP components that reflect diverse perceptual and cognitive processes and engage diverse cerebral locations confirms that the cerebral dysfunction in schizophrenia is widespread.

# Brain structure and schizophrenia

A variety of minor developmental anomalies, such as cavum septum pellucidum, have an increased prevalence in schizophrenia (Shioiri *et al*, 1996). Cavum septum is a splitting of the thin membranous septum that lies in the midline between the anterior horns of the lateral ventricles, beneath the corpus callosum. The most robust finding regarding abnormal brain structure in schizophrenia is enlargement of the cerebral ventricles, but the degree of enlargement is usually slight. Most sufferers have a ventricular size within the normal range. The enlargement can be detected reliably only by comparing a large number of schizophrenic patients with well matched control subjects. Meta-analysis of many studies reveals that the mean ventricular volume in schizophrenia is larger than that in healthy subjects by approximately 0.6 standard deviations (Raz & Raz, 1990). Ventricular enlargement is detectable at onset of the illness, and there is equivocal evidence indicating that it might progress during the illness (DeLisi, 1999).

There is evidence for a reduction in grey matter volume affecting all lobes of the brain (Zipursky *et al*, 1992) and, in addition, a more readily discernible reduction in volume of the hippocampus, especially on the left (Falkai & Bogerts, 1995), and of the thalamus (Andreasen *et al*, 1994). In discordant monozygotic twins, the affected twin almost always has the smaller hippocampal volume bilaterally, even when the volumes for both twins lie within the normal range (Suddath *et al*, 1990). This implies that there is at least a slight diminution in hippocampal volume in virtually all cases. It also indicates that genes alone cannot account for reduced hippocampal volume. Furthermore, there is preliminary evidence indicating that the transition from the prodromal phase to the first psychotic episode is associated with a detectable decrease in left hippocampal volume (Pantelis *et al*, 2000).

It is likely that some of the structural brain abnormalities in schizophrenia reflect abnormal early development. Woodruff *et al* (1997) found that the correlation between frontal lobe volume and temporal lobe volume, which is positive in healthy subjects, is reduced in schizophrenic patients. Since this correlation is thought to reflect the functional linkage between these areas during development, the reduced correlation in schizophrenia implies a lack of co-ordination between the neural activity in these areas during development.

Overall, the evidence indicates that there is a loss of brain tissue volume in schizophrenia that is determined partly by genetic risk and partly by factors associated with the development of overt illness. The loss of tissue volume occurs in many areas, but is most marked in the hippocampus and thalamus. The nature of the cellular process associated with this loss of tissue volume remains unknown. The evidence indicates that it is unlikely to be a substantial loss of neurons. It is more likely that the loss of volume reflects a decrease in neuropil, which includes dendrites, axons and synapses (Selemon & Goldman-Rakic, 1999). There is inconclusive evidence for a loss of white matter volume, and some evidence also for a decreased degree of myelination (Flynn *et al*, 1999).

# Regional cerebral activity in schizophrenia

The abnormal patterns of cerebral activity associated with the symptoms of schizophrenia have been described in Part II. In summary, the evidence indicates that each of the major groups of schizophrenic symptoms is associated with a distributed pattern of aberrant activity in the association cortex and associated subcortical nuclei. For each syndrome, the cerebral sites involved include the sites that are normally engaged during the aspects of mental processing implicated in each syndrome (Table 11.2, Plate 18). For example, reality distortion is associated with overactivity in the hippocampus, a brain structure which is involved in evaluating events in light of their context. Disorganisation is associated with overactivity in the anterior cingulate and adjacent medial prefrontal cortex, sites implicated in the selection of activity. Psychomotor poverty is associated with underactivity in the frontal cortex, including the left lateral and medial frontal sites involved in generating words (Liddle *et al*, 1992).

Schizophrenic patients also exhibit abnormal patterns of brain activity when engaged in a variety of tasks ranging from simple finger movements to complex tests of executive function. I have reviewed many of these studies elsewhere (Liddle, 2000a) and in this section will concentrate on a few illustrative studies.

Many studies have demonstrated a failure of the normal engagement of the frontal cortex during executive tasks. In a seminal study using the inhaled xenon technique to measure rCBF, Weinberger *et al* (1986) demonstrated that schizo-phrenic patients exhibited less activation of the dorsolateral prefrontal cortex than healthy control subjects during performance of the Wisconsin Card Sort Test. In this task, the participant is required to sort cards into four heaps according to a sorting rule that must be deduced from the feedback delivered after each trial. Once the participant has deduced the rule, it is changed arbitrarily without warning and the new sorting rule must be deduced. Satisfactory

**Table 11.2** Cognitive deficits and aberrant regional cerebral activity (measured using rCBF or regional cerebral glucose metabolism) associated with the characteristic syndromes of schizophrenia

| Syndrome | Cognitive deficit | Impaired tasks | Increased regional cerebral activity | Decreased regional cerebral activity |
|---|---|---|---|---|
| Reality distortion | Evaluation of mental activity | Internal monitoring[1,2] | Medial temporal lobe[9,10,11]<br>Left lateral frontal cortex[9,11]<br>Ventral striatum[9,10] | Posterior cingulate[9]<br>Left lateral temporo/parietal cortex[9,12] |
| Disorganisation | Selection of mental activity | Stroop[3,4,5,6]<br>Trails A[3]<br>Choice reaction time[5]<br>Unusual word choice[7]<br>Commission errors in CPT[8] | Right anterior cingulate anterior cingulate and adjacent medial prefrontal cortex[9,12,13]<br>Thalamus[9] | Right ventrolateral frontal cortex[9]<br>Bilateral parietal cortex[9,14] |
| Psychomotor poverty | Initiation of mental activity | Word generation[3,7,8]<br>Simple reaction time[5] | Basal ganglia[9,13] | Bilateral frontal cortex[9,12,15]<br>Left parietal cortex [9] |

[1] Frith & Done (1989).
[2] Mlakar et al (1994).
[3] Liddle & Morris (1991).
[4] Baxter & Liddle (1998).
[5] Ngan & Liddle (2000).
[6] McGrath (1992).
[7] Allen et al (1993).
[8] Frith et al (1991c).
[9] Liddle et al (1992).
[10] Silbersweig et al (1995).
[11] McGuire et al (1993).
[12] Ebmeier et al (1993).
[13] Yuasa et al (1995).
[14] Kaplan et al (1993).
[15] Wolkin et al (1992).

performance demands deployment of several cognitive skills, including working memory and cognitive flexibility. Schizophrenic patients tend to perform poorly. One of the issues in interpreting the abnormally low level of frontal activation exhibited by patients is the possibility that the relative underactivity merely reflects lack of engagement in the task. However, Weinberger and his colleagues have addressed this issue in several ways, such as selecting patients and healthy subjects who are matched in level of performance, and have demonstrated that the decrease in frontal activation cannot be accounted for simply by decreased engagement (Weinberger & Berman, 1996).

Furthermore, the reduction in prefrontal activity is correlated with decreased dopamine turnover, as indicated by decreased concentration of the dopamine metabolite HVA in the cerebrospinal fluid (Weinberger et al, 1988). In addition, the deficit can be partially alleviated by administration of the indirect dopamine agonist amphetamine (Daniel et al, 1991).

Schizophrenic patients do not exhibit decreased activation of the prefrontal cortex under all circumstances. For example, in a PET study of rCBF in medicated chronic schizophrenic patients during the performance of a paced word-generation task, my colleagues and I observed a normal magnitude of activation of the left prefrontal cortex in the patients (Frith et al, 1995). Word generation was paced by cues so that all participants produced words at the rate of one every five seconds, a rate that could be achieved even by schizophrenic patients with marked poverty of speech. Although the patients achieved a normal level of activation of the left lateral frontal cortex, there was evidence of impaired coordination between frontal lobe activity and activity at other sites. In healthy subjects, increased frontal activity during word generation is associated with suppression of rCBF in the lateral temporal cortex relative to that observed during the comparison task, which entailed the articulation of words provided by the experimenter. It is probable that this relative suppression of activity, in a part of the temporal cortex devoted to processing auditory information, reflects a mechanism for reducing interference from external auditory information during the internal generation of words. The patients failed to exhibit this relative suppression. Such a failure of coordination of cerebral activity in frontal and temporal sites would be expected to lead to an increased risk of distraction, and might even predispose to the misattribution of internally generated words to an external source. In a subsequent reanalysis of those data (Liddle, 2000a), we demonstrated not only abnormal coordination between activity in the frontal and temporal cortex, but also between activity in the frontal cortex and that in other brain sites, including the thalamus and the medial aspect of the parietal lobe (see Plate 19).

Such impaired coordination of activity between different brain sites can be described as disordered functional connectivity. The term 'functional connectivity' refers to the existence of a correlation in the variation over time of cerebral activity at spatially separated sites. In a study of unmedicated first-episode patients, Fletcher et al (1996) demonstrated a similar abnormality of frontotemporal functional connectivity during word generation. However, in a subsequent study of remitted patients, my colleagues and I did not find evidence of anomalous frontotemporal connectivity, although we did observe abnormal connectivity between the left lateral prefrontal cortex and right anterior cingulate cortex

(Spence *et al*, 2000). These findings suggest that anomalous frontotemporal connectivity is more pronounced in symptomatic patients. In that study we also examined a group of obligate carriers of the genetic predisposition to schizophrenia. Obligate carriers are unaffected individuals from families in which several family members have schizophrenia and the position of the obligate carrier in the family demonstrates that he or she must have transmitted the predisposition. The obligate carriers exhibited some abnormalities of connectivity similar to those seen in the remitted patients.

Overall, the functional imaging studies demonstrate that, under a variety of circumstances, schizophrenic patients fail to activate the frontal cortex despite adequate engagement in the relevant task. However, under other circumstances, such as during paced word generation, patients can activate the prefrontal cortex to a normal degree, but the coordination of activity between the prefrontal cortex and other brain areas is abnormal. The precise details of the pattern of abnormal functional connectivity appear to depend on clinical state, although the available evidence indicates that aberrant coordination of cerebral activity is an aspect of the genetic predisposition to schizophrenia.

# Neurochemistry and pharmacology of schizophrenia

## Dopamine

The observation that blockade of dopamine $D_2$ receptors alleviates psychotic symptoms while the administration of stimulants, such as amphetamine, that promote dopamine release precipitates psychosis suggests that dopamine is overactive in schizophrenia. Laruelle *et al* (1996) have employed SPET to assess the release of endogenous dopamine in schizophrenic patients. They measured the displacement of the dopamine $D_2$ ligand IBZM from receptors in the striatum following the administration of amphetamine. The amount of IBZM displaced provides an indicator of the amount of endogenous dopamine released by the action of amphetamine. They found that the displacement of IBZM was greater in patients than in healthy controls, and that the magnitude of the displacement was proportional to the severity of induced positive symptoms. Laruelle and colleagues interpreted these observations as evidence for excessive release of dopamine in the patients. Their finding has subsequently been confirmed by Breier *et al* (1997b) using PET with the similar $D_2$ ligand, raclopride.

Subsequently, Abi-Dargham *et al* (2000) used the displacement of IBZM to estimate the change in the number of available $D_2$ receptors after depletion of endogenous dopamine using alpha-methyl-para-tyrosine. They found that the depletion procedure led to a greater increase in IBZM binding in schizophrenic patients than in controls, which indicates a greater baseline level of endogenous dopamine in the synaptic cleft before depletion in schizophrenic patients.

Furthermore, they found that the number of available $D_2$ receptors after depletion was greater in patients than in healthy controls, which indicates that the total density of $D_2$ receptors in the striatum is abnormally high in patients. Overall, these findings provide substantial evidence that dopaminergic overactivity plays a role in schizophrenia, especially in the production of positive symptoms.

The relationship of levels of dopaminergic activity to psychomotor poverty symptoms is less clear. As discussed in Chapter 8, it is plausible that psychomotor poverty reflects dopamine underactivity in the prefrontal cortex. Furthermore, the observation that failure to activate the prefrontal cortex during the Wisconsin Card Sort Test is associated with low levels of HVA in the cerebrospinal fluid (Weinberger et al, 1988) implies that impaired prefrontal function during that test is related to dopaminergic underactivity. Under many circumstances, there is evidence of a reciprocal relationship between dopaminergic activity in the prefrontal cortex and that in the striatum (e.g. Simon et al, 1988). Thus it is possible that, in schizophrenia, dopaminergic underactivity in frontal cortex coexists with dopaminergic overactivity in ventral striatum. The frontal under-activity might lead to psychomotor poverty and/or impaired executive function, while striatal overactivity would predispose to reality distortion and dis-organisation.

## Serotonin

While dopamine remains the neurotransmitter most strongly implicated in schizophrenia, there is evidence that several other transmitters play a role. The atypical antipsychotic clozapine, which blocks many different neuroreceptors, is more effective than typical antipsychotics, which block dopamine receptors, for treating hitherto resistant symptoms (Kane et al, 1988). Examination of the receptor affinities of several antipsychotics with atypical properties led Meltzer et al (1989) to propose that the atypical action of clozapine might be due, at least in part, to blockade of serotonin 5-HT$_2$ receptors. There are conflicting findings regarding abnormalities of 5-HT$_2$ receptors in schizophrenia. The balance of evidence indicates that there is decreased receptor density in the frontal cortex. In a PET study of unmedicated first-episode patients, Ngan et al (2000) found a reduction in density of 5-HT$_2$ receptors in the frontal cortex. Such a decrease might reflect a compensatory down-regulation in response to intrinsic sero-tonergic overactivity. There is little evidence that blockade of 5-HT$_2$ receptors alone has an antipsychotic effect, but Duinkerke et al (1993) demonstrated that augmentation of typical antipsychotic treatment by addition of the 5-HT$_2$ receptor blocker ritanserin produced a moderate reduction in negative (psychomotor poverty) symptoms. Chaudhry et al (1997) reported that cyproheptadine, which also blocks 5-HT$_2$ receptors, improves verbal fluency and other aspects of executive function in schizophrenia.

The second generation of antipsychotic drugs, including risperidone and olanzapine, all block serotonin 5-HT$_2$ receptors in addition to blocking dopamine $D_2$ receptors. While the most clearly established clinical advantage of these novel drugs is the reduction in extrapyramidal side-effects compared with the typical

$D_2$-blocking drugs, it has also been claimed that the novel drugs are more effective in treating symptoms, especially the negative symptoms. These claims should be treated with caution because of flaws in several of the treatment trials, especially difficulties arising from differential rates of drop-out from the studies and, in some instances, inappropriate choice of dose of the typical antipsychotic used for comparison. It therefore remains uncertain whether or not the second-generation antipsychotics are more effective than typical antipsychotics, such as haloperidol, in treating either positive or negative symptoms. None the less, there is substantial evidence that both risperidone and olanzapine are more effective than haloperidol in alleviating cognitive impairment (Green *et al*, 1997; Meltzer & McGurk, 1999; Purdon *et al*, 2000). It is plausible that 5-HT$_2$ blockade accounts for at least some of this superiority.

## Glutamate

Pharmacological agents such as the anaesthetic agent ketamine and the recreational drug PCP, which block the NMDA glutamatergic receptor, generate symptoms that resemble the reality distortion, disorganisation and psychomotor poverty symptoms that occur in schizophrenia (Javitt & Zukin, 1991). Furthermore, NMDA receptor blockade reduces the amplitude of mismatch negativity, as is seen in schizophrenia. Thus the hypothesis that glutamatergic neurotransmission is underactive in schizophrenia is plausible. Since glutamate plays such a central role in excitatory neurotransmission in the thalamus, association cortex and limbic system, disturbance of glutamatergic neurotransmission might well account for the widespread disruptions of cerebral function observed in schizophrenia.

# Synthesis and hypothesis

The evidence that genes, together with environmental influences that disrupt cerebral development, play a role in the causation of schizophrenia suggests that the relevant genes create a vulnerability to disruption of neural development. It appears that this putative disruption can result in subtle but widespread brain dysfunction. Disturbance is most apparent in the functions that engage the multimodal association cortex, which raises the possibility that there is mal-development of long-distance connections between cerebral regions. There is a slight deficit in the volume of brain tissue, not accounted for by a reduced number of neurons, in many cerebral areas, and this deficit is most pronounced in the hippocampus and thalamus. Since these sites receive especially dense projections from all areas of the association cortex, the relatively pronounced decrease in hippocampal and thalamic volume, without overt loss of neurons, supports the hypothesis that the essential pathological process is maldevelopment of long-distance connections. The functional consequence of this damage is that the coordination of activity at multiple cerebral sites, which is essential for the efficient initiation and organisation of mental activity, is impaired. Furthermore, impaired long-distance connectivity might be expected to lead to impaired regulation of the modulatory monoamine neurotransmitters, creating a predisposition to florid psychosis at times of stress.

Breier et al (1993) demonstrated that schizophrenic patients exhibit excessive production of the dopamine metabolite HVA in response to the stress of transient glucose deprivation. The magnitude of the increase in HVA is inversely correlated with frontal lobe volume, which suggests that defective frontal lobe structure creates a predisposition to excessive dopamine release at times of stress. This would be consistent with the evidence from studies of animals (Chapter 5) that indicate that projections from the frontal lobes act to buffer stress-induced subcortical dopaminergic activity. Maldevelopment of these projections might therefore predispose to excessive dopamine transmission in the basal ganglia at times of stress. As discussed in Chapter 4, this would be expected to produce excessive positive feedback to the cortex, and so promote psychomotor excitation and increase the risk of reality distortion and disorganisation.

While increased dopamine transmission might account for florid psychotic episodes, the nature of the psychotic symptoms would be determined largely by the location of aberrant intracerebral connections. Increased subcortical dopaminergic transmission combined with aberrant connections from the neocortex to the hippocampus would be expected to produce reality distortion (Chapter 6). Increased dopaminergic transmission and aberrant connections between ventral frontal cortex and other neocortical areas might result in disorganisation (Chapter 7). It should be noted that in cases with severely aberrant connectivity, reality distortion or disorganisation might persist in the chronic phase of illness, independent of dopaminergic hyperactivity. Such persistent symptoms would not be expected to respond to treatment with dopamine blockers.

Impaired connectivity between frontal lobes and other cerebral areas would be expected to lead to difficulties in the initiation of mental activity, producing psychomotor poverty symptoms (Chapter 8). Failure of connections between cerebral areas might also account for sustained cognitive impairments. Insofar as the essential problem is aberrant connectivity rather than loss of neurons, appropriate modulation by monoaminergic neurotransmitters might alleviate cognitive defects and negative symptoms. The evidence reviewed above suggests that blockade of serotonin 5-HT$_2$ receptors can indeed have such an effect. Finally, by virtue of impaired regulation of limbic function and of monoaminergic neurotransmission, patients with schizophrenia would be more vulnerable to anxiety and mood disorders in response to stress or loss (Chapters 9 and 10).

Plate 20 provides a summary of this developmental dysregulation hypothesis, according to which interacting genetic and environmental influences lead to the maldevelopment of long-range intracerebral (glutamatergic) connections, resulting in dysregulation of monoaminergic neurotransmission, and ultimately to the multiplicity of symptoms that occur in schizophrenia.

# Chapter 12

# Bipolar affective disorder

## Clinical features of bipolar affective disorder

Bipolar affective disorder is characterised by episodes of mania and of depression. Individuals who suffer only manic episodes are also described as bipolar because the available evidence indicates that the cause of and pathological mechanisms in unipolar mania are similar to those in cases with mania and depression. However, many cases of depression have relatively little in common with bipolar illness, so unipolar depression is not included within bipolar disorder. DSM–IV (American Psychiatric Association, 1994) distinguishes between bipolar 1 disorder, in which fully fledged manic episodes occur, and bipolar 2 disorder, which is characterised by less severe, hypomanic episodes, together with episodes of depression.

The features of a manic episode include prominent psychomotor excitation together with elation or irritability. Speech is rapid and difficult to interrupt. Although the patient jumps from idea to idea, a degree of connection between ideas is usually more discernible than in the disorganised thinking typical of schizophrenia. The patient's thinking is expansive and often grandiose. Self-esteem is inflated. The grandiosity can evolve into grandiose and/or paranoid delusions. Hallucinations are usually of self-reinforcing voices addressing the patient in the second person. Third-person auditory hallucinations can occur but are relatively rare. The patient has a reduced need for sleep. Behaviour tends to be disinhibited and irresponsible.

The features of a depressive episode in bipolar disorder are generally similar to those of depressive episodes occurring in major depressive disorder (see Chapter 9), although there is an increased likelihood of marked psychomotor symptoms compared with typical unipolar depression. Mixed states that combine features of mania and depression are also quite common. In a mixed state, the mood is labile and can fluctuate between elation, with associated expansiveness and grandiosity, and depression, with tears and self-depreciation, during a single clinical interview.

### Time course

Typically, the illness is characterised by discrete episodes of mood disturbance with intervening periods of normal function. There is wide variation between cases in the interval between episodes. It usually lasts many months or even years, although in rapid-cycling cases the patient can switch from mania to depression within a few days. In the early phase of the illness, episodes tend to be precipitated by stressful events (Ambelas, 1987), but once the illness is well established the episodes tend to become more frequent and less clearly related to stressful precipitants. This pattern has prompted Post *et al* (1992) to propose that a form of 'kindling' may occur in bipolar disorder. Kindling is a phenomenon observed in animals subjected to artificially induced seizures. With repeated seizure induction, the seizure threshold is lowered, so that each successive seizure requires a lesser stimulus. It is noteworthy that anticonvulsants have mood-stabilising properties, and this suggests a possible overlap between the mechanism of seizures and of bipolar mood episodes.

# Overlap with schizophrenia

Patients with either bipolar mood disorder or schizophrenia can exhibit symptoms from any of the seven major clusters of psychiatric symptoms (depression; elation; psychomotor poverty; psychomotor excitation; disorganisation; reality distortion; anxiety). Furthermore, the pattern of correlations between symptoms is similar in each disorder (Maziade *et al*, 1995), which suggests that there are similarities in the underlying pathophysiological mechanisms. In bipolar disorder, the most characteristic symptom clusters are depression, psychomotor poverty, elation and psychomotor excitation, whereas in schizophrenia the characteristic clusters are psychomotor poverty, disorganisation and reality distortion. In bipolar disorder, there is more likely to be internal consistency between the clinical features, insofar as elated mood is likely to be accompanied by grandiosity and excitation, whereas depression is more likely to be associated with low self-esteem, guilt and psychomotor poverty. Most importantly, the symptoms of bipolar disorder tend to be episodic, with relatively normal function between episodes, whereas the symptoms of schizophrenia are more likely to persist beyond the florid episodes, and there is often enduring impairment of occupational and social function. This difference in time course was the cardinal feature that prompted Kraepelin (1919) to distinguish the two disorders.

However, these differences in clinical features are a matter of degree. As discussed in Chapter 11, there appears to be a spectrum of cases, extending from those typical of Kraepelin's concept of schizophrenia (dementia praecox) to classic manic–depressive individuals who enjoy normal function between episodes of acute illness. Use of the term schizoaffective disorder provides a pragmatic solution to the problem of assigning a diagnosis to cases that are near the mid-point of the spectrum, but, in the absence of identified natural boundaries that separate the condition from schizophrenia on the one hand and manic–depressive illness on the other, the definition of schizoaffective disorder is somewhat arbitrary.

There might be a single molecular disease process, modified by pathoplastic factors that determine the relative propensity to specific symptom clusters and to chronicity of symptoms. These pathoplastic factors might be genes or environmental factors that modify the expression of the illness. Alternatively, there might be two discrete disease processes that happen to affect somewhat similar brain systems. As we examine the evidence regarding the genetic, molecular and cerebral systems anomalies in bipolar disorder, we shall pay close attention to the similarities and differences between these two conditions.

# Secondary manic or bipolar mood disorders

There are several overt brain disorders in which either mania or bipolar mood disturbances are a recognised feature. These include stroke, multiple sclerosis and HIV infection.

Mania is much less common than depression following stroke. When mania occurs, it is usually following a stroke in the right limbic areas or in the paralimbic cortex (Starkstein & Robinson, 1989). The clinical features are very similar to those of mania in bipolar affective disorder, and include both elation and psychomotor excitation. In approximately one-third of cases, post-stroke mania occurs as part of a bipolar mood disorder, in which the first episode of depression usually precedes the first episode of mania (Robinson et al, 1988). In a study of nine patients with bipolar affective disorder associated with cerebrovascular lesions, Berthier et al (1996) found that only one had a family history of affective disorder. As in the cases studied by Starkstein & Robinson, the majority of cases studies by Berthier et al had suffered lesions in the right hemisphere that involved subcortical and midline structures. Two-thirds of the cases also exhibited dyskinetic movement disorders. Berthier et al concluded that damage to fronto-basal cortico-striato-thalamo-cortical circuits by subcortical vascular lesions may simultaneously provoke disorders of movement and of mood regulation.

Binswanger's disease is a cerebrovascular disorder that affects mainly periventricular and deep white matter. Its associated mental disturbances include depression, euphoria, irritability and anxiety. These symptoms respond to treatment with mood stabilisers (Joyce & Levy, 1989).

# Genetics of bipolar disorder

In a study of the concordance between twins for affective disorders diagnosed according to Kraepelinian criteria, Bertelson et al (1977) found that the concordance in monozygotic twins was 67% while that in dizygotic twins was 20%. In cases where at least one twin had bipolar disorder, the monozygotic concordance was 79%, compared with 24% for dizygotic pairs. Furthermore, of the 32 concordant pairs, 11 were concordant for unipolar depression and 14 concordant for bipolar disorder, while in seven pairs one twin was bipolar and one unipolar. This demonstrates that the genetic factors contributing to unipolar and bipolar disorder are partially distinguishable, but a minor proportion of unipolar cases have the genetic constitution of bipolar cases.

There is also evidence for overlap between the genetic constitution for bipolar disorder and that for schizophrenia. In some multiply affected families, cases of both schizophrenia and bipolar affective disorder occur (Maier *et al*, 1993). Furthermore, the presence of psychotic depression in a pedigree increases the risk of schizophrenia in later generations (Coryell *et al*, 1985).

## Linkage and gene association analyses

During the final decades of the twentieth century, a number of inconsistent findings emerged concerning the location of genes that predispose to bipolar disorder. For example, four groups of investigators found that bipolar disorder is linked to a locus on the long arm of chromosome 4 in the region of the loci DRD5 and D4S394, while five groups did not find linkage in this area (Kennedy & Macciardi, 1998).

Another site at which there have been conflicting findings is the monoamine oxidase A (MAO$_A$) gene. This gene is a candidate of special interest because monoamine oxidase catalyses the degradation of the neurotransmitters nor-adrenaline, dopamine and serotonin. In a meta-analysis of published data, Furlong *et al* (1999) found evidence of a significant association between bipolar affective disorder and a microsatellite in intron 2 of the MAO$_A$ gene in both Caucasian and Japanese populations.

With regard to the possible overlap between bipolar disorder and schizo-phrenia, there are several regions in the genome where there are prominent indications of linkage to both conditions (Wildenauer *et al*, 1999). These sites include a narrow region in the short arm of chromosome 10, the q32 region on chromosome 13 and the q11–q13 region of chromosome 22.

Schwab *et al* (1998) have examined both association and linkage studies based on an intronic polymorphism in the candidate gene *G-olf*, located on chromosome 18, in 59 families with schizophrenia. This gene codes for a G protein that is involved in transmembrane signalling (see Chapter 5). As we shall discuss below, there is accumulating evidence for excessive G-protein-coupled transmembrane signalling in bipolar disorder. Using transmission disequilibrium analysis, Schwab *et al* found evidence of an association between schizophrenia and this gene. However, the association became much stronger when they included bipolar affective disorder, schizoaffective disorder and schizophrenia in the phenotype. Similarly, linkage analysis demonstrated significant linkage to a locus adjacent to *G-olf*. This linkage was also much stronger when the phenotype included schizophrenia, schizoaffective disorder and bipolar disorder than when bipolar disorder was excluded from the phenotype. All affected cases were heterozygous for a particular single-nucleotide mutation in the intron of *G-olf*. Thus, in these 59 families, it appears that a single mutation confers susceptibility to both schizophrenia and bipolar affective disorder.

The existing evidence indicates that susceptibility to both bipolar disorder and schizophrenia is determined by many genes, each probably exerting only a relatively minor effect in many cases. Some of these genes appear to be relatively specific for one disorder or the other, while others are linked to both.

# Cognition and information processing in bipolar disorder

On the one hand, the clinical observation that patients with bipolar illness often function well between episodes indicates that enduring cognitive deficits are not a marked feature of the illness. One the other hand, there is a substantial body of evidence indicating an association between bipolar affective disorder and mild cognitive deficits. In their study of the antecedents of psychotic illnesses in the UK National Childhood Development Study birth cohort, born in 1958 and assessed on multiple occasions in childhood, Done et al (1994) found that children who subsequently developed affective psychosis exhibited a range of cognitive impairments, especially in language and arithmetic. The average severity of these deficits was less severe than that seen in pre-schizophrenic children, but the nature of the deficits was similar. Affective psychosis was also associated with clumsiness, grimaces and poor coordination in childhood. In a study of the UK National Survey of Health and Development birth cohort born in 1946, Van Os et al (1997) found that low educational achievement and motor abnormalities such as twitches and grimaces were associated with affective disorder in general. Delayed motor and language milestones were associated with childhood-onset affective disorder.

The Swedish Conscript Study (David et al, 1997), which examined the results of psychometric testing at age 18 in army conscripts who subsequently developed psychosis, found that those who subsequently developed affective psychosis had a lower than average IQ, but not as low as was observed in those who subsequently developed schizophrenia.

These findings suggest that psychotic affective illness, like schizophrenia, is associated with indices of brain dysfunction that are likely to be of developmental origin, although the association is less strong in affective illness. Unfortunately, these studies did not explicitly separate the antecedents of bipolar disorder from those of depressive psychosis. Many other studies have reported information-processing deficits in bipolar patients that resemble deficits seen in schizophrenia, although they are usually less severe and/or more transient in bipolar disorder. These include deficits in backward masking and increased latency of the P300 ERP during detection of oddball stimuli.

## Backward masking

When an informative visual stimulus is followed closely in time by an un-informative visual stimulus, there is interference with the processing of the informative stimulus. Masking arises because the transient and sustained visual pathways detect different characteristics of a visual stimulus at slightly differing times during the early stages of processing. The thalamic and thalamo-cortical projections involved in these stages of processing are well known. Backward masking is impaired in bipolar patients during manic episodes. It is not related to the severity of psychotic symptoms and persists when mania resolves (McClure, 1999). Backward masking deficits are also common in schizophrenia.

## Event-related potentials

The P300 component elicited by oddball stimuli is decreased in amplitude in bipolar disorder, but some evidence suggests that the spatial distribution of the abnormality differs from that seen in schizophrenia, with bipolar subjects showing anterior reduction and schizophrenic subjects showing posterior reduction (Salisbury et al, 1999).

# Brain structure and bipolar disorder

The early studies applying imaging techniques to assess brain structure in bipolar disorder revealed the existence of ventricular enlargement, similar to that seen in schizophrenia but less marked (Pearlson & Veroff, 1981). Subsequently, Strakowski et al (1993) observed increased size of the third ventricle, and a trend towards larger lateral ventricles in first-episode manic patients. Roy et al (1998) found enlargement of the temporal horn of the lateral ventricle in both bipolar disorder and schizophrenia. However, several studies that have examined total cerebral grey matter volume in bipolar patients and in schizophrenic patients have reported a significant reduction of grey matter in schizophrenia but not in bipolar disorder (Harvey et al, 1994; Zipursky et al, 1997).

Studies that have focused on specific brain regions have tended to find that the maximal changes in bipolar disorder occur at loci different from those where focal changes are reported most frequently in schizophrenia. In bipolar disorder, the most substantial focal change is decreased grey matter volume in the subgenual area of the anterior cingulate (Drevets et al, 1997). In a study of first-episode patients with affective psychosis, Hirayasu et al (1999) also found reduced grey matter volume in the left subgenual cingulate gyrus in patients with a family history of affective disorder. The most robust focal changes reported in schizophrenia are enlargement of the temporal horn of the lateral ventricle and deficits in tissue volume in the medial temporal lobe and thalamus (Chapter 11). The structure of the temporal lobe has been less intensively investigated in bipolar disorder, although enlargement of the temporal horn of the lateral ventricle has been reported (Roy *et al*, 1998). Furthermore, in an MRI study of patients in the first episode of psychosis, Velakoulis *et al* (1999) found that patients with affective psychosis and those with schizophrenia/schizophreniform psychosis had smaller left hippocampal volumes compared with controls.

Small regions of strongly increased signal strength in deep subcortical white matter visible on $T_2$-weighted MRI images are consistently reported in studies of bipolar patients (McDonald *et al*, 1999). The pathophysiological significance of these hyperintensities is unknown. These hyperintensities are much less common, but do occur, in schizophrenia.

Overall, the evidence from structural imaging studies in bipolar disorder demonstrates focal loss of grey matter in the subgenual cingulate gyrus, ventricular enlargement and hyperintensities in deep subcortical white matter. There is some overlap with the structural abnormalities reported in schizophrenia but, in contrast to schizophrenia, there is little evidence for widespread loss of cortical grey matter.

# Regional cerebral activity in bipolar disorder

As discussed in Chapter 9, functional imaging studies have demonstrated that both depression and elation are associated with abnormal regional cerebral activity in the prefrontal cortex and limbic structures. However, the evidence is difficult to interpret because of apparently paradoxical findings in the ventral and medial frontal cortex, and in the cingulate gyrus. The bulk of the evidence supports the conclusion that depression is associated with reduced rCBF or metabolism in these regions, yet treatment results in a further decrease. One possible interpretation is that the predisposition to depression is associated with decreased cerebral activity in these areas, but the actual experience of depressive symptoms is associated with a transient increase relative to the abnormally low baseline.

The evidence regarding regional cerebral activity associated with mania presents a similar apparent paradox. The first functional imaging study of patients with bipolar illness revealed widespread cortical hypometabolism during the depressed state, and a widespread increase in regional metabolism during the transition from depression to a euthymic or manic state (Baxter *et al*, 1985). Subsequently, several cross-sectional studies have shown that ventromedial rCBF is abnormally low in manic patients (Rubin *et al*, 1995; Blumberg *et al*, 1999). In contrast, Goodwin *et al* (1997) found that patients who suffered manic relapse following discontinuation of lithium exhibited a relative increase in rCBF in the anterior cingulate and a trend towards a significant increase in the orbital cortex. Thus, as in the case of depression, the balance of evidence indicates that the predisposition to mania is associated with a decrease in cerebral activity in the orbital frontal cortex and cingulate gyrus, but the actual experience of manic symptoms is associated with an increase in cerebral activity in these areas, relative to the reduced baseline.

This conclusion must be regarded as tentative in the light of factors such as the likelihood that those who can tolerate the scanning procedure might not be typical manic patients. Taking the evidence regarding the regional cerebral activity associated with mania together with the evidence regarding that associated with depression leads to the hypothesis that, in the euthymic state in bipolar disorder, there is decreased cerebral activity in the orbital frontal cortex and anterior cingulate, relative to that in healthy control subjects; the experience of both mania and depression is associated with a transient increase from this diminished baseline in these areas, while, in contrast, other neocortical areas, including the dorsolateral frontal cortex, exhibit decreased cerebral activity during the depressed phase and increased activity during the manic phase. A definitive answer to this issue might be provided by a longitudinal study extending through depressed, euthymic and manic phases.

# Neurochemistry and pharmacology of bipolar disorder

## Serotonin

A substantial body of evidence indicates that underactivity of serotonergic neurotransmission might be a permissive factor in bipolar illness – that is, it provides the circumstances that allow both manic and depressive episodes to develop. The majority of studies that have measured the level of the serotonin metabolite 5-HIAA in cerebrospinal fluid (after the administration of probenecid to block the active transport of 5-HIAA out of the cerebrospinal fluid) have found that it is decreased in both mania and depression (Goodwin *et al*, 1973), which indicates a decreased turnover of serotonin. Consistent with this evidence, Young *et al* (1994) demonstrated decreased 5-HIAA and a decreased ratio of serotonin to 5-HIAA in the frontal and parietal cortex of the brains of patients with bipolar disorder, in a post-mortem study.

Thakore *et al* (1996) demonstrated that the release of prolactin induced by the indirect serotonin agonist D-fenfluramine is blunted in mania, just as it is in patients with unipolar depression. However, not all studies have confirmed this finding. For example, Yatham (1996) found that a mixture of the D- and L-isomers of fenfluramine produced normal changes in prolactin and cortisol levels in a group of 10 manic patients.

If there is sustained underactivity of serotonergic transmission in bipolar illness, compensatory up-regulation of postsynaptic receptors might be antici-pated. Ipsapirone is a selective $5\text{-HT}_{1A}$ receptor agonist that can promote increased release of ACTH and cortisol via action at postsynaptic receptors.

**207**

Yatham *et al* (1999b) found that ACTH and cortisol responses to ipsapirone were significantly increased in mania when compared with those in healthy controls, which suggests that manic patients have enhanced postsynaptic 5-$HT_{1A}$ receptor sensitivity.

If serotonin underactivity is a permissive factor, the gene coding for the serotonin transporter, which regulates synaptic levels of serotonin, is a potential candidate for involvement in bipolar disorder. In a preliminary study of a polymorphism in intron 2 of the gene for the serotonin transporter in parent–offspring trios, Kirov *et al* (1999) found that a specific allele, allele 12, was preferentially transmitted from heterozygous parents to affected offspring, although the degree of bias was relatively small. This indicates that a variant of the serotonin transporter might increase the susceptibility to bipolar affective disorder. However, the genetic effect, even if real, is likely to be small.

## Dopamine

Evidence that has accumulated over several decades strongly implicates dopaminergic overactivity in the mechanism of mania. One of the most consistent findings is that dopamine precursor L-dopa precipitates hypomania in bipolar subjects (Murphy *et al*, 1971). The indirect dopamine agonist amphetamine, in single doses (e.g. 20 mg), increases arousal in healthy subjects, and precipitates hypomania in bipolar patients (Jacobs & Silverstone, 1986). Typical antipsychotics, which block dopamine $D_2$ receptors, are effective in alleviating mania. Furthermore, the degree of pre-treatment elevation of the dopamine metabolite HVA predicts response to antipsychotic treatment in mania (Mazure & Bowers, 1998).

While there is strong evidence for dopaminergic overactivity during episodes of mania, the cardinal mechanism that predisposes to the episodic mood disturbances in bipolar disorder is likely to involve additional processes. The effectiveness of lithium in stabilising mood is one of the striking clinical features of bipolar illness, but lithium does not attenuate the arousing effects of D-amphetamine in healthy volunteers (Silverstone *et al*, 1998). Furthermore, the therapeutic effect of haloperidol, administered at a dose that is adequate to produce a very high level of blockade of dopamine $D_2$ receptors (5 mg daily), is enhanced by augmentation with lithium (Chou *et al*, 1999), which implies that there is a pathophysiological process in addition to dopaminergic excess.

Moreover, there is some potentially paradoxical evidence. In particular, using PET with the $D_2$ ligand, N-methylspiperone, Pearlson *et al* (1995) found evidence of an increased density of dopamine $D_2$ receptors in patients with psychotic mania, similar to their findings in schizophrenia. In general, it would be expected that dopaminergic hyperactivity would lead to compensatory down-regulation of postsynaptic dopamine receptors, resulting in decreased receptor density. In the case of schizophrenia, where a similar potential paradox exists, it has been proposed that there is tonic dopamine underactivity, leading to up-regulation of receptors, together with excessive phasic bursts of dopamine release. Furthermore, it is possible that the abnormal elevation of $D_2$ receptors is a feature associated specifically with psychosis, rather than with mania *per se*.

## Noradrenaline

In a post-mortem study of the brains of patients who had suffered bipolar affective disorder, Young *et al* (1994) found that noradrenaline turnover – as estimated by the ratio of the major noradrenaline metabolite, MHPG, to noradrenaline – was increased in the frontal, temporal and occipital cortex and in the thalamus.

Because of the role of noradrenaline in arousal and in sensory gating (Chapter 5), it is plausible that elevated noradrenaline activity in bipolar disorder is correlated with the level of arousal. In a comparison between bipolar patients exhibiting mixed mania and bipolar patients exhibiting agitated depression, Swann *et al* (1994) found that the MHPG level in the cerebrospinal fluid and the urinary excretion of noradrenaline were higher in patients with mixed mania than in patients with agitated depression. These findings indicate that the noradrenergic abnormalities are related to the current clinical state, but not merely to the level of psychomotor agitation.

## GABA

GABA is the major inhibitory neurotransmitter in the human brain. In particular, it exerts an inhibitory influence on noradrenergic, dopaminergic and serotonergic neurotransmission. The observation that valproate, which is a GABA agonist, is effective in treating bipolar disorder led Emrich *et al* (1980) to propose that GABA neurotransmission may be diminished in bipolar disorder. A substantial body of evidence, reviewed by Shiah & Yatham (1998), indicates that GABA activity is diminished in depression, but few studies have examined GABA function in mania. Petty *et al* (1993) found that plasma GABA levels are significantly lower in patients with bipolar illness in both manic and depressed phases, when compared with healthy subjects. This is consistent with the hypothesis that decreased GABA neurotransmission occurs in both phases of the illness. Shiah *et al* (1999) assessed the function of $GABA_B$ receptors in mania by measuring the release of growth hormone in response to the $GABA_B$ receptor agonist baclofen. They found that the growth hormone response was significantly increased in manic patients relative to healthy controls, which indicates up-regulation of hypothalamic $GABA_B$ receptors, consistent with a deficit of GABA neurotransmission.

## Second messengers and PKC

Any adequate account of neurotransmission in bipolar disorder must take account of the efficacy of mood stabilisers such as lithium, both in prophylaxis and in treating acute symptoms. As discussed in Chapter 5, a growing body of evidence implicates second messenger systems in the mechanism of action of mood stabilisers. The majority of receptors for the monoamine neurotransmitters that are implicated in mood disorders are coupled to G-proteins in the postsynaptic cell membrane. Binding of a neurotransmitter molecule sets in train a cascade of signalling processes via second messenger systems, which mobilise a variety of metabolic processes within the postsynaptic neuron. Some of these metabolic processes are regulated via enzyme phosphorylation carried out by PKC. Some of the metabolic effects produce an immediate alteration of the function of the neuron. Other effects lead to the expression of genes and the synthesis of proteins, thereby producing slower adaptive changes.

In a post-mortem study of receptor-mediated activation of G proteins in the brains of people with bipolar affective disorder, Friedman & Wang (1996) found evidence of enhanced receptor–G-protein coupling, and an increase in the trimeric state of the G proteins. While it is difficult to exclude the possibility that these changes reflect treatment effects, they are none the less consistent with the hypothesis that exaggerated transmembrane signalling is a characteristic of bipolar affective disorder. Furthermore, as discussed above, Schwab *et al* (1998) identified an association between a variant of the gene *G-olf*, which specifies a transmembrane G protein, and schizophrenia-like psychotic disorder. This association was strongest when schizophrenia, schizoaffective disorder and affective disorder were included in the phenotype.

### The phosphatidyl inositol system

One of the second messenger systems is the phosphatidyl inositol system. The function of this system depends on cleavage of inositol phosphates by the enzyme inositol monophosphatase to form myo-inositol, which is a precursor of phosphatidyl inositol. The observation that lithium inhibits the enzyme inositol monophosphatase suggests that lithium can dampen down neurotransmission by reducing the rate of production of myo-inositol. By performing serial measurements of myo-inositol in the frontal cortex, Moore *et al* (1999) demonstrated that the reduction of myo-inositol in the right frontal cortex precedes the alleviation of symptoms, which indicates that if a reduction of myo-inositol is involved in the therapeutic effect, a subsequent step is necessary to achieve the full therapeutic effect.

Lithium and other mood stabilisers also affect later steps in the signal transduction cascade, including PKC. Manji *et al* (1999a) have shown that the chronic administration of the two structurally highly dissimilar agents lithium and valproate brings about a strikingly similar reduction in PKC alpha and epsilon isozymes in the rat frontal cortex and hippocampus. In view of PKC's critical role in regulating neuronal excitability and neurotransmitter release, they postulated that PKC inhibition may have an antimanic effect. They tested this hypothesis with a trial of treatment using tamoxifen, which is a PKC inhibitor, and found that taxomifen does indeed have antimanic action.

### The cAMP system

The other main second messenger system is the cAMP system. In a post-mortem study of the brains of patients with bipolar disorder, Fields *et al* (1999) found that maximal activity of the enzyme cAMP-dependent protein kinase was significantly higher (104%) in the temporal cortex cytosolic fractions from the brains of bipolar disorder patients than in matched controls. They found that the sensitivity of the enzyme to activation by cAMP was altered. They concluded that the higher cAMP-dependent protein kinase activity in bipolar disorder may be associated with a reduction of regulatory subunits of this enzyme, reflecting a possible adaptive response of this transducing enzyme to increased cAMP signalling.

Chen *et al* (1996) found that the mood stabiliser carbamazepine, in clinically relevant doses, diminishes the production of cAMP, and also attenuates the phosphorylation of CREB. Since CREB plays a role in cAMP-stimulated gene expression, this finding indicates that carbamazepine might reduce gene expression associated with increased signalling via the cAMP second messenger system.

Overall, there are several strands of evidence supporting the hypothesis that mood stabilisers achieve their effects through inhibition of postsynaptic signal transduction. In addition, all mood stabilisers tend to suppress kindling, which makes it plausible that inhibition of signal transduction and suppression of kindling are linked (Stoll & Severus, 1996). Both mechanisms dampen the excessive intracellular and intercellular signalling that may be a core feature of bipolar disorder.

# Mechanism of switching

A clue to the mechanism by which the switch from depression to mania may occur is provided by the observation that virtually all effective antidepressant treatments can trigger manic episodes in bipolar patients. However, not all antidepressant treatments are equally potent at inducing mania. Tricyclic antidepressants are among the most potent, while lamotrigine, paroxetine and moclobemide have a lower propensity to cause switching (Calabrese *et al*, 1999). Sustained treatment with tricyclics diminishes the sensitivity of dopamine autoreceptors (Chiodo & Antelman, 1980). Since autoreceptors inhibit dopamine release, down-regulation would be expected to promote dopaminergic over-activity. It is possible that an increase in dopaminergic transmission is the trigger for switching.

# The HPA axis in bipolar disorder

The disturbance of HPA axis function that is characteristic of depression tends to be more marked during the depressive phase of bipolar illness than in unipolar illness. For example, Rybakowski & Twardowska (1999) found that, during acute depressive episodes, cortisol concentration at 16 hours after the administration of dexamethasone and cortisol release after subsequent infusion of CRF were significantly elevated in bipolar patients compared with unipolar patients and with control subjects. During remission, significantly higher cortisol concentrations were recorded after CRF infusion in bipolar than in unipolar patients. They also found that the HPA axis dysregulation increased with increasing duration of illness in the unipolar patients.

These observations are consistent with the hypothesis that disturbances of the HPA axis, reflected in elevated cortisol levels, play a triggering role in episodes of depression in both unipolar and bipolar illness. In the early phase of a unipolar depressive illness, episodes would be expected only when stress causes an elevation of the cortisol level. However, in bipolar disorder, and in the later phases of unipolar illness, spontaneous elevation of the level of cortisol, unrelated to major stress, might precipitate episodes, consistent with the observation that, in bipolar disorder and in the late phases of unipolar depression, the episodes have a more endogenous character.

Dysregulation of the HPA axis might also precede manic episodes. In a study of the release of ACTH after CRF stimulation, Vieta *et al* (1999) found that bipolar patients showed higher baseline and peak ACTH concentrations than control subjects, and that greater stimulation of ACTH release by CRF predicted manic/hypomanic relapse within six months.

# Synthesis

There is overlap between bipolar disorder and schizophrenia, not only in clinical features, but also in genetic predisposition and in abnormalities of cerebral structure and function. None the less, there are clear-cut differences between typical bipolar disorder and typical schizophrenia. As might be expected from the much lower likelihood of substantial disability between episodes, bipolar disorder is associated with fewer neurodevelopmental anomalies, and less marked deficit in grey matter volume, although, paradoxically, there is a higher prevalence of white matter hyperintensities. While there is overlap in genetic predisposition, this overlap is only partial. There is overlap in treatment insofar as antipsychotics are effective in treating reality distortion, disorganisation and psychomotor excitation in both conditions. Tricyclic antidepressants can be effective for treating depression in both conditions, although, in practice, their use is limited in bipolar disorder by the risk of precipitating manic episodes. However, the mood stabilisers lithium, carbamazepine and valproate are effective in bipolar disorder, but have a lesser role to play in schizophrenia.

On balance, the evidence indicates that bipolar disorder and schizophrenia lie at two ends of a spectrum. It is valuable to distinguish between typical cases of each disorder because treatment options and prognosis are different. However, no natural boundary between the conditions is apparent, and it is probable that cases with intermediate clinical features share the pathophysiology of both conditions.

There is also overlap between bipolar affective disorder and unipolar disorder in clinical features and genetic predisposition. In general, HPA axis dysregulation is more marked in bipolar disorder. While depression is often a less severe illness than bipolar disorder, the degree of disability between episodes is often greater in unipolar depression. The genetic evidence indicates that unipolar depression lies between bipolar disorder and schizophrenia on the spectrum that extends from mood disorder to schizophrenia (Maier *et al*, 1993).

The evidence reviewed in this chapter indicates that bipolar disorder arises from subtle maldevelopment of the brain. This maldevelopment appears to have its strongest impact on the limbic and paralimbic areas of the brain. There is circumstantial evidence indicating that repeated mood episodes lead to further damage, including increasing malfunction of the limbic regulation of the HPA axis, resulting in a lowering of the threshold for relapse. Several monoamine neurotransmitters are implicated. In particular, serotonin underactivity appears to play a permissive role for both manic and depressive episodes. Acute manic episodes are associated with overactivity of the catecholamine transmitters, while it is likely that these transmitters are underactive during depressive episodes (see Chapter 9). Accumulating evidence, especially evidence regarding the mechanism of action of mood stabilisers, implicates abnormalities in second messenger systems.

# Chapter 13

# Obsessive–compulsive disorder

## Clinical features of OCD

Obsessions are persistent ideas, thoughts, impulses or images that are experienced as intrusive and cause anxiety or distress. They are recognised as a product of the patient's own mind, despite being unwelcome. Typical examples are intrusive thoughts about contamination and persistent doubts, for example about failing to switch off electrical appliances or to lock doors, or a preoccupation with the possibility of having performed an act such as knocking down a pedestrian while driving. A patient with obsessional doubts might repeatedly check electrical switches, in some cases for a period of hours. Obsessions about germs can lead to ritual hand washing, to such an extent that the skin becomes raw. Compulsions are repetitive behaviours or mental acts performed with the object of alleviating the anxiety or distress generated by obsessions. Typical mental compulsions include ritual counting and silent repetition of words.

The major feature distinguishing obsessional thoughts from delusions is insight. The person recognises that the obsessions and associated compulsions are unreasonable, at least at some point during the illness. However, in a particular episode the person might lose this ability.

Obsessive–compulsive disorder is relatively common. The lifetime risk is approximately 2–3%, and minor obsessional symptoms more common still (Bebbington, 1998). Onset can be in childhood. The course of OCD can be episodic but in most cases it is chronic. In a study of 135 cases with illness duration of at least 10 years, Perugi *et al* (1998) found that 27.4% were episodic and 72.6% chronic. A two-year follow-up study by Eisen *et al* (1999) revealed that over the two-year period only 12% achieved full remission, while 47% achieved partial remission. The probability of relapse after remission was 48%. This relatively poor outcome cannot be attributed to inadequate treatment, as approximately 80% of the sample had received at least 12 weeks of appropriate pharmacological treatment during the period of the study.

Some cases of OCD respond to serotonin reuptake inhibitors and/or to cognitive–behavioural therapy (Hand, 1998). These two treatments are about equally effective and produce substantial improvement in approximately 25–50%

of cases. Medication and psychological treatments can be synergistic in their effects (O'Connor *et al*, 1999). In those cases that are not responsive, augmentation with dopamine blockers or with clonazepam is sometimes beneficial. In those cases where severe, disabling symptoms persist despite thorough trials of pharmacological and psychological treatment, cingulotomy might be considered. In this neurosurgical procedure, the white matter tracts in the cingulate gyrus are severed. Cingulotomy is effective in approximately 50% of cases (Jenike, 1998).

## Comorbidity

Obsessive–compulsive disorder tends to coexist with other anxiety disorders or with mood disorders (see Chapter 10). Perugi *et al* (1998) found that patients with episodic OCD are more likely to have a family history of mood disorders and have a higher lifetime comorbidity with panic and bipolar 2 disorder. As was discussed in Chapter 6, it has long been recognised that features of OCD occur in schizophrenia. Estimates of the prevalence of clinically significant OCD features in schizophrenia, in large epidemiological samples diagnosed according to modern criteria, range from 12.2% for comorbid OCD (Karno *et al*, 1988) to 59.2% for a lifetime occurrence of obsessive–compulsive symptoms in patients with schizophrenia (Bland *et al*, 1987). Using a rigorous diagnosis of schizophrenia according to DSM–III criteria, and the Yale–Brown Obsessive Compulsive Scale to score OCD features, Eisen *et al* (1997) found that 7.8% of 77 schizophrenic patients also met criteria for OCD.

# Cognition and information processing in OCD

The majority of patients with OCD usually perform normally in tests of memory and concentration, apart from a tendency to be slow (Martin *et al*, 1995). They are not impaired on executive tasks such as the Wisconsin Card Sort Test, which reflects the function of the dorsolateral prefrontal cortex (Abbruzzese *et al*, 1995). However, they do show some executive deficits. For example, in a comprehensive assessment of many aspects of cognitive function in a group of patients with OCD, Purcell *et al* (1998) found that the patients performed within the normal range on tasks involving short-term memory capacity, delay-dependent visual memory, pattern recognition, attentional shifting or planning ability; however, the patient group exhibited specific cognitive deficits related to spatial working memory, spatial recognition and the initiation and execution of motor tasks.

A small number of studies have reported more marked cognitive deficits. For example, Martinot *et al* (1990) observed significant deficits in memory and attentional tasks in a group of 16 non-depressed OCD patients, who participated in a PET study of regional metabolism. In contrast to the majority of patients with OCD, these patients exhibited decreased rCBF in the prefrontal cortex (see below). It is possible that these cases represent a more severely impaired subgroup of cases with a poorer prognosis.

In a study of ERPs using the P300 oddball detection paradigm, Miyata *et al* (1998) found that patients with OCD have reduced latency and increased amplitude of the N2 component. This finding suggests that the patients were hyper-responsive to salient stimuli. In an investigation of brain-stem auditory evoked potentials, Nolfe *et al* (1998) demonstrated that patients with OCD, and patients with generalised anxiety disorder, had a significant increase of wave I–V inter-peak latency, which implies abnormal neurotransmission of sensory information in the brain-stem (see Chapter 10).

Patients with OCD exhibit moderate deficits in pre-pulse inhibition of the startle reflex. Pre-pulse inhibition is a measure of sensorimotor gating. When a stimulus that normally elicits a startle reflex is closely preceded by a weak stimulus (the pre-pulse), the processing of the pre-pulse interferes with processing of the startle stimulus. In patients with OCD, the reaction time to the startle stimulus is slower than normal (Schall *et al*, 1996).

# Autonomic arousal

Clinical observation suggests that patients with OCD exhibit overarousal when facing situations that prompt obsessional thoughts, impulses or images, and that this overarousal diminishes after completion of the compulsion. To explore these phenomena further, Hoehn-Saric *et al* (1995) compared OCD patients with healthy controls on a number of measures of arousal. These included self-reports and psychophysiological measures such as heart inter-beat interval, skin conductance, respiration, blood pressure and electromyographic activity, during rest and also during two psychologically stressful tasks. The patients rated themselves higher on both the mental and somatic aspects of anxiety. The psychophysiological measures were not elevated at rest. During the tasks, changes in electrodermal, cardiovascular (except blood pressure) and muscle activities were smaller in patients with OCD, indicating decreased physiological flexibility. The investigators concluded that hyperarousal, measured peripherally, is not an essential pathological feature of OCD. Rather, the patients exhibit less physiological flexibility in response to environmental demands.

# Regional cerebral activity in OCD

Functional imaging studies using PET have fairly consistently indicated increased rCBF or metabolism in the orbital frontal cortex and basal ganglia of patients with OCD. For example, the early studies by Baxter *et al* (1988) demonstrated that non-depressed patients with OCD have increased metabolism in the heads of the caudate nuclei and orbital gyri, compared with healthy subjects. Similarly, Nordahl *et al* (1989) observed increased glucose metabolism bilaterally in the orbital frontal cortex, although they did not find a significant increase in the basal ganglia. In a PET study of cases of childhood-onset OCD, Swedo *et al* (1989) demonstrated increased glucose metabolism in the left orbital frontal, right sensorimotor and bilateral prefrontal and anterior cingulate regions, compared with controls.

Studies that have examined the effects of treatment on the pattern of cerebral activity in OCD report reductions in the abnormalities. Benkelfat *et al* (1990) demonstrated that the increased metabolism in the orbital frontal cortex and the head of the left caudate resolved during treatment with clomipramine. Subsequently, Swedo *et al* (1992) demonstrated that during successful treatment with clomipramine or fluvoxamine (both of which block the reuptake of serotonin) there was a significant decrease in bilateral orbital frontal cerebral glucose metabolism, relative to global metabolism. Among the treated patients, the decrease in right orbital frontal metabolism was directly correlated with two measures of OCD improvement.

In a PET study of the effects of treatment with the serotonin reuptake inhibitor fluoxetine or with behavioural therapy, Baxter *et al* (1992) found that right caudate metabolism decreased significantly in those who responded to fluoxetine, while there was a trend towards significant reduction in right caudate metabolism in those treated with behaviour therapy. Furthermore, grouping all responders together, the investigators found that, before treatment, metabolism in the right orbital cortex and thalamus correlated significantly with metabolism in the right caudate, but these correlations were not significant after treatment; this implies overactivity in the relevant cortico-subcortical circuit prior to treatment. A similar pattern of correlations was observed in the left hemisphere.

McGuire *et al* (1994) performed PET scans while patients with OCD were exposed to one of a hierarchy of contaminants that elicited increasingly intense urges to engage in compulsive rituals. The patients showed significant positive correlations between symptom intensity and blood flow in the right inferior frontal gyrus, caudate nucleus, putamen, globus pallidus and thalamus, and the left hippocampus and posterior cingulate gyrus. Negative correlations were observed in the right superior prefrontal cortex, and the temporoparietal junction, particularly on the right side. They concluded that the increases in rCBF in the orbital frontal cortex, neostriatum, global pallidus and thalamus might be related to urges to perform compulsive movements, while those in the hippocampus and posterior cingulate cortex correspond to the anxiety that accompanies them.

Thus there is consistent evidence from several PET studies that indicates that OCD symptoms are associated with overactivity in a circuit that embraces the orbital cortex, caudate and thalamus. Successful treatment with serotonin reuptake inhibitors, including clomipramine, fluvoxamine and fluoxetine, abolishes this overactivity. Furthermore, the evidence indicates that successful behaviour therapy also abolishes the overactivity in this circuit. In contrast, the PET study by Martinot *et al* (1990) (mentioned in the section on cognitive function, above) found decreased regional metabolism in the frontal cortex. Since the subjects in this study exhibited atypically marked cognitive impairments, it is possible that they were a group of patients with especially severe brain disorder.

The SPET studies of regional cerebral activity in OCD show somewhat greater variability than the PET studies. Using SPET to measure rCBF in patients with OCD and in healthy control subjects, Machlin *et al* (1991) found that the patients had a significantly higher ratio of medial–frontal to whole-cortex blood flow, but they did not find any differences in orbital frontal blood flow. In a subsequent study, the same group of investigators (Hoehn-Saric *et al*, 1991) demonstrated that treatment with fluoxetine significantly reduced the patients' 'hyperfrontality' (as determined by the ratio of medial–frontal to whole-cortex blood flow) and significantly lowered ratings of obsessive–compulsive and anxiety symptoms.

In a SPET study comparing rCBF in OCD patients with that in healthy control subjects, Lucey *et al* (1995) found significant reductions in rCBF in the patients in seven brain regions: the right and left superior frontal cortex, right inferior frontal cortex, left temporal cortex, left parietal cortex, right caudate nucleus and right thalamus. Thus they observed a reduction of rCBF relative to healthy controls in the regions in which the majority of PET studies have reported overactivity. Furthermore, they performed a factor analysis of the symptoms of their patients and identified two factors: one factor reflecting OCD phenomena, and the other reflecting anxiety and avoidance symptoms. They found that the OCD factor was negatively correlated with rCBF in the left inferior frontal, medial frontal and right parietal cortex. The anxiety/avoidance factor was positively correlated with left and right superior frontal, right inferior frontal, medial frontal cortical, and right and left caudate and thalamic rCBF.

Also using SPET, Edmonstone *et al* (1994) found a bilateral reduction of rCBF in the basal ganglia in OCD patients, but noted a positive correlation between anxiety ratings and tracer uptake in the basal ganglia in the OCD group, while Crespo-Facorro *et al* (1999) demonstrated that patients with OCD have decreased rCBF in the right orbital frontal cortex.

Thus, in contrast to the majority of PET studies, the SPET studies report normal or reduced rCBF in the orbital frontal cortex and basal ganglia, including the caudate nuclei, in patients with OCD. Despite the discrepancies, virtually all the PET and SPET studies report abnormalities in the orbital frontal cortex and caudate nucleus. Furthermore, there is consistent evidence that effective treatment leads to a decrease in activity in these brain areas. In addition, two SPET studies (Edmonstone *et al*, 1994; Lucey *et al*, 1995) report that severity of anxiety is correlated positively with rCBF in the basal ganglia (including caudate nucleus) despite an overall reduction in patients with OCD relative to healthy controls. It is noteworthy that the only PET study to record decreased activity in the orbital cortex and basal ganglia in OCD relative to healthy subjects was a study of patients who had atypically severe cognitive impairment.

As in the functional imaging studies of depression (Chapter 9) and of anxiety (Chapter 10), the PET and SPET studies of OCD reveal the paradoxical situation in which some studies report underactivity while others report overactivity at medial frontal, limbic and/or basal ganglia locations. As we proposed in the case of both depression and anxiety, the most probable explanation is that the predisposition to the disorder is associated with underactivity in these brain areas, while the actual experience of symptoms (especially the anxiety associated with obsessions) is associated with an increase from this abnormally low baseline. An alternative possibility is that increased activity in the orbital frontal cortex and basal ganglia reflects a compensatory response to OCD.

# Brain structure and OCD

There have been few studies of brain structure in OCD. Using MRI, Szeszko *et al* (1999) compared brain structure in 26 patients with OCD with that in 26 healthy controls. They found that the patients had significant reductions in tissue volume bilaterally in the orbital frontal cortex and in the amygdala. The finding of reduced orbital frontal volume is consistent with the evidence from functional imaging studies implicating this area and the associated cortico-striato-thalamo-cortical loop. The abnormality of the amygdala is consistent with the evidence indicating that the amygdala plays a central role in anxiety disorders.

# Neurochemistry and pharmacology of OCD

Clomipramine and other serotonin reuptake inhibitors relieve OCD symptoms, although the therapeutic effect builds gradually, over about eight weeks. In contrast, specific noradrenaline reuptake inhibitors are not effective, despite their efficacy in treating other anxiety disorders. Among the serotonin reuptake inhibitors, clomipramine and fluvoxamine are the most effective, which suggests that the therapeutic effect is not merely a response to serotonin reuptake inhibition but depends on some specific feature of these two medications (Stein *et al*, 1995).

Serotonin agonists can exacerbate OCD symptoms. For example, the serotonin $5-HT_{1A}$ agonist sumatriptan can produce an acute exacerbation of OCD, although sustained treatment tends to alleviate the symptoms (Stern *et al*, 1998). In a study using SPET to examine the effects of sumatriptan on rCBF, Stein *et al* (1999) found that only half the subjects experienced exacerbation of OCD symptoms, and in these subjects exacerbation was associated with a decease in frontal rCBF. Furthermore, those who suffered such an exacerbation were less likely to respond to subsequent treatment with a selective serotonin reuptake inhibitor. They concluded that exacerbation in response to sumatriptan challenge identifies a subgroup with poor prognosis. Their finding suggests that the increase in frontal rCBF seen in many other imaging studies might represent a compensatory mechanism that is mounted by 'good prognosis' cases.

Stahl (1998) proposed that the explanation for the characteristic therapeutic effects of serotonin reuptake inhibitors may be found in delayed neurochemical adaptations. He suggested that the most likely mechanism is desensitisation of somatodendritic serotonin 5-HT$_{1A}$ autoreceptors in the midbrain raphe nucleus. However, indirect evidence also implicates other serotonin receptor types. Delgado & Moreno (1998) reported that patients with OCD can experience remission of symptoms during intoxication with psychedelic drugs that have potent 5-HT$_{2A/2C}$ agonist activity. Sargent *et al* (1998) found that after eight weeks of treatment, clomipramine increases the cortisol response to the serotonin precursor 5-hydroxytryptophan. This neuroendocrine response is mediated by 5-HT$_2$ receptors. Treatment with other serotonin reuptake inhibitors also enhances the cortisol response to 5-hydroxytryptophan, but treatment with other tricyclic antidepressants does not. Sargent *et al* interpreted their data as evidence that changes in 5-HT$_2$ receptors might be linked to the therapeutic effect on OCD symptoms of clomipramine and other serotonin reuptake inhibitors.

# Synthesis

Obsessive–compulsive disorder is associated with abnormal function of the cortico-subcortical circuit projecting from the orbital frontal cortex to the caudate nucleus, thence to the thalamus and ultimately projecting back to the orbital cortex. This feedback circuit plays a role in regulating the orbital frontal cortex. Underactivity of the orbital frontal cortex is associated with disinhibited or disorganised behaviour (Chapter 7). Therefore it is plausible that overactivity in the orbital cortex, and the subcortical loop that helps regulate it, might be associated with obsessionalism. While much of the evidence indicates that patients with OCD do have overactivity at sites in this circuit, several studies demonstrate that some patients with OCD have underactivity in these brain sites. These patients have more marked cognitive impairments and less anxiety. Some of the evidence suggests that the predisposition to OCD is associated with underactivity in this circuit, and the experience of symptoms is associated with an increase in activity, while other evidence suggests that overactivity in this circuit reflects a compensatory response to the disorder in cases with a good prognosis. The efficacy of cingulotomy in alleviating severe OCD supports the proposal that excessive neural activity in the paralimbic cortex is an essential component of the pathophysiology of the condition.

The pharmacological evidence indicates that serotonin plays a crucial role. Serotonin agonists can exacerbate OCD symptoms, while reuptake inhibitors are effective in treating the disorder. However, the long time lag between the initiation of treatment and the therapeutic effect suggests that the mechanism involves adaptive changes, such as changes in 5-HT$_{1A}$ or 5-HT$_2$ receptors.

# Chapter 14

# Psychopathy

## Introduction

In the earlier chapters of Part III we have dealt with conditions that are characterised by a change in mental state from that which is usual for the individual. It is widely accepted that such changes should be regarded as illnesses. However, in circumstances in which an individual habitually exhibits a pattern of mental activity or behaviour that is markedly different from normal throughout adult life, it is not usual to label such a condition as an illness; instead, it is regarded as a personality disorder. From a practical standpoint, it can be useful to distinguish personality disorders from illnesses because personality disorders are usually more resistant to treatment. Furthermore, from an ethical perspective, it is reasonable to question whether or not it is right for doctors to attempt to change the characteristics that make people who they are. In contrast, the treatment of illnesses is generally oriented towards allowing ill people to return to their premorbid 'natural' state. None the less, the distinction between mental illness and personality disorder is not clear cut. For example, in many cases, obsessive–compulsive disorder is a remarkable, enduring pattern of behaviour that arises in childhood.

Certain clusters of abnormal mental and behavioural phenomena occur together consistently in personality disorders. It is possible that these patterns of mental and behavioural phenomena reflect consistent patterns of brain malfunction. Therefore, in this chapter we will examine psychopathy, a personality disorder whose clinical definition has been refined gradually over nearly 200 years, to a stage where the definition is sufficiently reliable to give reasonable prospects of identifying underlying patterns of brain activity.

## Clinical features of psychopathy

The concept of psychopathy has evolved, via a controversial path, from Pinel's concept of *manie sans delire*, which he applied to patients who exhibited unexplained outbursts of rage or violence but without delusions (Pinel, 1806). Within this category, Pinel included both antisocial personalities and also non-psychotic manic patients. The next significant step in defining the concept was Prichard's description of moral insanity (Prichard, 1835). He defined moral insanity as "morbid perversion of the natural feelings, affections, inclinations, temper, habits, moral dispositions and natural impulses without any remarkable disorder or defect of the intellect or knowing or reasoning faculties and in particular without any insane delusion or hallucination". Noteworthy in Prichard's list of morbid perversions is perversion of moral dispositions.

By employing words such as 'habits' and 'dispositions', Prichard implied that moral insanity was an enduring trait rather than a transient state. Broadly speaking, abnormal enduring traits reflect disorders of the personality, whereas abnormal transient states reflect mental illnesses. However, even if Prichard's definition of 'moral insanity' does exclude transient states, it none the less embraces a diverse range of morbid personalities. Furthermore, the equating of moral deficiencies with insanity might open the door to the indiscriminate use of psychiatry to deal with behaviour deemed to be socially undesirable.

The decisive step in defining the modern concept of psychopathy was taken by Cleckley. He described a personality type characterised by lack of empathy for others and lack of ability to feel remorse or shame. He identified 16 characteristics of this personality type:

(1)  superficial charm and good intelligence;
(2)  absence of delusions and other signs of irrational thinking;
(3)  absence of nervousness or psychoneurotic manifestations;
(4)  unreliability;
(5)  untruthfulness and insincerity;
(6)  lack of remorse or shame;
(7)  inadequately motivated antisocial behaviour;
(8)  poor judgement and failure to learn from experience;
(9)  pathological egocentricity and incapacity for love;
(10) general poverty in major affective reactions;
(11) specific loss of insight;
(12) unresponsiveness in general interpersonal relations;
(13) fantastic and uninviting behaviour with drink and sometimes without;
(14) suicide rarely carried out;
(15) sex life impersonal, trivial and poorly integrated;
(16) failure to follow any life plan.
(Reproduced from Cleckley, 1988, with permission.)

Cleckley's claim that this personality type identifies a discrete category of individuals has been challenged on several grounds (Blackburn, 1988). First, several of the personality characteristics specified by Cleckley occur in other personality disorders. For example, superficial charm and egocentricity occur in narcissism, while poverty in affective reactions can occur in schizoid personality. Second, several of the 16 items refer to behaviours that are not in themselves personality traits but deviant behaviours that might arise from various origins.

For example, 'fantastic and uninviting behaviour with drink and sometimes without' might arise from a variety of causes. None the less, for the most part, Cleckley's items do refer to personal characteristics. Third, the traits identified by Cleckley might be regarded as dimensions of normal personality variation without any natural demarcation that distinguishes normal from pathological.

Despite these criticisms, Cleckley's contribution was the identification of a cluster of personality traits – including features such as lack of remorse or shame, untruthfulness and insincerity, poverty of affect, shallow relationships, poor judgement and failure to learn from experience, failure to follow any life plan, and lack of insight – that tend to cluster together and are associated with a propensity towards antisocial behaviour.

Subsequently, Hare (1980) devised a Psychopathy Checklist based on Cleckley's 16 items, with guidelines for scoring based on a semi-standardised interview. The revised version of this checklist (PCL–R) has well established reliability (Hare *et al*, 1990). The PCL–R comprises 20 items. These include several that might be regarded as social behaviours, possibly of multifactorial origin, rather than intrinsic personality traits. These items include juvenile delinquency; promiscuous sexual behaviour; criminal versatility; and 'many short-lived marital relationships'. None the less, the majority of the items are personality characteristics that lie at the heart of the concept of psychopathy proposed by Cleckley. These include: conning and manipulative; lack of remorse or guilt; shallow affect; callous and lacking empathy.

Factor analysis of the items in the PCL–R reveals two major clusters of clinical features loading on separate factors (Table 14.1). Factor 1 describes a cluster of affective/interpersonal traits, including callousness and lack of empathy, central to the concept of psychopathy. Factor 2 describes traits and behaviours associated with an unstable, unsocialised lifestyle, or social deviance (Hare *et al*, 1990). These factors are strongly correlated, at least in samples of incarcerated offenders.

**Table 14.1** Items on the Hare Psychopathy Checklist – Revised (PCL–R), arranged according to their loading on the interpersonal/affective and social deviance factors

| Factor 1: Interpersonal/affective | Factor 2: Social deviance | Not loading on either factor |
|---|---|---|
| 1 Glibness and superficial charm | 3 Need for stimulation/proneness to boredom | 11 Promiscuous sexual behaviour |
| 2 Grandiose sense of self-worth | 9 Parasitic lifestyle | 17 Many short-lived marital relationships |
| 4 Pathological lying | 10 Poor behavioural controls | 20 Criminal versatility |
| 5 Conning/manipulative | 12 Early behavioural problems | |
| 6 Lack of remorse or guilt | 13 Lack of realistic, long-term goals | |
| 7 Shallow affect | 14 Impulsivity | |
| 8 Callous/lack of empathy | 15 Irresponsibility | |
| 16 Failure to accept responsibility for own actions | 18 Juvenile delinquency | |
| | 19 Revocation of conditional release | |

Items are numbered as they occur in the PCL–R.
Adapted, with permission, from Hare (1998).

Among the personality disorders defined in the DSM–IV (American Psychiatric Association, 1994), the one closest to Cleckley's concept of psychopathy is antisocial personality disorder. The essential feature of antisocial personality disorder is a pervasive, enduring pattern of disregard for and violation of the rights of others. The specific features employed in making the diagnosis are a failure to conform to social norms with respect to lawful behaviours; deceitfulness; impulsivity; aggressiveness; recklessness; irresponsibility; and lack of remorse. Apart from lack of remorse, these features are predominantly weighted towards the second factor of the PCL–R. None the less, the description of antisocial personality disorder provided in DSM–IV does specify callousness and lack of empathy as associated features. The DSM–IV criteria also specify that the person exhibited conduct disorder before the age of 15.

Broadly speaking, Cleckley's concept of psychopathy places specific personality traits at the core of the concept while regarding socially deviant behaviour as an associated factor. The DSM–IV concept of antisocial personality places the emphasis on personality features that are immediately related to observable socially deviant behaviour, while treating less easily quantified personality traits such as callousness and lack of empathy as associated factors.

In this chapter, our goal is to identify the nature of the mental and neural mechanisms underlying the intrinsic personality traits that form the core of Cleckley's concept of psychopathy. On account of the good inter-rater reliability of the PCL–R, and its fidelity to the concept proposed by Cleckley, we shall, wherever possible, rely on studies that have used this scale. It should be borne in mind that a minority of the items in the PCL–R reflect socially deviant behaviour that might arise from many different causes, so total PCL–R score is likely to be a somewhat contaminated measure of the essential core of the disorder. None the less, the high correlations usually observed between the two factors of the PCL–R indicate that the contamination is not serious.

## Comparison with pseudo-psychopathy

Injury to the frontal lobes, especially the orbital frontal cortex can result in a cluster of clinical features that include irresponsible, disorganised behaviour, shallow affect and garrulous speech. This cluster of features has been labelled pseudo-psychopathy (Blumer & Benson, 1975), although it should be noted that behaviour tends to be feckless rather than callous. While pseudo-psychopathy includes features similar to the features that comprise the impulsive component of psychopathy, the analogy with psychopathy is imperfect.

## Psychopathic behaviour and the temporal lobes

Psychopathic behaviour is observed in patients with epilepsy arising in the anterior temporal lobe (Hill *et al*, 1957). Surgical removal of the anterior temporal lobe often alleviates these behaviours. In particular, hostility is reduced and there is increased empathy and warmth in interpersonal relationships. The improvement on removal of the anterior temporal lobe implies that the psychopathic behaviours are due to pathological overactivity in the temporal lobe, rather than to destruction of brain tissue in this region.

## Time course of psychopathy

Impulsivity, social deviance and antisocial behaviour tend to diminish by middle age, but the egocentric, manipulative and callous traits fundamental to psychopathy persist throughout adult life. Harpur & Hare (1994) assessed the severity of psychopathy in 889 male prison inmates in the age range 16–69. Factor 1, representing the affective/interpersonal traits central to psychopathy, was stable across the age range, while factor 2, which represents behaviours associated with an unstable, unsocialised lifestyle, declined with age.

Several investigators have attempted to trace the roots of psychopathy in childhood. On the basis of evidence indicating that children with hyperactivity/ impulsivity/attention problems together with conduct problems (e.g. aggressive conduct; deceitfulness or theft; violation of rules or of the rights of others) are at the greatest risk for chronic offending, Lynam (1996) proposed that this combination of features identified fledgling psychopaths. In a survey of 430 boys aged 12–13 years, he found that those with these features were serious and persistent offenders, impulsive and more prone to blame problems on factors external to themselves (Lynam, 1997). In a subsequent study of a large sample of boys, he found that those with hyperactivity/impulsivity/attention problems and conduct problems were more antisocial, more disinhibited and tended to be the more neuropsychologically impaired than those with only hyperactivity/impulsivity/ attention problems, or those with only conduct problems (Lynam, 1998). While the evidence assembled by Lynam indicates that the combination of hyperactivity, impulsive behaviour, attentional problems and conduct disorder comprises a substantial risk of antisocial behaviour, antisocial behaviour is not synonymous with psychopathy. It is not certain that these children have the callousness and lack of empathy that are the core features of psychopathy. Hence it is probably premature to identify these individuals as fledgling psychopaths.

Frick et al (1994) assessed psychopathic features in a sample of 95 children referred for the clinical evaluation of behavioural problems. Factor analysis of these features revealed two dimensions of behaviour, one associated with impulsivity and conduct problems, the other associated with the interpersonal and motivational aspects of psychopathy. Scores on the impulsivity factor were highly associated with traditional measures of conduct problems. In contrast, scores for the interpersonal factor were only moderately associated with traditional measures of conduct problems, but were associated more strongly with other features, such as sensation seeking. This study confirms that psychopath-like personality features occur in childhood and segregate into two clusters, similar to the findings in adults.

Fisher & Blair (1998) examined the relationships between risk-taking strategies, the ability to recognise moral transgression, and childhood conduct problems as measured by the Psychopathy Screening Device, in 39 children with emotional and behavioural difficulties. Risk-taking strategies were assessed using a card game. Ability to recognise moral transgressions was assessed using a moral/

conventional distinction scale that assesses the child's sensitivity to the difference between moral transgressions, which result in harm to others, from conventional transgressions, which usually result in social disorder. They found that risk-taking performance and the ability to make moral/conventional distinctions were correlated. Performance on both measures predicted the extent of behavioural disturbance. These findings provide further evidence that a cluster of features typical of adult psychopaths occurs in childhood. None the less, on the current evidence, it would be premature to make a diagnosis of psychopathy in childhood.

Af Klinteberg (1996) used longitudinal data from 82 male and 87 female subjects to determine the relationship of childhood vulnerability indicators, norm-breaking behaviour in adolescence, and personality traits and biochemical measures in adulthood, with violent and non-violent criminal offences up to the age of 40. The data included teacher ratings of behaviour at age 13; self-ratings of norm-breaking behaviours at age 15; scores on the Karolinska Scales of Personality; and biochemical measures at age 26–27 years. In both the male and female groups, criminal offences during the life span were associated with childhood externalising and adolescent norm-breaking behaviour. Furthermore, high levels of norm-breaking behaviour in adolescence were associated with high impulsiveness, low socialisation and low platelet monoamine oxidase activity in adulthood in both male and female subjects. Low platelet monoamine oxidase is a biochemical indicator of psychosocial maladjustment, which we shall discuss in greater detail below.

This evidence of continuity of psychopathic features from childhood and adolescence into adulthood raises the question of what type of causal events might operate during development. Marshall & Cooke (1999) compared the childhood experiences of 50 criminal psychopaths with those of 55 criminal non-psychopaths, to determine whether the groups differed in either the type or the intensity of adverse experiences in childhood. They used the PCL–R to assess psychopathy and the Childhood Experience of Care and Abuse interview to assess childhood experiences. Both assessment measures have been shown to be reliable. Corroborative material was obtained from adult and child service providers. Factor analysis of the childhood experience variables revealed two distinct factors, familial and societal, both of which were highly correlated with adult psychopathy scores. These findings suggest that childhood experiences play a role in determining the severity of psychopathy in adulthood.

However, it is also possible that events even earlier in the development of the nervous system play a role. Anderson *et al* (1999) described two informative cases of individuals who suffered damage to the prefrontal cortex before the age of 16 months. As in typical cases of pseudo-psychopathy arising from frontal lesions in adulthood, these two individuals exhibited severely impaired social behaviour, despite normal basic cognitive abilities, in adult life. They were insensitive regarding the future consequences of decisions, showed defective autonomic responses to threat of punishment and failed to respond to behavioural interventions. However, in contrast to people suffering orbital frontal damage in adulthood, who are typically fatuous rather than callous, the two patients had defective social and moral reasoning, which suggests an impaired ability to acquire complex social conventions and moral rules.

# Genetics of antisocial behaviour

Genetic studies have generally examined the contribution of genes to criminality or antisocial personality rather than to strictly defined psychopathy. Using pooled data from seven studies, McGuffin & Gottesman (1984) calculated that the concordance for adult criminal antisocial behaviour is 51% in monozygotic twins and 22% in dizygotic twins. While the higher concordance in monozygotic twins indicates that genes play a role, the effects of parental rearing contribute to the risk. In a study of adoptees, Cadoret & Stewart (1991) found that a combination of criminality on the part of the biological parents and low socio-economic status of the adoptive parents predisposed to antisocial personality disorder and criminality. On balance, it is likely that there is a genetic influence on psychopathy, although studies employing stricter diagnostic criteria are required before any definite conclusions can be drawn.

# Cognition and information processing in psychopathy

Psychopaths do not usually exhibit widespread cognitive impairments. For example, Hart *et al* (1990) administered a comprehensive battery of neuro-psychological tests to two separate groups of 90 and 167 male prison inmates who had been assessed using the PCL–R. When the prisoners were divided into groups with high, moderate or low scores for severity of psychopathy, there were no group differences in test performance in either of the samples.

However, there is evidence of impairment on tasks that are used to assess function of the orbital frontal cortex. Lapierre *et al* (1995) compared psychopathic criminals with non-psychopathic criminals on measures related to orbital frontal or ventromedial frontal functioning (e.g. olfaction; 'go'/'no go' task performance), as well as on control measures more strongly associated with function of the dorsolateral frontal cortex and/or the parietal cortex. While the two groups performed similarly on all the control measures, the psychopaths were significantly impaired on all the orbital and ventromedial frontal tasks.

## Response inhibition and risk taking

Further evidence of abnormal function during response inhibition tasks is revealed by ERP studies during 'go'/'no go' tasks. The difference between the scalp potential recorded during 'no go' trials and 'go' trials exhibits a negative peak at frontal electrode sites approximately 400 ms after the presentation of the stimulus. This frontal negativity is regarded as an indicator of the cerebral process associated with response inhibition. Kiehl *et al* (2000b) compared ERPs in criminal psychopaths with those in criminal non-psychopaths during perform-ance of a simple 'go'/'no go' task in which the subjects were required to respond to an arrow pointing in one direction, and to inhibit responding to an arrow pointing in the opposite direction. The task was so easy that neither non-psychopaths nor psychopaths made many errors, and there was no significant difference between the groups in error rate. Trials in which the participants made errors were excluded from the analysis. The non-psychopaths exhibited the predicted frontal negativity during 'no go' trials compared with 'go' trials. This frontal negativity was significantly reduced in psychopaths. Thus, even in trials during which the psychopaths performed correctly, they exhibited evidence of abnormal neural activity in the cerebral circuits implicated in response inhibition.

Howland *et al* (1993) found that psychopaths were more likely to make incorrect responses in a cued reaction time task when the cues were ambiguous, but only when responding with their right hand. They interpreted this as evidence that psychopaths are less likely to inhibit well established dominant responses.

In tasks that involve selective attention, psychopaths are prone to ignore warning cues in favour of stimuli that interest them (Jutai & Hare, 1983). Studies that assess risk-taking strategies indicate that adolescents with psychopathic traits are over-responsive to rewards (Quay, 1988). For example, Shapiro *et al* (1988) found that adolescents with high scores for conduct disorder continued to respond to the possibility of reward in a card-playing task under circumstances where the risk of punishment was increasing. Similarly, Scerbo *et al* (1990) found that adolescent psychopaths were more strongly influenced by the possibility of reward when participating in a game that involved learning when to respond to cards associated with either reward or penalty. Overall, the evidence indicates that psychopaths exhibit motivational biases that predispose to risk taking.

## Processing affective material

There is also evidence that psychopaths exhibit abnormal processing of affect-laden verbal material. Williamson *et al* (1991) administered a lexical decision task employing both affect-laden and neutral words, and pseudo-words (formed by substituting vowels), to both criminal psychopaths and a control group of criminal non-psychopaths. The subjects were required to judge whether or not each item presented was a word. Reaction time was measured. In addition, ERPs were recorded using scalp electrodes. The non-psychopaths were significantly faster in making the lexical decision for affective words than for neutral words, and the relevant ERP components were significantly larger. In sharp contrast, psychopaths failed to show either facilitation of reaction time or larger ERPs to affective words.

In a subsequent study, Kiehl *et al* (1999a) presented words with negative emotional connotations and emotionally neutral words and the participant was required to make a judgement about emotional significance. Both criminal psychopaths and criminal non-psychopaths responded more rapidly to the emotional words. However, the non-psychopaths exhibited ERPs for emotional words that differed significantly from those for neutral words, whereas this difference was not significant in psychopaths. While the observation that psychopaths responded more rapidly to emotional words implies some difference in their processing of emotional and neutral words, the lack of the normal ERP difference indicates less difference in the neural processing between emotional and neutral words than occurs in non-psychopaths.

## Semantic processing

Kiehl *et al* (1999a) also recorded ERPs in criminal psychopaths and criminal non-psychopaths during two more tasks that involved semantic processing. In the first task, abstract words, concrete words and pseudo-words were presented, and the participants were required to determine whether or not the presented item was a word or pseudo-word. All participants responded faster to concrete words than to abstract words. The non-psychopaths also exhibited ERPs for abstract words that differed significantly from the ERPs for concrete words, which implies different neural processing of abstract words, but the psychopaths failed to show this differentiation. In the second task, concrete and abstract words were presented and the participants were required to determine whether the word was concrete or abstract. The non-psychopaths exhibited ERPs for abstract words that differed from those for concrete words. The psychopaths made more errors and, furthermore, failed to exhibit significant differences between the ERPs for abstract and those for concrete words. Both of these studies indicate that psychopaths fail to process abstract words in a normal manner.

## Frontocentral negativity

In all three of the single-word processing tasks presented in the studies by Kiehl *et al* (1999a), the ERPs of the psychopaths included a large frontocentral negative-going electrical component (N350) irrespective of word type or content. This component was absent or very small in the non-psychopaths. In a separate study, Kiehl *et al* (1999b) recorded ERPs in criminal psychopaths and criminal non-psychopaths during a visual oddball stimulus detection task. In this task, too, the psychopaths exhibited a larger frontocentral negative component (N550) during the target condition than did non-psychopaths. This latter study not only confirmed that psychopaths exhibit abnormal neural processing, even in a very simple stimulus detection task, but also provides yet another instance in which psychopaths exhibit an aberrant frontocentral negative component in the time interval 300–600 ms after stimulus presentation. Furthermore, the occurrence of this frontocentral negative component during a simple, non-linguistic task implies that it is not confined to language tasks.

Large frontocentral negative components in this time window during trials that entail response to a stimulus are rarely observed in ERP studies. However, such components are seen in patients with lesions of the anterior temporal lobe (Johnson, 1988; Yamaguchi & Knight, 1993). This observation raises the possibility that psychopaths may have a malfunction of the anterior temporal lobe, and is consistent with several studies that have shown an association between localised temporal lobe electroencephalographic abnormalities and aggressive psychopathy. For example, Hill & Waterson (1942) found slow-wave activity localised to the temporal lobe in 14% of 194 habitually aggressive psychopaths. Kurland *et al* (1963) observed positive spiking in the temporal region in 40% of impulsive aggressive psychopaths. Howard (1984) found an association between posterior temporal slow-wave activity and high psychopathy scores on the Minnesota Multiphasic Personality Inventory.

## Hemispheric lateralisation

Several studies have found evidence of reduced hemispheric lateralisation for language in psychopaths. In a verbal dichotic listening task, Hare & McPherson (1984) found that criminal psychopaths had less right-ear advantage than criminal non-psychopaths. Raine *et al* (1990) observed a similar decrement in right-ear advantage in adolescent psychopaths. Hare & Jutai (1988) found that psychopaths exhibited a left-visual-field advantage during performance of a semantic categorisation task.

## Summary of cognition and information processing in psychopathy

While psychopaths do not usually exhibit widespread cognitive impairment, they do exhibit deficits in several specific domains, including response inhibition, as assessed in 'go'/'no go' tasks; in the processing of emotional information; and in processing abstract information. Furthermore, there is evidence indicating diminished hemispheric specialisation for language. These deficits implicate the frontal cortex and the temporal lobe.

# Regional cerebral activity in psychopathy

Intrator *et al* (1997) used SPET to measure rCBF during the processing of words with emotional connotations. They found that the psychopaths exhibited more activity than healthy subjects in the lateral temporal lobe during the processing of affective words. This apparently paradoxical result was confirmed by my colleagues and me in an fMRI study of regional cerebral activity during a task that entailed the learning, rehearsal and subsequent recognition of words (Kiehl *et al*, 2000c). Half the blocks of words were emotionally neutral while the other half were emotionally negative. In healthy subjects, learning the emotional words was associated with significantly greater activity in limbic and paralimbic areas, such as the amygdala and anterior cingulate. In contrast, psychopaths did not exhibit a significant increase in activity in limbic and paralimbic areas, but instead exhibited greater activity in the left temporal pole and inferior posterolateral frontal cortex (Plate 21). Thus psychopaths exhibit evidence of differences in cerebral activity when processing emotional words compared with neutral words, but, in contrast to healthy subjects, these differences are not in cerebral areas that have a recognised role in emotional processing.

In another fMRI study, we found that healthy subjects produced greater activation of the right anterior temporal lobe and posterolateral frontal cortex during the processing of abstract words relative to that during the processing of concrete words (Kiehl & Liddle, unpublished data). The amount of activation in these areas during the processing of abstract words relative to concrete words was significantly less in psychopaths. This finding is consistent with the evidence that psychopaths have an impaired ability to process abstract information. It might also be interpreted as evidence consistent with decreased hemispheric specialisation for linguistic processing.

# Autonomic reactivity

Psychopaths exhibit reduced autonomic arousal under at least some circumstances. For example, Hare (1978) found that criminals with high scores for psychopathy and low scores for socialisation exhibited smaller skin conductance responses to 120 dB sounds than did other groups, when presented with a random series of tones having either a fast or a slow rise time and ranging in intensity from 80 to 120 dB. He interpreted this as evidence that psychopaths are electrodermally hyporesponsive to intense stimuli that do not signal the need for a specified response.

# Neurochemistry and pharmacology of psychopathy

There is substantial evidence indicating disturbances of the modulatory mono-amine neurotransmitters in impulsive aggressive behaviour. In particular, low levels of the serotonin metabolite 5-HIAA are observed in the cerebrospinal fluid of patients with a propensity to impulsive aggression directed against either self or others (Linnolia et al, 1983; Lidberg et al, 1985a). Many studies have demonstrated a negative correlation between platelet monoamine oxidase activity and impulsivity and other antisocial behaviours (Lidberg et al, 1985b; Schalling et al, 1987; af Klinteberg, 1996). Platelet monoamine oxidase activity is weakly correlated with 5-HIAA levels in the cerebrospinal fluid. While the evidence implicating abnormalities of serotonin in impulsivity is strong, it is unclear whether psychopathy itself is associated with abnormal serotonergic neurotransmission.

Several studies have reported that prolactin release in response to the indirect serotonin agonist fenfluramine is decreased in individuals with impulsive aggressive personalities (Coccaro *et al*, 1989; Moss *et al*, 1990; O'Keane *et al*, 1992). In a study that attempted to tease apart possible abnormalities of serotonergic neurotransmission associated with impulsive aggressive behaviour from those associated with the callous and non-empathic aspects of psychopathic behaviour, Netter *et al* (1999) examined the relationships between psychopathic characteristics in healthy males and the results of four tests that reflect different aspects of serotonergic function. They measured prolactin and cortisol release following challenge with fenfluramine, and also following challenge with the serotonin 5-HT$_{1A}$ agonist ipsapirone. The cortisol response to ipsapirone reflects action at postsynaptic receptors. Fenfluramine promotes the release of serotonin from presynaptic nerve terminals. They related the neuroendocrine challenge results to each of two personality dimensions: impulsive aggression and psychoticism. In the personality inventory they employed, psychoticism referred to an emotionless, non-empathic personality style.

They found that in response to ipsapirone, cortisol release was blunted in those with high impulsive aggression whereas prolactin release was blunted in those with high psychoticism. Conversely, in response to fenfluramine, cortisol release was blunted in those with high psychoticism while prolactin release was blunted in those with high impulsive aggression. This complex pattern of results implies that abnormalities of serotonergic neurotransmission are associated with both impulsive aggression and with the emotionless, non-empathic aspects of psychopathy, but in different ways. However, the pattern of abnormalities revealed by currently available data is too complex to allow a simple interpretation.

Both testosterone and thyroid hormone levels are related to aspects of psychopathy. For example, Stalenheim *et al* (1998a) demonstrated that serum levels of total testosterone and sex hormone-binding globulin were correlated with socially deviant behaviour, reflected in factor 2 of the PCL–R. Alm *et al* (1996) demonstrated that serum levels of the thyroid hormone tri-iodothyronine were elevated in former juvenile delinquents who exhibited persistent criminal behaviour. Subsequently, Stalenheim *et al* (1998b) demonstrated that serum levels of tri-iodothyronine are elevated in criminals with high psychopathy scores, while, conversely, the free thyroxine level is decreased.

# Synthesis

The combined evidence from neuropsychological testing, electroencephalography, ERP recording and functional brain imaging clearly establishes that the function of circuits concerned with emotional processing, response inhibition and the processing of abstract language are impaired in psychopaths. These circuits embrace limbic structures such as the amygdala, paralimbic cortex, lateral frontal cortex and temporal polar cortex. Furthermore, the neurochemical evidence indicates that diminished serotonergic neurotransmission is associated with at least some of the clinical features of psychopathy.

The observation that diminished serotonergic function, as indicated by decreased levels of 5-HIAA in the cerebrospinal fluid, is associated with impulsive violence occurring in other mental conditions, such as suicidality in depressed patients (Lidberg *et al*, 1985a), suggests that this particular abnormality is associated with impulsive violence rather than with the core features of psychopathy. None the less, the finding by Netter *et al* (1999) that abnormalities of serotonergic neurotransmission are associated not only with impulsive aggression but also with the emotionless, non-empathic aspects of psychopathy suggests that serotonergic abnormalities are involved in all aspects of psychopathy.

At first sight, the observation that overt damage to the orbital frontal cortex in adult life produces a pseudo-psychopathic syndrome characterised by feckless behaviour and shallow emotions, but lacking callousness and lack of empathy, might suggest that the orbital cortex is involved only in the aspects of psychopathy that reflect behavioural and emotional dysregulation. However, the cases reported by Anderson *et al* (1999), in which damage to the prefrontal cortex occurring before 16 months led not only to pseudo-psychopathic features, but also to defective social and moral reasoning, raises the possibility that the crucial factor in the genesis of the full psychopathic syndrome is disruption of the frontal cortex at an early stage of development.

The evidence that we have reviewed suggests the hypothesis that the primary event causing psychopathy is disruption of the early development of frontotemporal circuits. This disruption might be determined by genes or by environmental factors that damage the brain *in utero* or during infancy. This hypothesis would not rule out the possibility that events later in childhood, such as economic deprivation (Cadoret & Stewart, 1991) or other adverse childhood experiences (Marshall & Cooke, 1999), might influence the expression of the condition.

Just as adverse childhood circumstances might have an adverse influence on the expression of psychopathy, it is possible that favourable circumstances might minimise the behavioural expression of the disorder. The performance of the psychopaths in our fMRI study of cerebral activity during the processing of emotional words suggests that they recognised, at least subliminally, the emotional significance of words (Kiehl *et al*, 2000c). The imaging data indicated that they recruited neocortical language processing areas to compensate for a deficit in limbic processing. These findings suggest that it is possible for psychopaths to minimise the behavioural manifestation of the disorder by employing alternative strategies. The evidence that psychopathy is associated with deficits in the processing of abstract language suggests that concrete strategies are likely to be most appropriate.

The evidence that the behavioural disorders represented by factor 2 of the PCL–R diminish with age suggests that these disorders might be treated by appropriate modification of modulatory neurotransmitters, such as serotonin. On the other hand, the interpersonal characteristics such as callousness tend to be more enduring and hence are likely to be less amenable to pharmacological modification. None the less, the evidence that even these attributes are associated with serotonergic abnormalities (Netter *et al*, 1999) provides some grounds for hope that they might be modified by pharmacological treatment.

# Epilogue

The immense complexity of the human mind and brain will continue to present major challenges. Substantial progress has been made in delineating the anatomical locations and the chemical neurotransmitters implicated in mental symptoms, although the details, at a molecular level, of the mechanisms by which brain systems facilitate the normal activities of the mind, and the processes that disrupt these mechanisms in mental illness, are still largely unknown. For many years, the barrier to progress was the inaccessibility of the human brain in life. While we still lack the ability to observe and measure the electrical and chemical events of neural signalling in the living human brain on the time scale of action potentials and the spatial scale of the individual synapse, currently available imaging techniques allow us to measure local brain activity in populations of neurons localised fairly well in either space or time.

In the last decade of the twentieth century, functional imaging techniques such as PET and fMRI provided images of the kaleidoscope of neural activity associated with mental processes. Initially, we were satisfied to identify which specific brain sites were engaged during a particular mental process, and which sites were under- or overactive in individuals with mental disorder. As we have seen in this book, mental symptoms reflect aberrant activity in circuits that are distributed widely in the brain. The next generation of progress is likely to include the delineation of the ways in which activity is coordinated in these distributed circuits, and how the coordination can be disrupted by disease.

The mapping of the human genome ranks as one other major contribution of the closing years of the twentieth century to our understanding of ourselves. Not only did the techniques of molecular genetics make it possible to read virtually the entire sequence of trinucleotide elements that form the code specifying the composition of all the proteins that make up the human body, but these techniques have also provided many tools for exploring the role that these proteins play in the function of the body. For example, the ability to knock out the expression of a particular gene during a particular phase of development, in laboratory animals, makes it possible to explore the role of the protein specified by that gene in both the developing and the mature brain. The genes that code for a human being have been decoded and, in principle at least, we can delineate the function of the animal homologues of the proteins specified by those genes.

Furthermore, the delineation of the mechanisms by which the brain activity associated with mental events modifies gene expression in the brain, and therefore changes the molecular composition of brain cells, has provided an understanding of how psychological processes are not only related to current brain activity, but can also modify future brain function.

The chasm that separated psychological descriptions of human function from descriptions in the terminology of neuroscience had a destructive influence on psychiatry in the middle years of the twentieth century. Modern neuroscience has not triumphed over psychology; indeed, *Hamlet* still provides more insight into some aspects of human behaviour than all the knowledge accumulated using the techniques of neuroscience. But we now have a bridge across the chasm.

The stigma of mental illness is likely to diminish as its mechanisms are understood, and increased understanding is likely to lead to more rational treatment strategies. However, this understanding will also create new challenges. The debate regarding the nature and extent of human autonomy and responsibility for one's own actions is no longer confined to a philosophical speculation on the nature of free will. As we begin to understand the ways in which brain abnormalities predispose to behaviour that is harmful to self or others, it will be necessary for individuals to re-evaluate the way in which they take responsibility for their own mental well-being, and for society to re-evaluate the way in which it deals with those who cause harm to others.

The depressed individual may find relief through treatment with medication that modifies neurotransmission directly, and or by psychological strategies that influence the same neurotransmitter pathways. It is likely that, in many circumstances, medication will provide relief more rapidly, and there may be a temptation to abdicate responsibility for one's own mental health. However, the understanding provided by neuroscience and by psychology suggests that full recovery requires far more than the resetting of the level of activity of a few neurotransmitters. It is unlikely that neuroscience will ever provide a blueprint that can predict every thought and every feeling in each individual. Consequently, the concept of autonomy is likely to continue to have a place in any adequate model of human behaviour. One of the goals of psychiatric practice should be the integration of neuroscience and psychology not only to promote the relief of a patient's symptoms, but also to help the patient acquire greater capability to influence his or her own mental function.

In the realm of personality disorders, the evidence that a disorder such as psychopathy arises from disordered development of the brain raises the question of whether or not psychopaths should be held accountable for their actions. The brain abnormalities associated with psychopathy may increase the propensity to act in an antisocial manner; they will not predict with certainty how an individual will behave in specific circumstances on a particular occasion. According to current legal criteria in the UK and in the USA, psychopaths have sufficient understanding of their behaviour to take responsibility for their actions. However, while society may reasonably hold a psychopath responsible for his or her actions, justice should perhaps be tempered by the evidence that disordered brain development may contribute to the individual's propensity to take that action. In the longer term, it is possible that the emerging neuroscientific understanding of psychopathy will not only inform these judgements, but also provide the basis for effective treatment and rehabilitation.

# Glossary

**acetylcholine**: A neurotransmitter molecule. In the central nervous system, it is employed by neurons with cell bodies located in nuclei in the basal forebrain area, whose axons project widely throughout the cerebral cortex and the basal ganglia. It acts as a modulator of neural activity, facilitating selective attention and promoting memory formation. It is also a major neurotransmitter in the peripheral nervous system, where it mediates the neural control of skeletal and smooth muscle.

**action potential**: The propagating wave of electrical depolarisation, which conveys information along the axon of a neuron. It is generated by the opening of ion channels that allow the passage of ions through the cell membrane, thereby reducing the polarisation of the membrane that exists in the resting state, due to differences in ion concentrations across the membrane.

**adrenaline**: A molecule consisting of a catechol ring structure and an attached amine group that is employed as a neurotransmitter in the sympathetic division of the autonomic nervous system. It is also a hormone released from the medulla of the adrenal gland. It mediates 'fight or flight' responses.

**adrenergic**: Pertaining to neuronal activity mediated by the neurotransmitter adrenaline (epinephrine) or noradrenaline (norepinephrine).

**adrenocorticotrophic hormone** (ACTH): A hormone produced in the anterior lobe of the pituitary gland. It acts on the adrenal gland to stimulate the release of glucocorticoid hormones, including cortisol.

**affect**: A person's immediate emotional state, experienced subjectively, and recognisable objectively by others. Mood is the predominant affect over a time interval.

**affective disorders**: Disorders of affect and mood. The principal affective disorders are major depressive disorder, dysthymia, and bipolar mood disorder.

**afferent**: Pertaining to input. Afferent fibres are axons conducting information toward a specified set of neurons.

**agitation**: Excessive motor activity accompanied by a feeling of inner tension. The activity is usually non-productive and repetitive. Typically, it consists of behaviour such as pacing, fidgeting or wringing of hands.

**agnosia**: Failure to recognise or identify objects despite intact sensory function.

**agonist**: A molecule that binds to a neuro-receptor and alters it in a way that brings about the action normally mediated by that receptor. A full agonist is capable of producing the maximal effect that can be produced by stimulating that receptor. A partial agonist is capable only of producing less than the maximal effect, even when administered in concentration sufficient to occupy all available receptors. An indirect agonist promotes the release of the endogenous agonist from presynaptic terminals. An inverse agonist is a molecule that binds to the relevant receptor, but produces a physiological effect opposite to that produced by the usual agonist.

**agoraphobia:** Anxiety about being in places or situations from which escape might be difficult or embarrassing or in which help may be unavailable in the event of a panic attack. (Typically, fear of leaving home, being in a crowd, or travelling in a train.)

**akathisia:** Continuous restless movements accompanied by a sense of inner restlessness, commonly produced by treatment with antipsychotic medication.

**akinesia:** A state of diminished or absent voluntary movement.

**akinetic mutism:** A state of apparent alertness but with no speech or voluntary motor responses, apart from eye movements.

**alogia:** An impoverishment of thinking that is inferred from a reduced amount of informative speech. Replies are typically brief and there is little spontaneous speech (poverty of speech), or, alternatively, speech conveys little information due to being too concrete, too abstract, repetitive, or stereotyped (poverty of content of speech).

**Alzheimer's disease:** A progressive dementia with characteristic pathological changes in cerebral tissue, including deposition of amyloid protein, senile plaques and neurofibrillary tangles, most marked in temporal and parietal cortex.

**amnesia:** Loss of memory.

**amygdala:** A component of the limbic system located adjacent to the uncus in the antero-medial part of the temporal lobe (plates 4,5,11). It is part of the neural system mediating fear.

**angular gyrus:** A portion of the inferior parietal lobule that arches over the posterior end of the superior temporal sulcus. Lesions result in difficulties with reading and writing.

**anhedonia:** Reduced ability to experience pleasure from activities that normally generate pleasure.

**antagonist:** A molecule that can bind to a neuro-receptor without producing the normal effect of stimulation of that receptor, while none the less preventing endogenous and exogenous ligands from binding effectively to the receptor.

**anterior commissure:** A white matter bundle that crosses the midline of the brain in the lamina terminalis, at the rostral end of the third ventricle. It connects the temporal lobes (plate 5).

**anxiety:** The apprehensive anticipation of danger or future misfortune, accompanied dysphoric mood and/or somatic symptoms of tension, including autonomic arousal. Anxiety is often distinguished from fear, in that fear is in due proportion to a real threat or danger, whereas anxiety arises from threat that is perceived rather than real, or is out of proportion to a real threat.

**apathy:** Lack of feeling, motivation, or interest.

**aphasia:** Impaired understanding or production of language, arising from damage to the brain.

**apraxia:** Inability to perform previously learned motor activities despite intact comprehension and motor function.

**aqueduct** (cerebral aqueduct): The narrow conduit for cerebrospinal fluid, connecting the third ventricle and fourth ventricle within the midbrain (plate 5).

**archicortex:** Three layered cerebral cortex, of early evolutionary origin, located in the limbic structures on the medial aspect of the cerebral hemispheres.

**articulatory loop:** A component of the working memory system, that holds material in mind by means of subvocal speech.

**association cortex:** Cerebral cortex that integrates information from diverse sources. Sensory association cortex processes complex features of a sensory stimulus. Multimodal association cortex integrates information from diverse sensory modalities and information reflecting motivation and goals.

**ataxia:** Impaired coordination of voluntary muscular movement.

**athetosis:** Slow, random, writhing movements, especially of the arms and legs, arising from dysfunction of the motor system. It can be a side-effect of dopamine-blocking antipsychotic medication.

**attention:** The ability to focus in a sustained manner on a particular stimulus or activity.

**auditory cortex:** Primary auditory cortex is located in the transverse temporal gyrus (Heschl's gyrus) on the superior aspect of the temporal lobe (plate 2). It receives auditory input from the medial geniculate nucleus of the thalamus, and projects to association auditory cortex on the superior temporal gyrus.

**auditory hallucination:** The perception of a sound, usually a voice or voices, not arising from a sensory stimulus. The term pseudo-hallucination is sometimes used when the person is aware that the sound arises from within.

**autonomic nervous system:** The neural system responsible for regulating vascular and visceral activity in the body. It consists of two divisions: the sympathetic system, which employs adrenaline as a neurotransmitter, and the parasympathetic system which employs acetylcholine. The sympathetic system increases readiness for fight or flight. The parasympathetic system promotes body-maintenance functions, such as digestion.

**autoreceptor:** A neurotransmitter receptor located on the presynaptic terminal or cell body of a neuron that binds the neurotransmitter that is produced by that neuron. Activation of an autoreceptor inhibits further release of the neurotransmitter, thereby allowing a neurotransmitter to regulate its own release.

**avolition:** An inability to initiate and sustain goal-directed voluntary activities.

**axon:** The filamentous portion of a neuron that transmits electrical action potentials carrying information from soma to the presynaptic terminal, where the neuron makes functional contact with other neurons, muscles, or glands.

**axon collateral:** A branch of an axon.

**backward masking:** The blocking of recognition of a sensory stimulus caused by a second sensory stimulus presented a brief time later (typically up to 100 milliseconds later).

**basal ganglia:** A collection of grey matter nuclei located deep in the brain, including the caudate nucleus, putamen and ventral striatum (together forming the corpus striatum), the globus pallidus, the subthalamic nucleus, and the substantia nigra.

**Basal Nucleus of Meynert:** A grey-matter nucleus of the basal forebrain, from which cholinergic neurons project widely to the cerebral cortex.

**beta-blocker:** A pharmaceutical agent that inhibits the action of beta-adrenergic receptors, and thereby lowers blood pressure, dilates blood vessels and decreases arousal. Used in the treatment of hypertension, cardiac arrhythmias, anxiety-related tremors, neuroleptic-induced akathisia, social phobias, panic states and alcohol withdrawal.

**bipolar affective disorder:** A mood disorder characterised by episodes of mania (or hypomania) and depression. Mood disorders with only manic episodes are also considered bipolar.

**bizarre delusion:** A delusion that involves a phenomenon that is totally implausible.

**blocking:** A transient obstruction or interruption of the spontaneous flow of thought or speech, perceived as an absence of thought.

**blunted affect:** A reduction in the intensity of emotional expression.

**bradykinesia:** Abnormal generalised slowness of motor activity.

**brain stem:** Subcortical portion of the central nervous system connecting the diencephalon to the spinal cord. It comprises the medulla (adjacent to the spinal cord), pons and midbrain (adjacent to the diencephalon).

**Broca's area:** The speech-area in the inferior frontal cortex of the dominant hemisphere, usually the left, that coordinates the production of fluent speech.

**Capgras' syndrome:** The delusion that others have been replaced by impostors.

**catalepsy** (waxy flexibility, cerea flexibilitas): A form of catatonic behaviour that involves maintenance of an unusual body or limb posture for an extended period.

**239**

**catatonic behaviour:** Abnormalities of voluntary motor function, including catalepsy; stupor; purposeless excessive motor activity unrelated to external stimuli; negativism; mutism; posturing or stereotyped movements; echolalia; and echopraxia.

**caudal:** Towards the tail.

**caudate nucleus:** A C-shaped component of the basal ganglia located adjacent to the lateral ventricle, and bounded by the internal capsule (plate 5), consisting of a head, body and tail. The head is in the frontal lobe while the tail is in the temporal lobe. The caudate nucleus, putamen and ventral striatum constitute the corpus striatum.

**cavum septum pellucidum:** An atypical space between the two membranous layers of the septum pellucidum. It can occur in healthy individuals and has no known functional consequence, but is regarded as a minor anomaly of development.

**central executive:** The component of working memory that directs the function of slave systems such as the articulatory loop and the visuo-spatial scratch pad.

**central sulcus:** A prominent fissure separating the frontal lobe and parietal lobe. Primary motor cortex is located in its anterior (frontal) bank, and primary somato-sensory cortex in its posterior bank. Also called the Rolandic fissure (plate 1).

**cerebellum:** A component of the brain lying in the posterior cranial fossa, below the fibrous sheet known as the tentorium cerebelli and posterior to the brain stem. It consists of a median vermis and two lateral hemispheres (plates 1 and 5). The cerebellum modifies, coordinates and regulates motor activity, and also participates in higher mental functions by virtue of its connections with prefrontal cortex.

**cerebral hemispheres:** Paired hemispherical structures that develop as vesicles extruded from the diencephalon at the rostral end of the central nervous system, and eventually envelop it. The hemispheres are covered by cerebral cortex, a sheet of grey matter that is indented by deep fissures (sulci). Beneath the cortex is white matter containing fibres travelling to and from the cortex, while yet deeper lie the basal ganglia.

**cholecystokinins:** A group of peptide molecules found in the brain and gastrointestinal tract. In the brain they can act as neurotransmitters.

**cholinergic neurons:** Neurons that release the neurotransmitter, acetylcholine. In the central nervous system, their cell bodies are located in basal forebrain nuclei, such as the Basal Nucleus of Meynert.

**chorea:** A movement disorder characterised by irregular, involuntary jerking movements involving mainly the distal limb muscles. It can be a side-effect of treatment with dopamine-blocking antipsychotic medication, or due to degenerative changes in the caudate and putamen.

**choroid plexus:** A composite layer of cells attached to the walls of the ventricles that are specialised to secrete cerebrospinal fluid (plate 5).

**cingulate gyrus:** A gyrus composed of paleocortex, on the medial aspect of each cerebral hemisphere. It arches over the corpus callosum (plate 3). The anterior part consists of an emotional division, located adjacent to and below the genu of the corpus callosum, and cognitive division involved in response selection, adjacent to the junction of the genu and body of the corpus callosum.

**circumstantiality:** Speech that is indirect and delayed in achieving its goal because of excessive or irrelevant detail or parenthetical remarks.

**clanging:** A disorder of thought form in which the sound of a word, rather than its meaning, directs subsequent associations.

**classical conditioning:** The acquisition of a conditioned response to a conditioned stimulus as a result of pairing of the conditioned stimulus with an unconditioned stimulus that produces the response automatically.

**claustrum:** A thin sheet of grey matter between the insula and the extreme capsule, in each cerebral hemisphere (plate 5). Its function is uncertain.

**cognitive:** Pertaining to thoughts or thinking.

**commissure:** A fibre tract that crosses the midline of the brain or spinal cord to connect homologous areas of grey matter.

240

**comorbidity:** The simultaneous occurrence of two or more illnesses, such as the co-occurrence of schizophrenia and OCD or of alcohol dependence and depression.

**compulsion:** An excessive, unreasonable repetitive behaviour (such as hand-washing) or mental act (such as counting) performed to minimise the risk of a dreaded event or situation. The behaviour is usually recognised by the patient as excessive or unreasonable.

**concrete thinking:** Thinking characterised by overly literal, non-abstract interpretation of language or events.

**continuous performance task** (CPT): A test of sustained attention in which a series of stimuli, including designated target stimuli, is presented. The participant is required to respond when the target is presented. In the widely used AX version, the target is X, but only when it follows the letter A.

**coronal plane:** A plane of section through the brain, orientated vertically and extending from left to right.

**corpus callosum:** The largest commissure connecting the cerebral hemispheres (plate 3). It has four parts: the rostrum, genu, body and splenium (at the caudal end).

**corpus striatum:** A term for the three contiguous masses of grey matter (caudate nucleus, putamen and ventral striatum) that receive the main afferent fibres from the frontal cortex to the basal ganglia. The myelinated (white) fibres of the internal capsule pass through the dorsal part of the corpus striatum, partially separating the caudate and putamen, which none the less remain connected by bridges of grey matter (plate 5).

**cortex, cerebral:** The sheet of grey matter on the surface of the cerebral hemisphere. It is folded into gyri in such a way that much of its area is buried in the fissures (sulci).

**corticotrophin-releasing factor** (CRF): A peptide molecule that acts as a modulator in the neural and humoral systems that mediate responses to stress. CRF produced in the paraventricular nucleus of the hypothalamus is secreted into the blood supplying the anterior lobe of the pituitary gland where it promotes the release of ACTH. CRF receptors are also located at many other sites in the brain, especially in the limbic system and in the locus coeruleus.

**cortisol:** A steroid hormone produced by the adrenal gland that regulates many physiological processes in the body. In particular, it promotes glucose metabolism at times of stress and regulates immune responses. An excess of cortisol damages body tissues.

**cyclic adenosine monophosphate** (cAMP): A phosphorylated compound produced from adenosine triphosphate by the enzyme adenylate cyclase. On account of the energy released on sundering the phosphate bond, cAMP is capable of initiating many metabolic processes. In particular, it acts as a second messenger initiating a cascade of metabolic processes in postsynaptic neurons (plate 13).

**declarative memory:** Memory for facts or propositions. Declarative memory includes episodic and semantic memories, but not procedural memories.

**déjà vu:** The unjustified sensation or illusion that one is seeing what one has seen before.

**delirium:** A state of confusion with disorientation, due to sudden disruption of brain function.

**delusion:** A firmly fixed belief based on incorrect inference or unjustified assumption that cannot be accounted for on the basis of culture or religion. Types of delusion (based on content) include: bizarre delusions; delusional jealousy; grandiose delusions; delusion of reference; persecutory delusions; somatic delusions; thought broadcasting; and thought insertion.

**delusion of reference:** A delusional belief that events, objects, or other persons in one's immediate environment have an unusual significance that is related to oneself. An idea of reference has similar content but is not as firmly held.

**delusional jealousy:** The delusion that one's sexual partner is unfaithful.

**delusional mood:** A feeling that something unusual is about to happen of special significance for that person.

**delusional perception:** The misinterpretation of a normal perception as proof of an unrelated idea.

**dendrite:** A branching assemblage of filamentous processes typically extending several hundred microns from the soma (body) of a neuron, which constitutes the principal receptive component of the neuron.

**dendritic spines:** Small spike-like appendages arising from the dendritic shaft onto which synaptic contact is made. A typical pyramidal cell in the cerebral cortex bears several thousand dendritic spines.

**dentate gyrus:** A component of the hippocampal formation, with macroscopic appearance resembling a row of teeth, which lies adjacent to the CA4 region of the hippocampus (plate 9). It is the source of mossy fibres, which are the fibres that transmit the major input into the hippocampus (plate 10).

**depersonalisation:** An alteration in the experience of the self so that one feels detached from, or an external observer of, one's mental processes or body.

**depressed mood:** A symptom characterised by feeling sad or low in spirits.

**depression syndrome:** A cluster of signs and symptoms that includes pervasive depressed mood, together with characteristic cognitions concerning low self-esteem, guilt, or hopelessness, and somatic symptoms including sleep and appetite disturbance.

**derailment** ('loosening of associations'): A pattern of speech in which a person's ideas slip off one track onto another that is completely unrelated or only obliquely related. The slippage occurs between clauses, in contrast to incoherence, in which the disturbance is within clauses.

**derealisation:** An alteration in the perception of the external world so that it seems strange or unreal (e.g. people may seem unfamiliar or mechanical).

**dichotic listening task:** A task in which different stimuli are presented simultaneously to left and right ears. Such tasks assess the degree to which processing in one hemisphere dominates over the other. There is normally a right ear (left hemisphere) advantage for processing speech.

**diencephalon:** The brain region that connects the cerebral hemispheres to the rest of the central nervous system. It lies at the rostral end of the developing central nervous system, and the vesicles that become the cerebral hemispheres are extruded from it. Its major components are the thalamus and hypothalamus. It also includes the epithalamus (consisting of the pineal body and habenula nucleus – a small component of the limbic system adjacent to the postero-medial aspect of the thalamus) and the subthalamus (a nucleus closely connected to the basal ganglia).

**disorganisation syndrome:** A cluster of symptoms including formal thought disorder, inappropriate affect and bizarre behaviour, which occurs in various psychotic disorders, especially in schizophrenia.

**disorientation:** Confusion about the time of day, date, or season (time); one's current location (place); or who one is (person).

**distractibility:** Impaired ability to maintain attention, due to attention being drawn to unimportant or irrelevant external stimuli.

**distributed representation:** A meaningful mental event (e.g. a perception or a memory) is represented by neural activity in a large number of processing units. A given unit can participate in the representation of more than one event.

**dopamine:** A catecholamine molecule comprising a catechol ring structure with a substituted amine group, which acts as a neurotransmitter that acts to modulate the level of cerebral activity. The main dopamine pathways project from the substantia nigra to the dorsal striatum (the nigrostriatal system that regulates motor function); from the VTA in the midbrain to the ventral striatum and frontal cortex (the mesolimbic and mesocortical systems that regulate motivation and responses to stress); and from the hypothalamus to the pituitary gland (the tubero-infundibular system that inhibits prolactin release).

**dyskinesia:** Involuntary, abnormal muscular activity.

**dysphoria:** An unpleasant mood, such as feeling sad, ill-at-ease, or anxious.

**dystonia:** Disordered muscle tone, typically involving sustained contraction of muscles. Commonly affects external ocular muscles, neck, or trunk musculature.

**echolalia:** The apparently senseless repetition (echoing) of a word or phrase just spoken by another person.

**echopraxia:** The involuntary imitation of the movements of another.

**efferent:** Pertaining to output. The efferent fibres of a neuron are its axon and axon collaterals. The efferent pathway of a nucleus or cortical area is the collection of axons carrying output from the nucleus or cortical area.

**elevated mood:** An exaggerated feeling of well-being, elation.

**endogenous:** Generated from within.

**enkephalin:** A neurotransmitter molecule consisting of a short to medium length amino acid chain, having opiate-like effects, located in many areas of the brain, such as the striatum, limbic cortex, paralimbic cortex and raphe nuclei.

**entorhinal cortex:** The anterior part of the parahippocampal gyrus that projects to the hippocampal formation. It receives its main input from the parahippocampal area in the posterior part of the parahippocampal gyrus. Macroscopically, it is distinguished by the presence of verucca-like lumps on its surface.

**episodic memory:** A long-term store of information about specific personal events.

**euthymic:** Mood in the 'normal' range.

**event-related potentials** (ERPs): Shifts in electrical potential relative to a baseline value (recorded from the scalp, or from the brain itself) that have a consistent temporal relationship to a specific perceptual, cognitive or motor event.

**executive mental function:** The management of mental activity, including the initiation, selection and monitoring of activity, and the contextual coding of events.

**expansive mood:** Lack of restraint in expressing one's feelings, frequently with an overvaluation of one's significance or importance.

**extrapyramidal signs:** Motor abnormalities arising from malfunction of the basal ganglia.

**fimbria:** A component of the hippocampal formation, which contains axons from the pyramidal cells of the hippocampus (plate 9). Posterior to the hippocampal commissure, these axons coalesce to form the fornix (plate 4).

**flat affect:** Decreased intensity of affect.

**flight of ideas:** Accelerated speech, with rapid changes of topic that are usually based on understandable associations, distracting stimuli, or plays on words.

**formal thought disorder:** Disturbance in the form of thinking typically seen in psychotic disorders. The most common types entail disruption of the connections between words or ideas (e.g. derailment, tangentiality, incoherence); peculiar sentence construction; or idiosyncratic use of words (e.g. neologisms).

**fornix:** A bundle of axons from the hippocampus that arch beneath the corpus callosum to terminate in the septal nuclei (located at the base of the septum pellucidum), mamillary body (on the posterior aspect of the hypothalamus) and ventral striatum (plates 3 and 4).

**frontal lobe:** The part of the cerebral hemisphere lying anterior to the central sulcus, and antero-medial to the Sylvian fissure. It contains the prefrontal cortex, anterior and mid-cingulate cortex, frontal eye fields, premotor and supplementary motor areas, and primary motor cortex (plate 1).

**frontal pole:** The rostral tip of the frontal lobe.

**functional magnetic resonance imaging** (fMRI): A technique for imaging brain function that employs the fact that local neural activity leads to a local change in concentration of deoxygenated haemoglobin. Since deoxyhaemoglobin is paramagnetic, this change alters the magnetic environment, and hence produces a local change in the intensity of the image.

**fusiform gyrus:** A gyrus located on the inferior aspect of the temporal and occipital lobes, lying between the parahippocampal gyrus, medially, and the inferior temporal gyrus, laterally (plate 3). It is also called the occipito-temporal gyrus. Its diverse functions include visual object recognition and semantic processing (in the dominant hemisphere).

**gamma-aminobutyric acid** (GABA): An amino acid that acts as an inhibitory neurotransmitter. GABAergic neurons are the predominant inhibitory local circuit neurons in the cerebral cortex.

**gamma oscillations:** High frequency (25–80 Hertz) oscillations in electrical potential that can be recorded in the brain (or from the overlying scalp) and reflect the coordinated firing of assemblies of neurons.

**glia:** Non-neuronal cells in the nervous system. Glial cells include oligodendrocytes and Schwann cells that make myelin, and microglia that can transform into phagocytes.

**globus pallidus:** A component of the basal ganglia medial to the putamen (plate 5). It receives input from the putamen and sends output to the thalamus or to the sub-thalamic nucleus.

**glutamic acid:** An amino acid that functions as an excitatory neurotransmitter. Glutamatergic neurons, which use glutamate as their transmitter, are the most prevalent neurons in the cerebral cortex. They include pyramidal cells, which project from cerebral cortex to distant regions, and also excitatory local circuit neurons.

**go/no go tasks:** Tasks in which the participant is required to make a response to designated stimuli and refrain from responding to other stimuli. Such tasks are employed to test the ability to inhibit contextually inappropriate responses.

**G-protein:** A protein associated with a metabotropic neurotransmitter receptor in the membrane of a postsynaptic neuron, which initiates a cascade of metabolic processes in the neuron following binding of the relevant neurotransmitter molecule to the receptor (plates 13 and 14).

**grandiose delusion:** A delusion of inflated worth, power, identity, or special relationship to a famous person or deity.

**grandiosity:** An over-estimation of one's worth, power, importance, or identity.

**granular cells:** Non-pyramidal cells in the cerebral cortex. Most have relatively short axons and participate in local circuits.

**grey matter:** The tissue comprising the bodies (soma) of nerve cells and their non-myelinated processes, together with glia. It forms a folded sheet (the cerebral cortex) on the surface of the brain, and is also found in sub-cortical nuclei, such as the basal ganglia and thalamus.

**habituation:** A change in the response to a stimulus (usually a diminution of response) as a result of continuing or repeated exposure to the stimulus.

**hallucination:** A sensory perception with the sense of reality of a true perception occurring without external stimulation of the relevant sensory organ.

**hippocampal formation:** A folded sheet of tissue located mainly in the medial temporal lobe, containing the subiculum, hippocampus, dentate gyrus and fimbria (plate 9).

**hippocampus:** An elongated roll of three-layered archicortex, lying mainly in the medial part of the temporal lobe, adjacent to the inferior horn of the lateral ventricle (plates 4,5,9). It plays a role in declarative memory, in the control of the autonomic functions, and in emotional expression.

**homovanillic acid** (HVA): A major metabolite of the neurotransmitter, dopamine.

**hydroxyindole acetic acid** (5-HIAA): A major metabolite of the neurotransmitter, serotonin.

**hypnagogic:** Pertaining to the semiconscious state immediately preceding sleep; hypnagogic hallucinations can occur in healthy individuals.

**hypnopompic:** Pertaining to the state immediately preceding awakening; hypnopompic hallucinations can occur in healthy individuals.

**hypothalamic-pituitary-adrenal axis** (HPA axis): The system comprising hypothalamus, pituitary gland and adrenal gland that regulates the secretion of hormones from the adrenal gland to adjust the level of physiological activity throughout the body to meet current needs.

**hypothalamus:** The part of the diencephalon beneath the hypothalamic sulcus (plate 5). It coordinates the activity of the sympathetic and parasympathetic autonomic system that regulates visceral functions such as drinking and feeding, and also regulates the endocrine output of the pituitary gland.

**ideas of reference:** Incorrect interpretations of casual incidents and external events as having direct reference to oneself.

**illusion:** A misperception or misinterpretation of a real external stimulus, such as hearing the sound of a car engine as the sound of voices.

**inappropriate affect:** An abnormal affect that does not match the content of what is being said or thought.

**incoherence:** Speech or thinking that is essentially incomprehensible to others because words or phrases within a clause are combined without a logical or meaningful connection. (Also called word salad).

**inferior temporal gyrus:** An area of association cortex on the infero-lateral aspect of the temporal lobe that receives input from visual association cortex and other areas of association cortex (plate 1).

**inositol triphosphate** ($IP_3$): A molecule containing inositol, together with three phosphate groups, that acts as a second messenger in the phosphatidyl inositol system, which mediates a cascade of metabolic events in a postsynaptic neuron following binding of a neurotransmitter molecule to a receptor on the cell membrane (plate 14).

**insomnia:** A complaint of difficulty falling or staying asleep or poor sleep quality.

**insula:** The region of cerebral cortex buried within the lateral (Sylvian) fissure (plate 5).

**interhemispheric fissure** (or longitudinal fissure): The midline space separating the two cerebral hemispheres.

**internal capsule:** A band of white matter composed of axons entering and leaving the cerebral cortex. Its posterior limb separates the thalamus (medially) from the basal ganglia (laterally) while its anterior limb separates the caudate nucleus from the putamen (plate 5).

**interneuron:** A local-circuit neuron whose short axon provides excitatory or inhibitory connections within a grey matter region.

**ionotropic receptors:** Neurotransmitter receptors that change in conformation on binding of the relevant neurotransmitter in such a way as to open a channel for the passage of ions through the postsynaptic cell membrane.

**labile affect:** An affective state characterised by abnormal sudden rapid shifts.

**lateral fissure** (Sylvian fissure): The deep fissure on the lateral aspect of the cerebral hemisphere separating the temporal lobe from the frontal lobe (anteriorly) and from the parietal lobe (posteriorly) (plates 1 and 5).

**lateral geniculate body or nucleus:** A nucleus on the postero-lateral aspect of the thalamus that relays visual information from the ganglion cells of the retina to the primary visual cortex.

**L-dopa:** (levo-dihydroxyphenylalanine): The levo isomer of the hydroxylated amino acid, phenylalanine. In dopaminergic nerve terminals, a carboxyl group is removed from L-dopa to form the neurotransmitter, dopamine.

**245**

**learning:** The acquisition and storage of information, or the improvement in performance of some task with practice. Categories of learning include verbal, visuo-spatial, affective, cognitive and motor.

**lexical decision task:** A task in which the participant is required to decide whether a stimulus is a word or not. The non-word stimuli might be either pseudo-words that obey the orthographic rules of the language or letter strings that violate the orthographic rules.

**lexicon:** The stored representation of words and their meanings.

**ligand:** A molecule that binds to a specific receptor.

**limbic system:** A collection of archi-cortical areas and sub-cortical nuclei on the medial aspect of the cerebral hemispheres that play a major role in emotion and in declarative memory. Its major components are the septo-hippocampal and the amygdala/basal forebrain systems (plate 4).

**local-circuit neurons** (interneurons): Neurons with short axons that participate in circuits confined to a local brain region.

**locus coeruleus:** A nucleus in the rostral pons containing noradrenaline (norepinephrine) neurons that project widely in the brain, and mediate arousal.

**long-term memory:** The maintenance of information about past events and experiences in a store that is outside of consciousness.

**loosening of associations:** A disturbance of thinking made manifest by speech in which ideas shift from one subject to another that is unrelated or minimally related to the first.

**mamillary bodies:** Bilateral protuberances on the caudal aspect of the hypothalamus, which receive input from the hippocampus via the fornix and project via the mamillo-thalamic tract to the anterior nucleus of the thalamus. They play a role in declarative memory.

**manic–depressive disorder:** See bipolar disorder.

**medial forebrain bundle:** A pathway in the lateral hypothalamus, connecting the basal forebrain with the midbrain. Its fibres project indirectly via the reticular formation to pre-ganglionic sympathetic and parasympathetic viscero-motor neurons.

**medial geniculate nucleus or body:** A nucleus on the ventro-posterior aspect of the thalamus that relays auditory information from the inferior colliculus to primary auditory cortex located in the transverse gyrus of Heschl in the temporal lobe.

**memory:** A mental process that acquires and maintains information over a sustained period, and allows its retrieval at a later time. Types of memory include declarative memory (episodic and semantic) and procedural memory.

**metabotropic receptors:** Neurotransmitter receptors that are linked to membrane bound G-proteins in such a way that binding of the relevant neurotransmitter molecule to the receptor leads to a cascade of intracellular metabolic processes.

**3-methoxy-4-hydroxyphenylglycol** (MHPG): A major metabolite of noradrenaline.

**midbrain** (mesencephalon): The rostral portion of the brain stem, containing the tectum, aqueduct, tegmentum and cerebral peduncles. Anterior to the aqueduct lies the ventral tegmentum, which contains dopaminergic neurons that project to the ventral striatum and cortex; and the substantia nigra, which contains dopaminergic neurons projecting to the dorsal striatum. The midbrain also contains the rostral raphe nuclei from which serotonergic neurons project to the cerebral cortex.

**middle temporal gyrus:** The middle gyrus of the three gyri on the lateral surface of the temporal lobe (plate 1).

**monoamine neurotransmitters:** Neurotransmitter substances whose chemical structure includes an amine group. Monoamine transmitters include the catecholamines, noradrenaline (norepinephrine) and dopamine; and the indoleamine, serotonin. They largely act as modulators that adjust the tone of neural activity.

**mood:** A pervasive and sustained emotional state that colours the perception of the world, and influences motivation. In contrast to affect, which constitutes the fluctuating moment-to-moment emotional 'weather', mood is the more pervasive and sustained underlying emotional 'climate'. Types of mood include: euthymic (normal), dysphoric, depressed, elevated, elated, expansive and irritable.

**myelin:** A multi-layered sheath surrounding axons, which acts as an electrical insulator and facilitates rapid conduction of electrical signals.

**myo-inositol:** A form of inositol that is the precursor for the phosphorylated inositol compounds involved in the phosphatidyl inositol intracellular signalling pathway. The second messenger, inositol triphosphate, is de-phosphorylated to form myo-inositol, which is subsequently incorporated in phosphatidyl inositol. Eventually, with the binding of a neurotransmitter molecule, the phosphatidyl inositol is further phosphorylated to form inositol triphosphate again (plate 14).

**negative symptoms:** Symptoms that reflect the diminution or absence of a function that is present in normal individuals. The core negative symptoms characteristic of schizophrenia include poverty of speech, flat affect and decreased voluntary movement.

**negativism:** Apparently motiveless resistance to instructions or to being moved.

**neocortex:** Six-layered cortex of relatively recent evolutionary origin that covers 95% of the surface of the cerebral hemispheres.

**neologism:** an invented word, not in the normal lexicon, arising from a disorder of thought or language.

**neuron:** A cell capable of receiving, processing and transmitting the electrical signals that carry information in the nervous system.

**neuropil:** The packing between nerve cell bodies in grey matter. It contains axons, dendrites, synapses and glial cell processes.

**neurotransmitter:** A chemical that mediates transmission of signals between neurons. Propagation of an action potential to the terminal of the presynaptic neuron triggers the release of neurotransmitter molecules into the synaptic cleft between the neurons. Binding of the neurotransmitter molecules to a receptor on the surface of the postsynaptic neuron results in electrical and/or chemical changes in the postsynaptic neuron.

**N-methyl-D-aspartate** (NMDA): An amino acid that binds preferentially to a specific class of excitatory neurotransmitter receptors (known as NMDA receptors) that play a diverse range of roles in the brain. The usual endogenous agonist at NMDA receptors is glutamate. Activation of NMDA receptors allows the influx of calcium ions and sodium ions into the postsynaptic terminal. Under some circumstances, activation can have a toxic effect on the postsynaptic neuron.

**noradrenaline:** A molecule comprising a catechol ring structure with an amine group attached, that acts as a neurotransmitter in the central nervous system. It is employed by neurons with cell bodies in or near the locus coeruleus, in the brain stem, and projects widely to cerebral cortex. It acts as a modulator that increases the level of arousal in response to stimuli.

**nucleus accumbens:** The nucleus accumbens is a distinct mass of grey matter on the inferior, medial aspect of the head of the caudate nucleus, in rodents. It plays a role in converting motivation to action. The human homologue is the ventral striatum.

**obsession:** A recurrent, intrusive and distressing thought, impulse, or image, that is recognised as being an excessive and unreasonable product of one's own mind.

**obsessive–compulsive disorder** (OCD): A mental disorder characterised by obsessive thoughts, impulses or images, that tend to generate anxiety; and compulsions, which are repetitive behaviours or mental acts that the person feels obliged to perform to alleviate the anxiety.

**occipital lobe:** Cerebral cortex beneath the occipital bone and posterior to the parieto-occipital sulcus (plate 1). It is mainly involved in processing visual information.

**oddball stimulus:** A sparsely distributed stimulus interposed at irregular intervals in a series of regular stimuli. The oddball stimulus differs from the regular stimuli in a characteristic such as pitch.

**olfactory bulb:** A grey matter protuberance at the end of the olfactory tract, on the orbital surface of the brain. The bulb and tract arise as an evagination from the developing cerebral hemisphere. The bulb receives input from the olfactory epithelium and projects via the olfactory tract to olfactory cortex.

**olfactory cortex:** Cortex involved in perception of odour. It includes the anterior perforated substance anterior to the optic tract on the brain's basal surface (perforated by small blood vessels supplying the basal ganglia); the parolfactory area and adjacent subcallosal gyrus below the genu of the corpus callosum; and the periamygdaloid cortex in the uncus.

**olfactory hallucination:** A hallucination involving the perception of odour in the absence of an external olfactory stimulus.

**operant conditioning:** The acquisition of a specific response to a stimulus mediated by receipt of a reward that reinforces the response to the stimulus.

**orbitofrontal cortex:** The ventral surface of the prefrontal cortex (plates 3 and 5).

**overvalued idea:** An unreasonable and sustained belief, not ordinarily accepted by other members of the person's culture; it is held with less conviction than a delusion.

**paleocortex:** Six layered cortex located mainly on the medial aspect of each cerebral hemisphere that is of evolutionary origin intermediate between three layered archicortex and six layered neocortex.

**panic attacks:** Discrete episodes with sudden onset of intense apprehension, fear, or terror, often associated with fear of losing control or going crazy, and with somatic symptoms such as shortness of breath, palpitations, pounding heart or accelerated heart rate, chest pain or discomfort, or a sensation of being smothered or choking. Uncued panic attacks occur without an identified situational trigger; cued panic attacks occur on exposure to, or in anticipation of, a situational trigger.

**parahippocampal gyrus:** The most medial gyrus on the inferior surface of the temporal lobe (plate 3). It receives input from all modes of sensory association cortex, and from multimodal association cortex and the cingulate gyrus. Its anterior portion, the entorhinal cortex, projects to the dentate gyrus of the hippocampal formation.

**parallel processing:** Processing occurs simultaneously in multiple processing units.

**paranoid ideation:** Ideation involving suspiciousness, or the unreasonable belief that one is being harassed, persecuted, or treated unfairly.

**paraventricular nucleus** (PVN): A nucleus in the hypothalamus adjacent to the third ventricle, that projects via the hypothalamohypophyseal tract to the posterior lobe of the pituitary gland.

**parietal lobe:** The region of cortex posterior to the central sulcus, superior to the lateral (Sylvian) fissure, and anterior to the line joining the pre-occipital notch to the parieto-occipital notch (plate 1).

**Parkinson's disease:** A degenerative disease in which the dopaminergic fibres projecting from the substantia nigra to the dorsal part of the corpus striatum are lost, leading to tremor, rigidity and difficulty initiating movement.

**peptides:** Molecules consisting of short chains of amino acids. In the brain they are found in neurons and have many of the properties of neurotransmitters. They often coexist in the same presynaptic terminal with GABA or with a monoamine neurotransmitter.

**periamygdaloid cortex:** Cortex in the vicinity of the uncus (plate 3) that receives olfactory input from the olfactory bulb, together with input from other modalities.

**persecutory delusion:** A delusion in which the central theme is concerned with being attacked, harassed, cheated, persecuted, or the subject of a conspiracy.

**perseveration:** Unwarranted repetition of the same verbal or motor response.

personality: The enduring patterns of perceiving, evaluating and relating to the environment and oneself, that are characteristic of the individual, and are exhibited in a wide range of contexts. When personality traits are inflexible and cause either significant functional impairment or subjective distress, they constitute a personality disorder.

phobia: A persistent, irrational fear of a specific object, activity, or situation (the phobic stimulus) that results in a compelling desire to avoid it. This often leads to avoidance of the phobic stimulus.

pineal gland or body: An endocrine gland located behind the third ventricle, that arises as an evagination of the diencephalon. It secretes the hormone melatonin, and plays a role in maintaining circadian rhythms.

pituitary gland: An endocrine gland at the base of the brain, whose posterior lobe is formed by evagination of the brain, and anterior lobe by evagination of the roof of the mouth. It produces hormones (e.g. ACTH, gonadotophic hormones) whose roles include regulation of peripheral endocrine glands, such as the adrenal gland and the gonads. It is subject to regulation by neural input from the hypothalamus and to regulatory feedback via adrenal and gonadal hormones.

pons: The region of the brain-stem that encloses the fourth ventricle. Its posterior aspect is covered by the cerebellum.

positive symptoms: Mental symptoms that reflect the presence of mental activity that is not normally present in healthy individuals. Hallucinations and delusions are considered positive symptoms.

positron emission tomography: A technique that provides images of the spatial distribution of a tracer chemical that has been injected into the body after labelling with a positron-emitting isotope. The tracer chemical may be a molecule that binds to a specific receptor in the body, or takes part in a physiological process of interest. When the radioactive isotope decays, a positron is emitted and then annihilated on contact with a nearby electron, generating two gamma rays that travel in opposite directions. Coincident detection of the two gamma rays by detectors external to the body provides information of the direction of travel of the gamma rays and facilitates construction of an image of the spatial distribution of the tracer chemical. If the tracer is water labelled with a positron-emitting isotope of oxygen, the image represents regional cerebral blood flow, which is strongly correlated with local neural activity.

postcentral gyrus: The gyrus posterior to the central sulcus (plate 1). It contains primary somato-sensory cortex.

posterior commissure: White matter crossing the midline at the junction of the midbrain and thalamus, carrying fibres connecting the pre-tectal regions of the midbrain.

poverty of speech: A pathological decrease in the amount of speech generated.

precentral gyrus: The gyrus immediately anterior to the central sulcus (plate 1). It contains primary motor cortex, organised in a somatotopic manner, with the area representing the face inferiorly, near the lateral (Sylvian) fissure, while the lower parts of the body are represented superiorly. Parts below the knee are represented on the medial surface, in the paracentral lobule. The axons projecting from the precentral gyrus form a part of the cortico-spinal and cortico-bulbar motor tracts.

prefrontal cortex: The anterior part of frontal cortex, including all cortex anterior to the frontal eye-fields and premotor cortex.

premotor cortex: The somatotopically-organised motor area immediately anterior to the precentral sulcus (plate 2). It projects to primary motor cortex, and also contributes axons directly to the cortico-spinal tract.

pressured speech: Rapid speech that is difficult or impossible to interrupt.

prevalence: The total number of cases of a disorder existing within a unit of population at a given time or over a specified period.

**priming:** Facilitation of the processing of a stimulus by presentation of another related stimulus. The relationship can be based on habitual proximity (e.g. the word 'table' can facilitate processing of the word 'chair') or on meaning (semantic priming – e.g. the word 'hot' can facilitate processing of the word 'cold').

**procedural memory:** The establishment of facility in a behavioural skill by virtue of practice. (Contrast with declarative memory.)

**prodrome:** An early or premonitory phase of a disorder, prior to the onset of specific clinical features characteristic of the disorder.

**prolactin:** A hormone secreted by the anterior lobe of the pituitary gland that promotes lactation and also helps maintain the menstrual luteal phase. Its secretion is inhibited by dopamine.

**proprioception:** A sense of the position and condition of muscles, tendons and other deep structures relayed to the brain from receptors called proprioceptors.

**prosopagnosia:** Inability to recognise familiar faces, not accounted for by defective visual acuity or reduced consciousness or alertness.

**protein kinase C** (PKC): An enzyme in the phosphatidyl inositol signalling pathway that is activated by the second messenger, diacyl glycerol. It catalyses the phosphorylation of intracellular proteins, thereby rendering them metabolically active (plate 14).

**pseudo-dementia:** A syndrome in which the cognitive impairment typical of degenerative dementia arises from a potentially reversible mental disorder, such as depression.

**pseudo-word:** Letter string that is composed following the rules of English orthography, but is not a word (e.g. grat).

**psychomotor excitation:** Excessive motor activity and speech, together with labile affect.

**psychomotor poverty:** Abnormally diminished or slowed movement, speech and affect.

**psychopathy:** A personality disorder characterised by lack of conscience and behaviour that is irresponsible and impulsive.

**psychosis:** A mental disorder in which there is markedly impaired ability to evaluate reality. A strict definition demands the presence of delusions and/or hallucinations, and loss of insight. A broader definition embraces other positive symptoms of schizophrenia (i.e., disorganised speech, grossly disorganised or catatonic behaviour).

**psychotropic medication:** Medication that affects perception, thought, emotion, or volition.

**pulvinar:** The large protuberance on the posterior aspect of the thalamus, overhanging the midbrain. It has reciprocal connections with association cortex of the parietal, occipital and temporal lobes.

**putamen:** The component nucleus of the corpus striatum lying posterolaterally to the head of caudate nucleus, and separated from it by the anterior limb of the internal capsule (plate 5). It receives input from premotor areas of the frontal cortex, and projects to the globus pallidus.

**pyramidal cells:** Large, approximately conical neurons, especially prevalent in layers 3 and 5 of the cerebral cortex, which are the source of the long axons that project to distant parts of the nervous system. Pyramidal cells typically have an apical dendrite that extends towards the surface of the cortex and arborises in the superficial layers (plates 6 and 7).

**raphe nuclei:** Nuclei adjacent to the midline of the midbrain, pons and medulla, which contain serotonergic neurons.

**reality distortion syndrome:** A cluster of symptoms, comprising delusions and hallucinations, that occur in psychotic illnesses.

**reinforcement:** The strengthening of a response by obtaining reward or avoiding punishment.

**resonance:** The process whereby rhythmical activity at a particular frequency in one oscillatory system promotes similarly rhythmical activity in another oscillatory system that has a natural tendency to oscillate at the same frequency.

**retrieval:** The process of recall or recognition of information that is stored in memory.

**reuptake inhibitors:** Drugs that block the re-uptake of a neurotransmitter from the synaptic cleft into the presynaptic terminal, thereby sustaining the action of the neurotransmitter at postsynaptic receptors.

**rostral:** Towards the front of the nervous system.

**saccades:** Small, step-wise, rapid and coordinated movements of the eyes, that adjust the point of fixation.

**schizophrenia:** A psychotic mental disorder that entails relatively persistent disruption of mental activity. The characteristic symptoms include delusions and hallucinations (especially bizarre delusions and hallucinations such as the Schneiderian first rank symptoms), and also include symptoms of disorganisation and psychomotor poverty. Diagnostic criteria require that these symptoms cannot be accounted for by affective disorder or a general medical condition. It is associated with substantial impairment of occupational and/or social function persisting for at least 6 months.

**semantic memory:** A long-term store of meaningful generalised information. The information is generalised insofar as it is not the representation of a particular event experienced by the person (an episodic memory).

**semantics:** The meaning of linguistic signs (i.e. words).

**septal nuclei:** Nuclei embedded in the base of the septum pellucidum, which, together with the hippocampus, constitute the septo-hippocampal system (plate 4).

**septum pellucidum:** The membranous partition between the two lateral ventricles, beneath the corpus callosum.

**serial processing:** Processing that occurs in sequential stages.

**serotonin:** An indole-amine, also known as 5-hydoxytryptamine (5-HT), whose chemical structure contains a five-membered, nitrogen-containing indole ring and an amine group. It acts as a modulatory neurotransmitter in the central nervous system, and in the gastrointestinal tract.

**sign:** An objective manifestation of a pathological condition. Signs are observable by an examiner, and do not rely on the report of the affected individual.

**somatic delusion:** A delusion whose theme concerns the appearance or functioning of one's body.

**somatic hallucination:** The perception of a physical experience localised within the body that is not based on the stimulation of internal sensory organs. It is distinct from hypochondriacal preoccupation with normal physical sensations, and from a tactile hallucination, which entails a perception of being touched or having something on or under the skin.

**somatotopy:** An orderly representation of the body in an area of the brain, such that adjacent body parts are represented in adjacent locations.

**stereotyped movements:** Repetitive, non-functional motor behaviour (e.g. body rocking, head banging, mouthing of objects, picking at skin, or hitting one's own body).

**stressor:** Any life event or life change that places unusual demands on the coping ability of the individual. A stressor may be associated with the onset, exacerbation, or maintenance of a mental disorder.

**stria terminalis:** A collection of axons, together with embedded grey nuclei, that extends from the amygdala in the temporal lobe, and arches over the thalamus to reach the lamina terminalis, which is located at the rostral end of the third ventricle.

**striatum:** See corpus striatum.

**Stroop effect:** Slowing of the reporting of the ink-colour in which a word is printed, when the word itself is the name of a different colour (e.g. reporting the ink-colour 'blue' will tend to be slower when the stimulus is the word 'RED' printed in blue ink than when the stimulus is 'XXX' printed in blue ink).

**stupor:** An altered state of consciousness in which the individual exhibits immobility, mutism and reduced responsiveness to stimuli.

**subarachnoid space:** The space filled with cerebrospinal fluid, between the arachnoid membrane and the pia mater, which invests the cortical surface.

**subiculum:** A part of the hippocampal formation that contains cortex that is transitional between the three layered cortex of the hippocampus and the six layered cortex of the adjacent parahippocampal gyrus (plate 9).

**substantia nigra:** A region in the ventral midbrain containing the cell bodies of dopaminergic neurons that project to the dorsal part of the corpus striatum and play a role in modulating motor activity. These neurons degenerate in Parkinson's disease.

**subthalamic nucleus:** A grey matter mass between the cerebral peduncle and the thalamus, which has reciprocal connections with the globus pallidus.

**sulcus:** A deep indention between gyri of the cerebral cortex.

**superior temporal gyrus:** The gyrus on the supero-lateral aspect of the temporal lobe. In the dominant hemisphere, the posterior portion is part of Wernicke's area, which plays a cardinal role in the comprehension of speech (plates 1 and 2).

**supervisory mental processes:** Mental processes that manage the performance of mental or motor actions under circumstances in which the optimal action is not dictated uniquely by external circumstances. The supervisory processes include the planning, initiation, selection and monitoring of self-generated action.

**supplementary motor area** (SMA): A region of cerebral cortex on the medial aspect of the frontal lobe, anterior to the area of primary motor cortex in the paracentral lobule and superior to the cingulate sulcus. It plays a role in the preparation of motor activity.

**supramarginal gyrus:** Area of parietal cortex adjacent to the posterior-superior end of the superior temporal sulcus and anterior to the angular gyrus. Together with the angular gyrus and superior temporal gyrus, it plays an important role in the comprehension of speech.

**Sylvian fissure:** See lateral fissure.

**symptom:** A subjectively experienced manifestation of a pathological condition. While strict usage distinguishes symptoms from signs, it is common to use the term symptoms to include both symptoms and signs of illness.

**synapse:** A connection between two neurons; usually between an axon of the presynaptic neuron and either a dendrite or cell body of the postsynaptic neuron. Axo-axonal synapses, between two axons, are less common.

**syndrome:** A group of signs and symptoms that frequently occur together in a way that suggests a common underlying pathogenesis.

**syntax:** The rules of a language that govern how words are combined to produce phrases and sentences.

**tactile hallucination:** A perception of being touched, or of having something under one's skin, that does not arise from the stimulation of a sense organ.

**tangentiality:** Replying to a question in an oblique or irrelevant way.

**tegmentum:** The core of the midbrain, including the grey matter lying ventral to the cerebral aqueduct.

**temporal lobe:** The region of cerebral hemisphere inferior and lateral to the lateral (Sylvian) fissure (plate 1).

**temporal pole:** The anterior tip of the temporal lobe.

**thalamus:** The thalami are a pair of grey masses separated by the third ventricle in the diencephalon (plate 5). Each has reciprocal connections with all areas of ipsilateral cerebral cortex. They relay tactile, somatic, visual and auditory sensory information travelling to the cortex, and play a cardinal role in the coordination of cortical function.

**thought broadcasting:** The delusion that one's thoughts are being broadcast out loud so that they can be perceived by others.

**thought insertion:** The delusion that one's thoughts are not one's own, but rather are inserted into one's mind by an alien agency.

**tic:** An involuntary, sudden, recurrent, non-rhythmic, stereotyped motor movement or vocalisation.

**top-down processing:** A mechanism by which prior knowledge or conscious decision can influence the processing of information derived through the senses.

**transverse temporal gyrus** (of Heschl): A gyrus on the superior aspect of the temporal lobe, lying within the lateral (Sylvian) fissure, that contains primary auditory cortex (plate 2).

**unconscious:** Aspects of mental functioning that are outside of subjective awareness.

**uncus:** A protuberance of cerebral cortex on the antero-medial aspect of the temporal lobe containing periamygdaloid cortex overlying the amygdala (plate 3).

**ventral striatum:** The human homologue of the nucleus accumbens in rodents. It is a component of the corpus striatum located below the lower boundary of the anterior limb of the internal capsule, contiguous with the putamen and the head of the caudate nucleus above. It receives its main input from the ventral and medial frontal cortex, and a regulatory input from hippocampus and amygdala. It projects to a ventral extension of the globus pallidus (the ventral pallidum).

**ventricles:** Fluid-filled spaces within the brain. The lateral ventricle in each cerebral hemisphere connects via the interventricular foramen with the unpaired third ventricle lying between the two thalami (plate 5). At its caudal end, the third ventricle is connected via the aqueduct to the fourth ventricle located in the brainstem.

**vermis:** The midline region of the cerebellum (plate 5).

**visual cortex:** The primary visual cortex surrounds the calcarine fissure (plate 3). It receives input from the lateral geniculate nucleus, via the optic radiation. It projects to visual association cortex (Brodman areas 18 and 19) on the medial and lateral aspect of the occipital lobe.

**visual hallucination:** A visual perception that does not arise from a visual stimulus. It may be of a formed image of an object, such as a person, or unformed images, such as flashes of light.

**visuo-spatial scratch pad:** A component of working memory that maintains information in the form of visual images.

**Wernicke's area:** An area in the posterior portion of the superior temporal gyrus and adjacent supramarginal gyrus and angular gyrus of the dominant hemisphere. It plays a cardinal role in the comprehension of speech (plate 2).

**white matter:** Tissue of the central nervous system that appears white because it contains axons coated with layers of lipid-rich myelin.

**working memory:** A mechanism for maintaining and manipulating information in conscious awareness. Its components include an articulatory loop, a visuo-spatial scratch pad, and a central executive, responsible for directing the other components.

# References

Aarsland, D., Larsen, J. P., Lim, N. G., *et al* (1999) Range of neuropsychiatric disturbances in patients with Parkinson's disease. *Journal of Neurology, Neurosurgery and Psychiatry*, **67**, 492–496.

Abadie, P., Boulenger, J. P., Benali, K., *et al* (1999) Relationships between trait and state anxiety and the central benzodiazepine receptor: a PET study. *European Journal of Neuroscience*, **11**, 1470–1478.

Abbruzzese, M., Ferri, S. & Scarone, S. (1995) Wisconsin Card Sorting Test performance in obsessive–compulsive disorder: no evidence for involvement of dorsolateral prefrontal cortex. *Psychiatry Research*, **58**, 37–43.

Abercrombie, E. D., Wilkinson, L. O. & Jacobs, B. L. (1986) Environmental stress and activity of the locus coeruleus noradrenergic neurons in freely moving rats. *Society for Neuroscience Abstracts*, **12**, 1134.

Abi-Dargham, A., Rodenhiser, J., Printz, D., *et al* (2000) From the cover: increased baseline occupancy of D2 receptors by dopamine in schizophrenia. *Proceedings of the National Academy of Sciences USA*, **97**, 8104–8109.

Achte, K., Jarho, L., Kyykka, T., *et al* (1991) Paranoid disorders following war brain damage. Preliminary report. *Psychopathology*, **24**, 309–315.

Adams, W., Kendall, R. E., Hare, E. H., *et al* (1993) Epidemiological evidence that maternal influenza contributes to the aetiology of schizophrenia: an analysis of Scottish, English and Danish data. *British Journal of Psychiatry*, **163**, 522–534.

Adler, C. M., Goldberg, T. E., Malhotra, A. K., *et al* (1998) Effects of ketamine on thought disorder, working memory, and semantic memory in healthy volunteers. *Biological Psychiatry*, **43**, 811–816.

Adler, C. M., Malhotra, A. K., Elman, I., *et al* (1999) A comparison of ketamine-induced thought disorder in healthy volunteers and thought disorder in schizophrenia. *American Journal of Psychiatry*, **156**, 1646–1649.

Adolphs, R., Tranel, D., Damasio, H., *et al* (1994) Impaired recognition of emotion in facial expressions following bilateral damage to the human amygdala. *Nature*, **372**, 669–672.

Adolphs, R., Tranel, D. & Damasio, A. (1998) The human amygdala in social judgement. *Nature*, **393**, 470–474.

af Klinteberg, B. (1996) Biology, norms, and personality: a developmental perspective. *Neuropsychobiology*, **34**, 146–154.

Albus, M., Hubmann, W., Scherer, J., *et al* (2000) Neuropsychological functioning in first-episode schizophrenia: a 2-year follow-up. *Schizophrenia Research*, **41**, 36.

Alexander, G. E. & Crutcher, M. D. (1990a) Functional architecture of basal ganglia circuits: neural substrates of parallel processing. *Trends in Neurosciences*, **13**, 266–271.

Alexander, G. E. & Crutcher, M. D. (1990b) Neural representations of the target (goal) of visually guided arm movements in three motor areas of the monkey. *Journal of Neurophysiology*, **64**, 164–178.

Alexander, G. E. & Crutcher, M. D. (1990c) Preparation for movement: neural representations of intended direction in three motor areas of the monkey. *Journal of Neurophysiology*, **64**, 133–150.

Alexander, G. E., DeLong, M. R. & Strick, P. L. (1986) Parallel organization of functionally segregated circuits linking basal ganglia and cortex. *Annual Review of Neuroscience*, **9**, 357–381.

Alexander, G. E., Crutcher, M. D. & DeLong, M. R. (1990) Basal ganglia–thalamocortical circuits: parallel substrates for motor, oculomotor, 'prefrontal' and 'limbic' functions. *Progress in Brain Research*, **85**, 119–146.

Alexander, J. E., Porjesz, B., Bauer, L. O., *et al* (1995) P300 hemispheric amplitude asymmetries from a visual oddball task. *Psychophysiology*, **32**, 467–475.

Alexander, J. E., Bauer, L. O., Kuperman, S., *et al* (1996) Hemispheric differences for P300 amplitude from an auditory oddball task. *International Journal of Psychophysiology*, **21**, 189–196.

Alheid, G. F. & Heimer, L. (1988) New perspectives in basal forebrain organization of special relevance for neuropsychiatric disorders: the striatopallidal, amygdaloid, and corticopetal components of substantia innominata. *Neuroscience*, **27**, 1–39.

Allen, H. A., Frith, C. D. & Liddle, P. F. (1993) Negative features, retrieval processes and verbal fluency in schizophrenia. *British Journal of Psychiatry*, **163**, 769–775.

Alm, P. O., af Klinteberg, B., Humble, K., *et al* (1996) Criminality and psychopathy as related to thyroid activity in former juvenile delinquents. *Acta Psychiatrica Scandinavica*, **94**, 112–117.

Amaral, D. G., Price, J. L., Pitkanen, A., *et al* (1992) Anatomical organization of the primate amygdaloid complex. In *The Amygdala: Neurobiological Aspects of Emotion, Memory, and Mental Dysfunction* (ed. J. P. Aggleton), pp. 1–66. New York: Wiley-Liss.

Ambelas, A. (1987) Life events and mania: a special relationship? *British Journal of Psychiatry*, **150**, 235–240.

Ameri, A. (1999) The effects of cannabinoids on the brain. *Progress in Neurobiology*, **58**, 315–348.

American Psychiatric Association (1994) *Diagnostic and Statistical Manual of Mental Disorders* (4th edn) (DSM–IV). Washington, DC: APA.

Anderson, S. W., Bechara, A., Damasio, H., *et al* (1999) Impairment of social and moral behavior related to early damage in human prefrontal cortex. *Nature Neuroscience*, **2**, 1032–1037.

Andrade, L., Eaton, W. W. & Chilcoat, H. (1994) Lifetime comorbidity of panic attacks and major depression in a population based study. *British Journal of Psychiatry*, **165**, 363–369.

Andreasen, N. C. (1979a) Thought, language, and communication disorders: 1. Clinical assessment, definition of terms, and evaluation of their reliability *Archives of General Psychiatry*, **36**, 1315–1321.

Andreasen, N. C. (1979b) Thought, language, and communication disorders: 2. Diagnostic significance. *Archives of General Psychiatry*, **36**, 1325–1330.

Andreasen, N. C. (1982) Negative symptoms in schizophrenia: definition and reliability. *Archives of General Psychiatry*, **39**, 784–788.

Andreasen, N. C. (1986) *Comprehensive Assessment of Symptoms and History*. Iowa: University of Iowa.

Andreasen, N. C. & Grove, W. M. (1986) Thought, language and communication in schizophrenia: diagnosis and prognosis. *Schizophrenia Bulletin*, **12**, 348–359.

Andreasen, N. C. & Olsen, S. (1982) Negative v. positive schizophrenia: definition and validation. *Archives of General Psychiatry*, **39**, 789–794.

Andreasen N. C., Rezai, K., Alliger R., *et al* (1992) Hypofrontality in neuroleptic-naive patients and in patients with chronic schizophrenia. Assessment with xenon 133 single-photon emission computed tomography and the Tower of London. *Archives of General Psychiatry*, **49**, 943–958.

Andreasen, N. C., Arndt, S., Swayze, V. 2nd, *et al* (1994) Thalamic abnormalities in schizophrenia visualized through magnetic resonance image averaging. *Science*, **266**, 294–298.

Arndt, S., Alliger, R. J. & Andreasen, N. C. (1991) The distinction of positive and negative symptoms. The failure of a two dimensional model. *British Journal of Psychiatry*, **158**, 317–322.

Awh, E., Jonides, J., Smith, E. E., *et al* (1996) Dissociation of storage and rehearsal in verbal working memory: evidence from positron emission tomography. *Psychological Science*, **7**, 25–31.

Baddeley, A. D. & Hitch, G. J. (1974) Working memory. In *The Psychology of Learning and Motivation: Advances in Research and Theory*, vol. 8 (ed. G. H. Bower), pp. 47–90. New York: Academic Press.

Banki, C. M., Molnar, G. & Vojnik, M. (1981) Cerebrospinal fluid amine metabolites, tryptophan and clinical parameters in depression. *Journal of Affective Disorders*, 3, 91–99.

Barlow, H. B. (1972) Single units and sensation: a neuron doctrine for perceptual psychology? *Perception*, 1, 371–394.

Barnes, T. R. E., Curson, D., Liddle, P. F., *et al* (1989) The nature and prevalence of depression in chronic schizophrenic in-patients. *British Journal of Psychiatry*, 154, 486–491.

Barris, R. W. & Schuman, H. R. (1953) Bilateral anterior cingulate gyrus lesions. *Neurology*, 3, 44–52.

Baxter, R. & Liddle, P. F. (1998) Neuropsychological deficits associated with schizophrenic syndromes. *Schizophrenia Research*, 30, 239–249.

Baxter, L. R. Jr, Phelps, M. E., Mazziotta, J. C., *et al* (1985) Cerebral metabolic rates for glucose in mood disorders. Studies with positron emission tomography and fluorodeoxyglucose $F^{18}$. *Archives of General Psychiatry*, 42, 441–447.

Baxter, L. R. Jr, Schwartz, J. M., Mazziotta, J. C., *et al* (1988) Cerebral glucose metabolic rates in nondepressed patients with obsessive–compulsive disorder. *American Journal of Psychiatry*, 145, 1560–1563.

Baxter, L. R. Jr, Schwartz, J. M., Phelps, M. E., *et al* (1989) Reduction of prefrontal cortex glucose metabolism common in three types of depression. *Archives of General Psychiatry*, 46, 243–250.

Baxter, L. R. Jr, Schwartz, J. M., Bergman, K. S., *et al* (1992) Caudate glucose metabolic rate changes with both drug and behavior therapy for obsessive–compulsive disorder. *Archives of General Psychiatry*, 49, 681–689.

Beato, M. (1989) Gene regulation by steriod hormones. *Cell*, 56, 335–344.

Beaulieu, C., Kisvarday, Z., Somogyi, P., *et al* (1992) Quantitative distribution of GABA-immunopositive and -immunonegative neurons and synapses in the monkey striate cortex (area 17). *Cerebral Cortex*, 2, 295–309.

Bebbington, P. E. (1998) Epidemiology of obsessive–compulsive disorder. *British Journal of Psychiatry*, 173 (suppl. 35), 2–6.

Bebbington, P. E., Bowen, J., Hirsch, S. R., *et al* (1995) Schizophrenia and social stresses. In *Schizophrenia* (eds S. R. Hirsch & D. R. Weinberger), pp. 587–604. Oxford: Blackwell.

Beck, A. T. (1976) *Cognitive Therapy and the Emotional Disorders*. New York: International Universities Press.

Beck, A. T., Rush, J. A., Shaw, B. F., *et al* (1979) *Cognitive Therapy of Depression*. New York: Guilford.

Becker, E. S., Roth, W. T., Andrich, M., *et al* (1999) Explicit memory in anxiety disorders. *Journal of Abnormal Psychology*, 108, 153–163.

Behrman, M., Winocur, G. & Moscovitch, M. (1992) Dissociation between mental imagery and object recognition in a brain-damaged patient. *Nature*, 359, 636–637.

Bell, M. D., Lysaker, P. H., Beam-Goulet, J. L., *et al* (1994) Five component model of schizophrenia: assessing the factorial invariance of the positive and negative syndrome scale. *Psychiatry Research*, 52, 295–303.

Belluzzi, J. D. & Stein, L. (1977) Enkephalin may mediate euphoria and drive-reduction reward. *Nature*, 266, 556–558.

Bench, C. J., Friston, K. J., Brown, R. G., *et al* (1992) The anatomy of melancholia – focal abnormalities of cerebral blood flow in major depression. *Psychological Medicine*, 22, 607–615.

Bench, C. J., Friston, K. J., Brown, R. G., *et al* (1993) Regional cerebral blood flow in depression measured by positron emission tomography: the relationship with clinical dimensions. *Psychological Medicine*, 23, 579–590.

Benkelfat, C., Nordahl, T. E., Semple, W. E., *et al* (1990) Local cerebral glucose metabolic rates in obsessive–compulsive disorder. Patients treated with clomipramine. *Archives of General Psychiatry*, 47, 840–848.

Benkelfat, C., Bradwejn, J., Meyer, E., *et al* (1995) Functional neuroanatomy of CCK4-induced anxiety in normal healthy volunteers. *American Journal of Psychiatry*, 152, 1180–1184.

Bentall, R. P. (1994) Cognitive biases and abnormal beliefs: towards a model of persecutory delusions. In *The Neuropsychology of Schizophrenia* (eds A. S. David & J. C. Cutting), pp. 337–360. Hove: Lawrence Erlbaum.

Bentall, R. P. & Slade, P. D. (1985) Reality testing and auditory hallucinations: a signal detection analysis. *British Journal of Clinical Psychology*, **24**, 159–171.

Bertelson, A., Harvlad, B. & Huage, M. (1977) A Danish twin study of manic–depressive disorders. *British Journal of Psychiatry*, **130**, 350–351.

Berthier, M. L., Kulisevsky, J., Gironell, A., *et al* (1996) Poststroke bipolar affective disorder: clinical subtypes, concurrent movement disorders, and anatomical correlates. *Journal of Neuropsychiatry and Clinical Neuroscience*, **8**, 160–167.

Bilder, R. M., Mukherjee, S., Rieder, R. O., *et al* (1985) Symptomatic and neuropsychological components of defect states. *Schizophrenia Bulletin*, **11**, 409–419.

Blackburn, R. (1988) On moral judgements and personality disorders. The myth of psychopathic personality revisited. *British Journal of Psychiatry*, **153**, 505–512.

Bland, B. H., Seto, M. & Sinclair, B. R. (1981) Selective abolishment of type 2 unit rhythmicity of physiologically identified hippocampal formation neurons. *Experimental Brain Research*, **38**, 205–219.

Bland, R. C., Newman, S. C. & Orn, H. (1987) Schizophrenia: lifetime comorbidity in a community sample. *Acta Psychiatrica Scandinavica*, **75**, 383–391.

Bleuler, E. (1911) *Dementia Praecox or the Group of Schizophrenias* (trans. J. Zinkin). New York: International Universities Press (1950).

Blumberg, H. P., Stern, E., Ricketts, S., *et al* (1999) Rostral and orbital prefrontal cortex dysfunction in the manic state of bipolar disorder. *American Journal of Psychiatry*, **156**, 1986–1988.

Blumer, D. & Benson, D. F. (1975) Personality changes with frontal lobe lesions. In *Psychiatric Aspects of Neurological Disease* (eds D. Blumer & D. F. Benson), pp. 151–170. New York: Grune & Stratton.

Braengaard, J., Evans, S. M., Howard, C. V., *et al* (1990) The total number of neurons in the human neocortex unbiasedly estimated using optical dissectors. *Journal of Microscopy*, **157**, 285–304.

Brauer, L. H. & De Wit, H. (1997) High dose pimozide does not block amphetamine-induced euphoria in normal volunteers. *Pharmacology and Biochemistry of Behavior*, **56**, 265–272.

Breeze, G. P., Smith, R. D., Meuleler, R. A., *et al* (1973) Induction of adrenal catecholamine-synthesising enzymes following mother–infant separation. *Nature: New Biology*, **246**, 94–96.

Breier, A., Davis, O. R., Buchanan, R. W., *et al* (1993) Effects of metabolic perturbation on plasma homovanillic acid in schizophrenia: relationship to prefrontal cortex volume. *Archives of General Psychiatry*, **50**, 541–547.

Breier, A., Malhotra, A. K., Pinals, D. A., *et al* (1997a) Association of ketamine-induced psychosis with focal activation of the prefrontal cortex in healthy volunteers. *American Journal of Psychiatry*, **154**, 805–811.

Breier, A., Su, T. P., Saunders, R., *et al* (1997b) Schizophrenia is associated with elevated amphetamine-induced synaptic dopamine concentrations: evidence from a novel positron emission tomography method. *Proceedings of the National Academy of Sciences USA*, **94**, 2569–2574.

Breier, A., Adler, C. M., Weisenfeld, N., *et al* (1998) Effects of NMDA antagonism on striatal dopamine release in healthy subjects: application of a novel PET approach. *Synapse*, **29**, 142–147.

Breiter, H. C., Gollub, R. L., Weisskoff, R. M., *et al* (1997) Acute effects of cocaine on human brain activity and emotion. *Neuron*, **19**, 591–611.

Breitholtz, E., Johansson, B. & Ost, L. G. (1999) Cognitions in generalized anxiety disorder and panic disorder patients. A prospective approach. *Behaviour Research and Therapy*, **37**, 533–544.

Bremner, J. D., Innis, R. B., Ng, C. K., *et al* (1997) Positron emission tomography measurement of cerebral metabolic correlates of yohimbine administration in combat-related posttraumatic stress disorder. *Archives of General Psychiatry*, **54**, 246–254.

Broadbent, D. E. (1958) *Perception and Communication*. Oxford: Pergamon Press.

Broca, P. (1861) *Sur le volume et la forme du cerveau suivant les individus et suivant les races*. Paris: Hennuyer.

Brown, A. S. & Gershon, S. (1993) Dopamine and depression. *Journal of Neural Transmission, Genetics Section*, **91**, 75–109.

Brzustowicz, L. M., Honer, W. G., Chow, E. W. C., *et al* (1999) Linkage of familial schizophrenia to chromosome 13q32. *American Journal of Human Genetics*, **65**, 1096–1103.

Brzustowicz, L. M., Hodgkinson, K. A., Chow, E. W., *et al* (2000) Location of a major susceptibility locus for familial schizophrenia on chromosome 1q21–q22. *Science*, **288**, 678–682.

Buchan, H., Johnstone, E., McPherson, K., *et al* (1992) Who benefits from electroconvulsive therapy? Combined results of the Leicester and Northwick Park trials. *British Journal of Psychiatry*, **160**, 355–359.

Buchsbaum, M. S., Wu, J., DeLisi, L. E., *et al* (1986) Frontal cortex and basal ganglia metabolic rates assessed by positron emission tomography with [18F]2-deoxyglucose in affective illness. *Journal of Affective Disorders*, **10**, 137–152.

Byrne, M., Hodges, A., Grant, E., *et al* (1999) Neuropsychological assessment of young people at high genetic risk for developing schizophrenia compared with controls: preliminary findings of the Edinburgh High Risk Study (EHRS). *Psychological Medicine*, **29**, 1161–1173.

Byrne, M., Cosway, R., Hodges, A., *et al* (2000) The association between neuropsychology and psychotic symptoms in the Edinburgh high risk for schizophrenia study. *Schizophrenia Research*, **41**, 36.

Cador, M., Robbins, T. W.& Everitt, B. J. (1989) Involvement of the amygdala in stimulus–reward associations: interaction with the ventral striatum. *Neuroscience*, **30**, 77–86.

Cadoret, R. J. & Stewart, M. A. (1991) An adoption study of attention deficit/hyperactivity/aggression and their relationship to adult antisocial personality. *Comprehensive Psychiatry*, **32**, 73–82.

Cahusac, P. M. B., Miyashita, Y. & Rolls, E. T. (1989) Responses of hippocampal neurons in the monkey related to delayed response and object-place memory tasks. *Behavior and Brain Research*, **33**, 229–240.

Calabrese, J. R., Rapport, D. J., Kimmel, S. E., *et al* (1999) Controlled trials in bipolar I depression: focus on switch rates and efficacy. *European Neuropsychopharmacology*, **9** (suppl. 4), S109–S112.

Cannon, M., Cotter, D., Coffey, V. P., *et al* (1996) Prenatal exposure to the 1957 influenza epidemic and adult schizophrenia: a follow-up study. *British Journal of Psychiatry*, **168**, 368–371.

Carlson, G. A. & Goodwin, F. K. (1973) The stages of mania: a longitudinal analysis of the manic episode. *Archives of General Psychiatry*, **28**, 221–228.

Carlsson, M. & Carlsson, A. (1990) Interactions between glutamatergic and monoaminergic systems within the basal ganglia – implications for schizophrenia and Parkinson's disease. *Trends in Neurosciences*, **13**, 272–276.

Carr, D. B. & Sheehan, D. V. (1984) Panic anxiety: a new biological model. *Journal of Clinical Psychiatry*, **45**, 323–330.

Carter, C. S., Braver, T. S., Barch, D. M., *et al* (1998) Anterior cingulate cortex, error detection, and the online monitoring of performance. *Science*, **280**, 747–749.

Castillo, C. S., Starkstein, S. E., Fedoroff, J. P., *et al* (1993) Generalized anxiety disorder after stroke. *Journal of Nervous and Mental Diseases*, **181**, 102–108.

Chapman, L. J., Chapman, J. P. & Miller, G. A. (1964) A theory of verbal behaviour in schizophrenia. In *Progress in Experimental Personality Research*, vol. 1 (ed. B. A. Maher). New York: Academic Press.

Charney, D. S., Heninger, G. R. & Breier, A. (1984) Noradrenergic function in panic anxiety. Effects of yohimbine in healthy subjects and patients with agoraphobia and panic disorder. *Archives of General Psychiatry*, **41**, 751–763.

Charney, D. S., Woods, S. W., Goodman, W. K. & Heninger, G. R. (1987) Serotonin function in anxiety. II. Effects of the serotonin agonist MCPP in panic disorder patients and healthy subjects. *Psychopharmacology (Berlin)*, **92**, 14–24.

Charpark, S., Pare, D. & Llinas, R. (1995) The entorhinal cortex entrains fast CA1 hippocampal oscillations in the anaesthetized guinea pig: role of the monosynaptic component of the perforant path. *European Journal of Neuroscience*, **7**, 1548–1557.

Chaudhry, I. B., Soni, S. D., Hellewell, J. S. E., *et al* (1997) Antisaccade, clinical and motor executive functions in schizophrenia: effects of 5HT2 antagonist cyproheptadine. *Schizophrenia Research*, **24**, 212.

Checkley, S. (1992) Neuroendocrine mechanisms and the precipitation of depression by life events. *British Journal of Psychiatry*, **160** (suppl. 15), 7–17.

Chen, G., Pan, B., Hawver, D. B., *et al* (1996) Attenuation of cyclic AMP production by carbamazepine. *Journal of Neurochemistry*, **67**, 2079–2086.

Chen, B., Wang, J. F., Hill, B. C., *et al* (1999) Lithium and valproate differentially regulate brain regional expression of phosphorylated CREB and c-Fos. *Brain Research, Molecular Brain Research*, **70**, 45–53.

Chiodo, L. A. & Antelman, S. M. (1980) Tricyclic antidepressants induce subsensitivity of presynaptic dopamine autoreceptors. *European Journal of Psychopharmacology*, **64**, 203–204.

Chou, J. C., Czobor, P., Charles, O., *et al* (1999) Acute mania: haloperidol dose and augmentation with lithium or lorazepam. *Journal of Clinical Psychopharmacology*, **19**, 500–505.

Chua, S. E., Wright, I. C., Poline, J-B., *et al* (1997) Grey matter correlates of syndromes in schizophrenia: a semi-automated analysis of structural magnetic resonance images. *British Journal of Psychiatry*, **170**, 406–410.

Chua, P., Krams, M., Toni, I., *et al* (1999) A functional anatomy of anticipatory anxiety. *Neuroimage*, **9**, 563–571.

Chun, M. M. & Phelps, E. A. (1999) Memory deficits for implicit contextual information in amnesic subjects with hippocampal damage. *Nature Neuroscience*, **2**, 844–847.

Churchill, L., Austin, M. C. & Kalivas, P. W. (1992) Dopamine and endogenous opioid regulation of picrotoxin-induced locomotion in the ventral pallidum after dopamine depletion in the nucleus accumbens. *Psychopharmacology (Berlin)*, **108**, 141–146.

Clark, D. M. (1986) A cognitive approach to panic. *Behavioural Research and Therapy*, **24**, 461–470.

Clark, C. R., McFarlane, A. C., Weber, D. L., *et al* (1996) Enlarged frontal P300 to stimulus change in panic disorder. *Biological Psychiatry*, **39**, 845–856.

Cleckley, H. (1988). *The Mask of Sanity* (5th edn). Augusta: Cleckley.

Clow, A., Glover, V., Sandler, M., *et al* (1988) Increased urinary tribulin output in generalised anxiety disorder. *Psychopharmacology*, **95**, 378–380.

Coccaro, E. F., Siever, L. J., Klar, H. M., *et al* (1989) Serotonergic studies in patients with affective and personality disorders. *Archives of General Psychiatry*, **46**, 587–599.

Cohen, B. D., Nachmani, G. & Rosenberg S. (1974) Referent communication disturbances in acute schizophrenia. *Journal of Abnormal Psychology*, **83**, 1–13.

Cohen, J. D. & Servan-Schreiber, D. (1992) Context, cortex, and dopamine: a connectionist approach to behavior and biology in schizophrenia. *Psychological Reviews*, **99**, 45–77.

Cohen, J. D., Forman, S. D., Braver, T. S., *et al* (1994) Activation of the prefrontal cortex in a non-spatial working memory task with functional memory task with functional MRI. *Human Brain Mapping*, **1**, 293–304.

Cohen, J. D., Barch, D. M., Carter, C., *et al* (1999) Context-processing deficits in schizophrenia: converging evidence from three theoretically motivated cognitive tasks. *Journal of Abnormal Psychology*, **108**, 120–133.

Collicut, J. R. & Hemsley, D. R. (1981) A psychophysical investigation of auditory functioning in schizophrenia. *British Journal of Clinical Psychology*, **20**, 199–204.

Cools, A. R., Van Den Bos, R., Ploeger, G., *et al* (1991) Gating function of noradrenaline in the ventral striatum: its role in behavioural responses to environmental and pharmacological challenges. In *The Mesolimbic Dopamine System: From Motivation to Action* (eds P. Willner & J. Scheel-Kruger), pp. 141–173. Chichester: John Wiley.

Cooper, L. A. & Shephard, R. N. (1973) Chronometric studies of the rotation of mental images. In *Visual Information Processing* (ed. W. G. Chase), pp. 75–176. New York: Academic Press.

Coplan, J. D., Andrews, M. W., Rosenblum, L. A., *et al* (1996) Persistent elevations of cerebrospinal fluid concentrations of corticotropin releasing factor in adult non-human primates exposed to early life stressors: implications for the pathophysiology of mood and anxiety disorders. *Proceedings of the National Academy of Sciences USA*, **93**, 1619–1623.

Coplan, J. D., Trost, R. C., Owens, M. J., *et al* (1998) Cerebrospinal fluid concentrations of somatostatin and biogenic amines in grown primates reared by mothers exposed to manipulated foraging conditions. *Archives of General Psychiatry*, **55**, 473–477.

Corbetta, M., Miezen, F. M., Dobmeyer, S., *et al* (1991) Selective and divided attention during visual discrimination of shape, color and speed. Functional anatomy by positron emission tomography. *Journal of Neuroscience*, **11**, 2383–2402.

Corbetta, M., Miezen, F. M., Shulman, G. L., *et al* (1993) A PET study of visuospatial attention. *Journal of Neuroscience*, **13**, 1202–1226.

Cornblatt, B. A., Lenzenweger, M., Dworkin, R., *et al* (1985) Positive and negative schizophrenic symptoms, attention and information processing. *Schizophrenia Bulletin*, **11**, 397–408.

Coryell, W., Endicott, J., Keller, M., *et al* (1985) Phenomenology and family history in DSM–III psychotic depression. *Journal of Affective Disorder*, **9**, 13–18.

Craig, A. H., Cummings, J. L., Fairbanks, L., *et al* (1996) Cerebral blood flow correlates of apathy in Alzheimer disease. *Archives of Neurology*, **53**, 1116–1120.

Crespo-Facorro, B., Cabranes, J. A., Lopez-Ibor, J. J., *et al* (1999) Regional cerebral blood flow in obsessive–compulsive patients with and without a chronic tic disorder. A SPECT study. *European Archives of Psychiatry and Clinical Neuroscience*, **249**, 156–161.

Crow, T. J. (1980) The molecular pathology of schizophrenia: more than one disease process. *British Medical Journal*, **280**, 66–68.

Crow, T. J. (1985) The two syndrome concept: origins and current status. *Schizophrenia Bulletin*, **11**, 471–486.

Crutcher, M. D. & Alexander, G. E. (1990) Movement-related neuronal activity selectively coding either direction or muscle pattern in three motor areas of the monkey. *Journal of Neurophysiology*, **64**, 151–163.

Cummings, J. L. & Benson, F. (1984) Subcortical dementia. Review of an emerging concept. *Archives of Neurology*, **41**, 874–879.

D'Souza, D. C., Abi-Saab, W., Madonick, S., *et al* (2000) Cannabinoids and psychosis: evidence from studies with I.V. THC in schizophrenic patients and controls. *Schizophrenia Research*, **41**, 33.

Damasio, A. R., Damasio, H., Tranel, D., *et al* (1990) Neural regionalization of knowledge access: preliminary evidence. *Cold Spring Harbour Symposia on Quantantive Biology*, **55**, 1039–1047.

Daniel, D. G., Weinberger, D. R., Jones, D. W., *et al* (1991) The effect of amphetamine on regional cerebral blood flow during cognitive activation in schizophrenia. *Journal of Neuroscience*, **11**, 1907–1917.

David, A. S., Malmberg, A., Brandt, L., *et al* (1997) IQ and risk for schizophrenia: a population based cohort study. *Psychological Medicine*, **27**, 1311–1323.

Davis, M. & Shi, C. (1999) The extended amygdala: are the central nucleus of the amygdala and the bed nucleus of the stria terminalis differentially involved in fear versus anxiety? *Annals of the New York Academy of Sciences*, **877**, 281–291.

Davison, K. & Bagley, C. R. (1969) Schizophrenia-like psychoses associated with organic disorders of the central nervous system: a review of the literature. In *Current Problems in Neuropsychiatry. British Journal of Psychiatry, Special Publication 4* (ed. R. N. Herrington). Ashford, Kent: Headley Brothers.

Deeke, L., Scheid, P. & Kornhuber, H. H. (1969) Distribution of the readiness potential, pre-motion positivity, and motor potential of the human cerebral cortex preceding voluntary finger movements. *Experimental Brain Research*, **7**, 158–168.

Degl'Innocenti, A., Agren, H. & Backman, L. (1998) Executive deficits in major depression. *Acta Psychiatrica Scandinavica*, **97**, 182–188.

D'haenen, H. A. & Bossuyt, A. (1994) Dopamine D2 receptors in depression measured with single photon emission computed tomography. *Biological Psychiatry*, **35**, 128–132.

Delgado, P. L. & Moreno, F. A. (1998) Different roles for serotonin in anti-obsessional drug action and the pathophysiology of obsessive–compulsive disorder. *British Journal of Psychiatry*, **173** (suppl. 35), 21–25.

DeLisi, L. E. (1999) Regional brain volume change over the life-time course of schizophrenia. *Journal of Psychiatric Research*, **33**, 535–541.

DeLong, M. R. (1990) Primate models of movement disorders of basal ganglia origin. *Trends in Neurosciences*, **13**, 281–285.

de Montigny, C. (1989) Cholecystokinin tetrapeptide induces panic-like attacks in healthy volunteers. Preliminary findings. *Archives of General Psychiatry*, **46**, 511–517.

Desmedt, J. E. & Tomberg, C. (1994) Transient phase-locking of 40 Hz electrical oscillations in prefrontal and parietal human cortex reflects the process of conscious somatic perception. *Neuroscience Letters*, **168**, 126–129.

Deuchars, J., West, D. C. & Thomson, A. M. (1994) Relationships between morphology and physiology of pyramid–pyramid single axon connections in rat neocortex in vitro. *Journal of Physiology (London)*, **478**, 423–435.

Deutch, A. Y., Clark, W. A. & Roth, R. H. (1990) Prefrontal cortical dopamine depletion enhances the responsiveness of mesolimbic dopamine neurons to stress. *Brain Research*, **521**, 311–315.

Deutch, A. Y., Bourdelais, A. J. & Zahm, D. S. (1993) The nucleus accumbens core and shell: accumbal compartments and their functional attributes. In *Limbic Motor Circuits and Neuropsychiatry* (eds P. W. Kalivas & C. D. Barnes), pp. 45–77. Boca Raton, FL: CRC Press.

Dolan, R. J., Bench, C. J., Liddle, P. F., *et al* (1993) Dorsolateral prefrontal cortex dysfunction in the major psychoses: symptom or disease specificity? *Journal of Neurology, Neurosurgery and Psychiatry*, **56**, 1290–1294.

Dollfus, S. & Petit, M. (1995) Negative symptoms in schizophrenia: their evolution during an acute phase. *Schizophrenia Research*, **17**, 187–194.

Donchin, E. & Coles, M. G. H. (1988) Is the P300 component a manifestation of context updating? *Brain and Behaviour Sciences*, **11**, 357–374.

Done, D. J., Crow, T. J., Johnstone, E. C., *et al* (1994) Childhood antecedents of schizophrenia and affective illness: social adjustment at ages 7 and 11. *British Medical Journal*, **309**, 699–703.

Donlon, P. T., Rada, R. T. & Arora, K. K. (1976) Depression and the reintegration phase of acute schizophrenia. *American Journal of Psychiatry*, **133**, 1265–1268.

Dorow, R., Horowski, R., Paschelke, G., *et al* (1983) Severe anxiety induced by FG 7142, a beta-carboline ligand for benzodiazepine receptors. *Lancet*, **ii**, 98–99.

Douglas, R. J. & Martin, K. A. (1991) Opening the grey box. *Trends in Neurosciences*, **14**, 286–293.

Drevets, W. C., Videen, T. O., Price, J. L., *et al* (1992) A functional anatomical study of unipolar depression. *Journal of Neuroscience*, **12**, 3628–3641.

Drevets, W. C., Price, J. L., Simpson, J. R. Jr, *et al* (1997) Subgenual prefrontal cortex abnormalities in mood disorders. *Nature*, **386**, 824–827.

Drevets, W. C., Frank, E., Price, J. C., *et al* (1999) PET imaging of serotonin 1A receptor binding in depression. *Biological Psychiatry*, **46**, 1375–1387.

Duinkerke, S. J., Botter, P. A., Jansen, A. A., *et al* (1993) Ritanserin, a selective 5-HT2/1C antagonist, and negative symptoms in schizophrenia. A placebo-controlled double-blind trial. *British Journal of Psychiatry*, **163**, 451–455.

Eaton, W. W., Thara, R., Federman, B., *et al* (1995) Structure and course of positive and negative symptoms in schizophrenia. *Archives of General Psychiatry*, **52**, 127–134.

Ebmeier, K. P., Blackwood, D. H. R., Murray, C., *et al* (1993) Single photon emission tomography with 99mTc-exametazime in unmedicated schizophrenic patients. *Biological Psychiatry*, **33**, 487–495.

Ebmeier, K. P., Cavanagh, J. T., Moffoot, A. P., *et al* (1997) Cerebral perfusion correlates of depressed mood. *British Journal of Psychiatry*, **170**, 77–81.

Edmonstone, Y., Austin, M. P., Prentice, N., *et al* (1994) Uptake of 99mTc-exametazime shown by single photon emission computerized tomography in obsessive–compulsive disorder compared with major depression and normal controls. *Acta Psychiatrica Scandinavica*, **90**, 298–303.

Eisen, J. L. & Rasmussen, S. A. (1993) Obsessive–compulsive disorder with psychotic features. *Journal of Clinical Psychiatry*, **54**, 373–379.

Eisen, J. L., Beer, D. A., Pato, M. T., *et al* (1997) Obsessive–compulsive disorder in patients with schizophrenia and schizoaffective disorder. *American Journal of Psychiatry*, **154**, 271–273.

**261**

Eisen, J. L., Goodman, W. K., Keller, M. B., *et al* (1999) Patterns of remission and relapse in obsessive–compulsive disorder: a 2-year prospective study. *Journal of Clinical Psychiatry*, **60**, 346–351.

Elam, M., Yao, T., Thoren, P., *et al* (1981) Hypercapnia and hypoxia: chemoreceptor-mediated control of locus coeruleus neurons and splanchnic, sympathetic nerves. *Brain Research*, **222**, 373–381.

Emrich, H. M., Zersson, D. V., Kissling, H. J., *et al* (1980) Effect of sodium valproate on mania: the GABA hypothesis of affective disorders. *Archives für Psychiatrie und Nervenkrankenheit*, **229**, 1–16.

Ernst, M., Zametkin, A. J., Matochik, J., *et al* (1997) Intravenous dextroamphetamine and brain glucose metabolism. *Neuropsychopharmacology*, **17**, 391–401.

Etcoff, N. L., Freeman, R. & Cave, K. R. (1991) Can we lose memories of faces? Content awareness and awareness in a propagnosic. *Journal of Cognitive Neuroscience*, **3**, 25–41.

Falkai, P. & Bogerts, B. (1995) The neuropathology of schizophrenia. In *Schizophrenia* (eds S. R. Hirsh & D. R. Weinberger), pp. 275–292. Oxford: Blackwell Science.

Farde, L., Weisel, F-A., Stone-Elander, S., *et al* (1988) $D_2$ dopamine receptors in neuroleptic naïve schizophrenic patients. *Archives of General Psychiatry*, **47**, 213–219.

Fedoroff, J. P., Starkstein, S. E., Forrester, A. W., *et al* (1992) Depression in patients with acute traumatic brain injury. *American Journal of Psychiatry*, **149**, 918–923.

Feldman, S. & Weidenfeld, J. (1999) Glucocorticoid receptor antagonists in the hippocampus modify the negative feedback following neural stimuli. *Brain Research*, **821**, 33–37.

Fetoni, V., Soliveri, P., Monza, D., *et al* (1999) Affective symptoms in multiple system atrophy and Parkinson's disease: response to levodopa therapy. *Journal of Neurology, Neurosurgery and Psychiatry*, **66**, 541–544.

Fields, A., Li, P. P., Kish, S. J., *et al* (1999) Increased cyclic AMP-dependent protein kinase activity in postmortem brain from patients with bipolar affective disorder. *Journal of Neurochemistry*, **73**, 1704–1710.

Fischer, H., Andersson, J. L., Furmark, T., *et al* (1998) Brain correlates of an unexpected panic attack: a human positron emission tomographic study. *Neuroscience Letters*, **251**, 137–140.

Fisher, L. & Blair, R. J. (1998) Cognitive impairment and its relationship to psychopathic tendencies in children with emotional and behavioral difficulties. *Journal of Abnormal Childhood Psychology*, **26**, 511–519.

Fletcher, P. C., Frith, C. D., Grasby, P. M., *et al* (1996) Local and distributed effects of apomorphine on fronto-temporal function in acute unmedicated schizophrenia. *Journal of Neuroscience*, **16**, 7055–7062.

Flynn, S. W., MacKay, A. L., Vavasour, I. M., *et al* (1999) Abnormalities of myelin in schizophrenia demonstrated with 32-echo MRI technology. *Schizophrenia Research*, **36**, 196.

Ford, J. M. (1999) Schizophrenia: the broken P300 and beyond. *Psychophysiology*, **36**, 667–682.

Forstl, H., Burns, A., Levy, R., *et al* (1994) Neuropathological correlates of psychotic phenomena in confirmed Alzheimer's disease. *British Journal of Psychiatry*, **165**, 53–59.

Freedman, R., Coon, H., Myles-Worsley, M., *et al* (1997) Linkage of a neurophysiological deficit in schizophrenia to a chromosome 15 locus. *Proceedings of the National Academy of Sciences USA*, **94**, 587–592.

Frick, P. J., O'Brien, B. S., Wootton, J. M., *et al* (1994) Psychopathy and conduct problems in children. *Journal of Abnormal Psychology*, **103**, 700–707.

Friedman, E. & Wang, H. (1996) Receptor-mediated activation of G proteins is increased in postmortem brains of bipolar affective disorder subjects. *Journal of Neurochemistry*, **67**, 1145–1152.

Frith, C. D. (1992) *The Cognitive Neuropsychology of Schizophrenia*. Hove: Lawrence Erlbaum.

Frith, C. D. & Done, D. J. (1989) Experiences of alien control in schizophrenia reflect a disorder in the central monitoring of action. *Psychological Medicine*, **19**, 359–363.

Frith, C. D., Friston, K. J., Liddle, P. F., *et al* (1991a) A PET study of word finding. *Neuropsychologia*, **29**, 1137–1148.

Frith, C. D., Friston, K. J., Liddle, P. F., *et al* (1991b) Willed action and the prefrontal cortex in man: a study with PET. *Proceedings of the Royal Society (London) B*, **244**, 241–246.

Frith, C. D., Leary, J., Cahill, C., et al (1991c) Disabilities and circumstances of schizophrenic patients – a follow-up study. IV. Performance on psychological tests. *British Journal of Psychiatry*, **159** (suppl. 13), 26–29.

Frith, C. D., Friston, K. J., Liddle, P. F., et al (1992) PET imaging and cognition in schizophrenia. *Journal of the Royal Society of Medicine*, **85**, 222–224.

Frith, C. D., Friston, K. J., Herold, S., et al (1995) Regional brain activity in chronic schizophrenic patients during the performance of a verbal fluency task. *British Journal of Psychiatry*, **167**, 343–349.

Fuchs, E. & Flugge, G. (1995) Modulation of binding sites for corticotropin-releasing hormone by chronic psychosocial stress. *Psychoneuroendocrinology*, **20**, 33–51.

Furlong, R. A., Ho, L., Rubinsztein, J. S., et al (1999) Analysis of the monoamine oxidase A (MAOA) gene in bipolar affective disorder by association studies, meta-analyses, and sequencing of the promoter. *American Journal of Medical Genetics*, **88**, 398–406.

Fuster, J. M. (1997) *The Prefrontal Cortex: Anatomy, Physiology and Neuropsychology of the Frontal Lobe*. New York: Lippinscott-Raven.

Gaffan, D. (1994) Scene-specific memory for objects: a model of episodic memory impairment in monkeys with fornix transection. *Journal of Cognitive Neuroscience*, **6**, 305–320.

Garcia, R., Vouimba, R. M., Baudry, M., et al (1999) The amygdala modulates prefrontal cortex activity relative to conditioned fear. *Nature*, **402**, 294–296.

Geddes, J. R. & Lawrie, S. M. (1995) Obstetric complications and schizophrenia: a meta-analysis. *British Journal of Psychiatry*, **167**, 786–793.

Gerfen, C. R. (1989) The neostriatal mosaic: striatal patch-matrix organization is related to cortical lamination. *Science*, **246**, 385–388.

Gloor, P. (1997) *The Temporal Lobe and Limbic System*. Oxford: Oxford University Press.

Gloor, P., Olivier, A., Quesney, L. F., et al (1982) The role of the limbic system in experiential phenomena of temporal lobe epilepsy. *Annals of Neurology*, **12**, 129–144.

Goddard, A. W., Charney, D. S., Germine, M., et al (1995) Effects of tryptophan depletion on responses to yohimbine in healthy human subjects. *Biological Psychiatry*, **38**, 4–85.

Goldberg, G., Mayer, N. H. & Toglia, J. U. (1981) Medial frontal cortex infarction and the alien hand sign. *Archives of Neurology*, **38**, 683–686.

Goldberg, T. E., Ragland, D. R., Gold, J., et al (1990) Neuropsychological assessment of monozygotic twins discordant for schizophrenia. *Archives of General Psychiatry*, **47**, 1066–1072.

Goldberg, T. E., Greenberg, R. & Griffin, S. (1993) The impact of clozapine on cognition and psychiatric symptoms in patients with schizophrenia. *British Journal of Psychiatry*, **162**, 43–48.

Goldman-Rakic, P. S. (1987) Circuitry of primate prefrontal cortex and regulation of behaviour by representational memory. In *Handbook of Physiology: The Nervous System*, vol. 5 (eds F. Plum & V. Mountcastle). Baltimore: Williams & Wilkins.

Goldman-Rakic, P. S. (1988) Topography of cognition: parallel distributed networks in primate association cortex. *Annual Review of Neuroscience*, **11**, 137–156.

Goldman-Rakic, P. S. (1992) Working memory and the mind. *Scientific American*, September, 73–79.

Goodwin, D. W., Anderson, P. & Rosenthal, R. (1971) Clinical significance of hallucinations in psychiatric disorders. *Archives of General Psychiatry*, **24**, 76–80.

Goodwin, F. K., Post, R. M. Dunner, E. L., et al (1973) CSF amine metabolites in affective illness: the probenecid technique. *American Journal of Psychiatry*, **130**, 73–79.

Goodwin, G. M., Cavanagh, J. T., Glabus, M. F., et al (1997) Uptake of $^{99m}$Tc-exametazime shown by single photon emission computed tomography before and after lithium withdrawal in bipolar patients: associations with mania. *British Journal of Psychiatry*, **170**, 426–430.

Gotlib, L. H. (1981) Self-reinforcement and recall: differential deficits in depressed and non-depressed psychiatric patients. *Journal of Abnormal Psychology*, **90**, 512–530.

Gottesman, I. I. & Shields, J. (1982) *Schizophrenia: The Epigenetic Puzzle*. New York: Cambridge University Press.

Grace, A. A., Moore, H. & O'Donnell, P. (1998) The modulation of corticoaccumbens transmission by limbic afferents and dopamine: a model for the pathophysiology of schizophrenia. *Advances in Pharmacology*, **42**, 721–724.

Graeff, F. G., Guimaraes, F. S., De Andrade, T. G., et al (1996) Role of 5-HT in stress, anxiety, and depression. *Pharmacology and Biochemistry of Behaviour*, **54**, 129–141.

Graeff, F. G., Netto, C. F. & Zangrossi, H. Jr (1998) The elevated T-maze as an experimental model of anxiety. *Neuroscience and Biobehaviour Reviews*, **23**, 237–246.

Gray, J. A. (1982) *The Neuropsychology of Anxiety: An Enquiry into the Functions of the Septo-hippocampal System*. Oxford: Oxford University Press.

Gray, T. S. & Bingaman, E. W. (1996) The amygdala: corticotropin-releasing factor, steroids, and stress. *Critical Reviews in Neurobiology*, **10**, 155–168.

Gray, C. M., Konig, P., Engel, A. K., et al (1989) Oscillatory responses in cat visual cortex exhibit inter-columnar synchronization which reflects global stimulus properties. *Nature*, **338**, 334–337.

Green, M. F. (1998) *Schizophrenia from a Neurocognitive Perspective*. Boston: Allyn and Bacon.

Green, M. F., Marshall, B. D. Jr, Wirshing, W. C., et al (1997) Does risperidone improve verbal working memory in treatment-resistant schizophrenia? *American Journal of Psychiatry*, **154**, 799–804.

Grove, W. M. & Andreasen, N. C. (1985) Language and thinking in psychosis. Is there an input abnormality? *Archives of General Psychiatry*, **42**, 26–32.

Hafner, H., Maurer, K., Loffler, W., et al (1994) The epidemiology of early schizophrenia: influence of age and gender on onset and early course. *British Journal of Psychiatry*, **164** (suppl. 23), 29–38.

Halgren, E., Walter, R. D., Cherlow, D. G., et al (1978) Mental phenomena evoked by electrical stimulation of the human hippocampus and amygdala. *Brain*, **101**, 83–117.

Halgren, E., Marinkovic, K. & Chauvel, P. (1998) Generators of the late cognitive potentials in auditory and visual oddball tasks. *Electroencephalography and Clinical Neurophysiology*, **106**, 156–164.

Hand, I. (1998) Out-patient, multi-modal behaviour therapy for obsessive–compulsive disorder. *British Journal of Psychiatry*, **173** (suppl. 35), 45–52.

Harding, C. M., Zubin, J. & Strauss, J. S. (1992) Chronicity in schizophrenia: revisited. *British Journal of Psychiatry*, **161** (suppl. 18), 27–37.

Hare, R. D. (1978) Psychopathy and electrodermal responses to nonsignal stimulation. *Biological Psychology*, **6**, 237–246.

Hare, R. D. (1980) A research scale for the assessment of psychopathy in criminal populations. *Personality and Individual Differences*, **1**, 111–119.

Hare, R. D. (1998) Psychopathy, affect and behavior. In *Psychopathy: Theory, Research and Implications for Society* (eds D. J. Cooke, A. E. Forth & R. D. Hare), p. 106. Dordrecht: Kluwer.

Hare, R. D. & Jutai, J. W. (1988) Psychopathy and cerebral asymmetry in semantic processing. *Personality and Individual Differences*, **9**, 329–337.

Hare, R. D. & McPherson, L. M. (1984) Psychopathy and perceptual asymmetry during verbal dichotic listening. *Journal of Abnormal Psychology*, **93**, 141–149.

Hare, R. D., Harpur, T. J., Hakstian, A. R., et al (1990). The revised Psychopathy Checklist: reliability and factor structure. *Psychological Assessment*, **2**, 338–341.

Harlow, J. M. (1848) Passage of an iron rod through the head. *Boston Medical and Surgical Journal*, **39**, 389–393.

Harpur, J. & Hare, R. D. (1994) Assessment of psychopathy as a function of age. *Journal of Abnormal Psychology*, **103**, 604–609.

Harrow, M., Silverstein, M. & Marengo, J. (1983) Disordered thinking: does it identify nuclear schizophrenia? *Archives of General Psychiatry*, **40**, 765–771.

Hart, S. D., Forth, A. E. & Hare, R. D. (1990) Performance of criminal psychopaths on selected neuropsychological tests. *Journal of Abnormal Psychology*, **99**, 374–379.

Harvey, P. D., Earle-Boyer, E. A. & Levinson, J. C. (1986) Distractibility and discourse failure: their association in mania and schizophrenia. *Journal of Nervous and Mental Diseases*, **174**, 274–279.

Harvey, P. D., Earle-Boyer, E. A. & Levinson, J. C. (1988) Cognitive deficits and thought disorder: a retest study. *Schizophrenia Bulletin*, **14**, 57–66.

Harvey, I., Persaud, R., Ron, M. A., et al (1994) Volumetric MRI measurements in bipolars compared with schizophrenics and healthy controls. *Psychological Medicine*, **24**, 689–699.

Hazrati, L-N. & Parent, A. (1992) Differential patterns of arborization of striatal and subthalamic fibers in the two pallidal segments in primates. *Brain Research*, **598**, 311–315.

Hebb, D. O. (1949) *The Organization of Behavior: A Neuropsychological Theory*. New York: Wiley.

Heilbrun, A. B. (1980) Impaired recognition of self-expressed thought in patients with auditory hallucinations. *Journal of Abnormal Psychology*, **89**, 728–736.

Hellhammer, D. H., Hingtgen, J. N., Wade, S. E., *et al* (1983) Serotonergic changes in specific areas of rat brain associated with activity-stress gastric lesions. *Psychosomatic Medicine*, **45**, 115–122.

Hemby, S. E., Co, C., Dworkin, S. I., *et al* (1999) Synergistic elevations in nucleus accumbens extracellular dopamine concentrations during self-administration of cocaine/heroin combinations (speedball) in rats. *Journal of Pharmacology and Experimental Therapeutics*, **288**, 274–280.

Herman, J. P., Cullinan, W. E., Young, E. A., *et al* (1992) Selective forebrain fiber tract lesions implicate ventral hippocampal structures in tonic regulation of paraventricular nucleus corticotropin-releasing hormone (CRH) and arginine vasopressin (AVP) mRNA expression. *Brain Research*, **592**, 228–238.

Herman, J. P., Cullinan, W. E., Morano, M. I., *et al* (1995) Contribution of the ventral subiculum to inhibitory regulation of the hypothalamo-pituitary-adrenocortical axis. *Journal of Neuroendocrinology*, **7**, 475–482.

Herman, J. P., Prewitt, C. M. & Cullinan, W. E. (1996) Neuronal circuit regulation of the hypothalamo-pituitary-adrenocortical stress axis. *Critical Reviews of Neurobiology*, **10**, 371–394.

Herve, D., Blanc, G., Glowinski, J., *et al* (1982) Reduction of dopamine utilization in the prefrontal cortex but not in the nucleus accumbens after selective destruction of noradrenergic fibres innervating the ventral tegmental area in the rat. *Brain Research*, **237**, 510–516.

Hill, J. D. & Waterson, D. (1942) EEG studies of psychopathic personalities. *Journal of Neurology, Neurosurgery and Psychiatry*, **5**, 47–65.

Hill, J. D., Pond, D. A., Mitchell, W., *et al* (1957) Personality changes following temporal lobectomy for epilepsy. *Journal of Mental Science*, **103**, 18–27.

Hinde, R. A., Spencer-Booth, Y. & Bruce, M. (1966) Effects of 6-day maternal deprivation on rhesus monkey infants. *Nature*, **210**, 1021–1023.

Hinde, R. A. & Spencer-Booth, Y. (1970) Individual differences in the responses of rhesus monkeys to a period of separation from their mothers. *Journal of Child Psychology and Psychiatry*, **11**, 159–176.

Hirayasu, Y., Shenton, M. E., Salisbury, D. F., *et al* (1999) Subgenual cingulate cortex volume in first-episode psychosis. *American Journal of Psychiatry*, **156**, 1091–1093.

Hirsch, S. R., Jolley, A. G., Barnes, T. R., *et al* (1989) Dysphoric and depressive symptoms in chronic schizophrenia. *Schizophrenia Research*, **2**, 259–264.

Hoehn-Saric, R., Pearlson, G. D., Harris, G. J., *et al* (1991) Effects of fluoxetine on regional cerebral blood flow in obsessive–compulsive patients. *American Journal of Psychiatry*, **148**, 1243–1245.

Hoehn-Saric, R., McLeod, D. R. & Hipsley, P. (1995) Is hyperarousal essential to obsessive–compulsive disorder? Diminished physiologic flexibility, but not hyperarousal, characterizes patients with obsessive–compulsive disorder. *Archives of General Psychiatry*, **52**, 688–693.

Hoffman, R. E., Stopek, S. & Andreasen, N. C. (1986) A comparative study of manic vs schizophrenic speech disorganization. *Archives of General Psychiatry*, **43**, 831–838.

Holmes, M. C., French, K. L. & Seckl, J. R. (1995) Modulation of serotonin and corticosteroid receptor gene expression in the rat hippocampus with circadian rhythm and stress. *Brain Research, Molecular Brain Research*, **28**, 186–192.

Holsboer, F. (1999) The rationale for corticotropin-releasing hormone receptor (CRH-R) antagonists to treat depression and anxiety. *Journal of Psychiatric Research*, **33**, 181–214.

Horger, B. A. & Roth, R. H. (1996) The role of mesoprefrontal dopamine neurons in stress. *Critical Reviews of Neurobiology*, **10**, 395–418.

Howard, R. C. (1984) The clinical EEG and personality in mentally abnormal offenders. *Psychological Medicine*, **14**, 569–580.

**265**

Howland, E. W., Kosson, D. S., Patterson, C. M., *et al* (1993) Altering a dominant response: performance of psychopaths and low-socialization college students on a cued reaction time task. *Journal of Abnormal Psychology*, **102**, 379–387.

Hubbard, B. M. & Anderson, J. N. (1981) A quantitative study of cerebral atrophy in old age and senile dementia. *Journal of Neurological Science*, **50**, 135–145.

Huttunen, M. O. & Niskanen, P. (1973) Prenatal loss of father and psychiatric disorders. *Archives of General Psychiatry*, **35**, 429–431.

Huq, S. F., Garety, P. A. & Helmsley, D. R. (1988) Probabalistic judgments in deluded and non-deluded subjects. *Quarterly Journal of Experimental Psychology*, **40**, 801–812.

Iles, S. (1989) The loss of early pregnancy. *Baillieres Clinical Obstetrics and Gynaecology*, **3**, 769–790.

Ilsley, J. E., Moffoot, A. P. & O'Carroll, R. E. (1995) An analysis of memory dysfunction in major depression. *Journal of Affective Disorders*, **35**, 1–9.

Intrator, J., Hare, R., Stritzke, P., *et al* (1997) A brain imaging (single photon emission computerized tomography) study of semantic and affective processing in psychopaths. *Biological Psychiatry*, **42**, 96–103.

Jablensky, A. (1995) Schizophrenia: the epidemiological horizon. In *Schizophrenia* (eds S. R. Hirsch & D. R. Weinberger), pp. 206–252. Oxford: Blackwell.

Jacobs, D. & Silverstone, T. (1986) Dextroamphetamine-induced arousal in human subjects as a model for mania. *Psychological Medicine*, **16**, 323–329.

Jampala, V. C., Taylor, M. A. & Abrams, R. (1989) The diagnostic implications of formal thought disorder in mania and schizophrenia: a reassessment. *American Journal of Psychiatry*, **146**, 459–463.

Javanmard, M., Shlik, J., Kennedy, S. H., *et al* (1999) Neuroanatomic correlates of CCK-4-induced panic attacks in healthy humans: a comparison of two time points. *Biological Psychiatry*, **45**, 872–882.

Javitt, D. & Zukin, S. R. (1991) Recent advances in the phencyclidine model of schizophrenia. *American Journal of Psychiatry*, **148**, 1301–1308.

Jenike, M. A. (1998) Neurosurgical treatment of obsessive–compulsive disorder. *British Journal of Psychiatry*, **173** (suppl. 35), 79–90.

Johnson, R. Jr (1988) Scalp-recorded P300 activity in patients following unilateral temporal lobectomy. *Brain*, **111**, 1517–1529.

Johnston, M. H. & Holzman, P. S. (1979) *Assessing Schizophrenic Thinking*. San Francisco: Jossey-Bass.

Johnstone, E. C., Crow, T. J., Frith, C. D., *et al* (1976) Cerebral ventricular size and cognitive impairment in chronic schizophrenia. *Lancet*, **ii**, 924–926.

Johnstone, E. C, Crow, T. J., Frith, C. D., *et al* (1978a) Mechanism of the antipsychotic effect in the treatment of acute schizophrenia. *Lancet*, **i**, 848–851.

Johnstone, E. C., Crow, T. J., Frith, C. D., *et al* (1978b) The dementia of dementia praecox. *Acta Psychiatrica Scandinavica*, **57**, 305–324.

Johnstone, E. C, Owens, D. G. C., Frith, C. D., *et al* (1991) Disabilities and circumstances of schizophrenic patients – a follow-up study. III. Clinical findings. *British Journal of Psychiatry*, **159** (suppl. 13), 21–25.

Jones, P., Rodgers, B. & Murray, R. (1994) Child development risk factors for adult schizophrenia in the British 1946 birth cohort. *Lancet*, **344**, 1398–1402.

Jonides, J., Schumacher, E. H., Smith, E. E., *et al* (1997) Verbal working memory load affects regional brain activation as measured by PET. *Journal of Cognitive Neuroscience*, **9**, 462–475.

Jorge, R. E., Robinson, R. G., Arndt, S. V., *et al* (1993) Comparison between acute- and delayed-onset depression following traumatic brain injury. *Journal of Neuropsychiatry and Clinical Neuroscience*, **5**, 43–49.

Joyce, E. M. & Levy, R. (1989) Treatment of mood disorder associated with Binswanger's disease. *British Journal of Psychiatry*, **154**, 259–261.

Jutai, J. W. & Hare, R. D. (1983) Psychopathy and selective attention during performance of a complex-perceptual-motor task. *Psychophysiology*, **20**, 146–151.

Kaczmarek, B. L. J. (1987) The frontal lobes revisited. In *The Frontal Lobes* (ed. E. Perecman), pp. 225–240. New York: IRBN Press.

Kahlbaum, K. (1874) *Die Katatonie oder das Spannungs-Irresein*. Berlin: Hirschwald.

Kane, J. M., Honigfeld, G., Singer, J., *et al* (1988) Clozapine for the treatment resistant schizophrenic. *Archives of General Psychiatry*, **45**, 789–796.

Kaplan, R. D., Szechtman, H., Franco, S., *et al* (1993) Three clinical syndromes of schizophrenia in untreated subjects: relation to brain glucose activity measured by positron emission tomography (PET). *Schizophrenia Research*, **11**, 47–54.

Kapp, B. S., Pascoe, J. P. & Bixler, M. A. (1984) The amygdala: a neuroanatomical systems approach to its contributions to aversive conditioning. In *Neuropsychology of Memory* (eds N. Butters & L. R. Squire), pp. 473–488. New York: Guilford.

Kapur, S. & Remington, G. (1996) Serotonin–dopamine interaction and its relevance to schizophrenia. *American Journal of Psychiatry*, **153**, 466–476.

Karno, M., Golding, J. M., Sorenson, S. B., *et al* (1988) The epidemiology of obsessive–compulsive disorder in 5 US communities. *Archives of General Psychiatry*, **45**, 1094–1099.

Kaschka, W., Feistel, H. & Ebert, D. (1995) Reduced benzodiazepine receptor binding in panic disorders measured by iomazenil SPECT. *Journal of Psychiatric Research*, **29**, 427–434.

Kawanishi, Y., Harada, S., Tachikawa, H., *et al* (1999) Novel variants in the promoter region of the CREB gene in schizophrenic patients. *Journal of Human Genetics*, **44**, 428–430.

Kay, S. R. (1991) *Positive and Negative Symptoms in Schizophrenia*. New York: Brunner/Mazel.

Kay, S. R. & Sevy, S. (1990) Pyramidical model of schizophrenia. *Schizophrenia Bulletin*, **16**, 537–545.

Keck, P. E. Jr, McElroy, S. L., Tugrul, K. C., *et al* (1993) Valproate oral loading in the treatment of acute mania. *Journal of Clinical Psychiatry*, **54**, 305–308.

Keefe, R. S., Silva, S. G., Perkins, D. O., *et al* (1999) The effects of atypical antipsychotic drugs on neurocognitive impairment in schizophrenia: a review and meta-analysis. *Schizophrenia Bulletin*, **25**, 201–222.

Kelley, A. E. & Domesick, V. B. (1982) The distribution of the projection from the hippocampal formation to the nucleus accumbens in the rat: an anterograde and retrograde horseradish peroxidase study. *Neuroscience*, **7**, 2321–2335.

Kelley, A. E. & Stinus, L. (1985) Disappearance of hoarding behaviour after 6-hydroxydopamine lesions of mesolimbic dopamine neurons and its reinstatement with L-dopa. *Behavioural Neuroscience*, **99**, 531–545.

Kelly, W. F., Checkley, S. A., Bender, D. A., *et al* (1983) Cushing's syndrome and depression – a prospective study of 26 patients. *British Journal of Psychiatry*, **142**, 16–19.

Kendler, K. S., Neale, M. C., Kessler, R. C., *et al* (1993) A longitudinal twin study of personality and major depression in women. *Archives of General Psychiatry*, **50**, 853–862.

Kennedy, J. L. & Macciardi, F. M. (1998) Chromosome 4 workshop. *Psychiatric Genetics*, **8**, 67–71.

Kibel, D. A., Laffont, I. & Liddle, P. F. (1993) The composition of the negative syndrome of chronic schizophrenia. *British Journal of Psychiatry*, **162**, 744–750.

Kiehl, K. K. & Liddle, P. F. (2001) An event-related functional magnetic resonance imaging study of an auditory oddball task in schizophrenia. *Schizophrenia Research*, **48**, 159–171.

Kiehl, K. A., Smith, A. M., Mendrek, A., *et al* (1998) Activation of the amygdala during an affective memory task. *NeuroImage*, **7**, S902.

Kiehl, K. A., Hare, R. D., McDonald, J. J., *et al* (1999a) Semantic and affective processing in psychopaths: an event-related potential (ERP) study. *Psychophysiology*, **36**, 765–774.

Kiehl, K. A., Hare, R. D., Liddle, P. F., *et al* (1999b) Reduced P300 responses in criminal psychopaths during a visual oddball task. *Biological Psychiatry*, **45**, 1498–1507.

Kiehl, K. A., Liddle, P. F. & Hopfinger, J. B. (2000a) Error processing and the rostral anterior cingulate: an event-related fMRI study. *Psychophysiology*, **37**, 216–223.

Kiehl, K. A., Smith, A. M., Hare, R. D., *et al* (2000b) An event-related potential (ERP) investigation of response inhibition in schizophrenia and psychopathy. *Biological Psychiatry*, **48**, 210–221.

Kiehl, K. A., Smith, A. M., Hare, R. D., *et al* (2000c) Limbic abnormalities in affective processing by criminal psychopaths as revealed by fMRI. *NeuroImage*, **11**, S223.

Kiehl, K. A., Laurens, K. R., Duty, T. L., *et al* (2001) Neural sources involved in auditory target detection and novelty processing: an event-related fMRI study. *Psychophysiology*, **38**, 133–142.

Kimbrell, T. A., George, M. S., Parekh, P. I., *et al* (1999) Regional brain activity during transient self-induced anxiety and anger in healthy adults. *Biological Psychiatry*, **46**, 454–465.

Kircher, T., Liddle, P., Brammer, M., *et al* (2000) Production of thought disordered speech in schizophrenia is negatively correlated with activation in the left superior temporal gyrus. *Neuroimage*, **11**, S210.

Kirov, G., Rees, M., Jones, I., *et al* (1999) Bipolar disorder and the serotonin transporter gene: a family-based association study. *Psychological Medicine*, **29**, 1249–1254.

Kirschbaum, C., Wolf, O. T., May, M., *et al* (1996) Stress- and treatment-induced elevations of cortisol levels associated with impaired declarative memory performance in healthy adults. *Life Sciences*, **58**, 1475–1483.

Kleist, K. (1934) *Gehirnpathologie*. Leipzig: Barth.

Kluver, H. & Bucy, P. (1937) 'Psychic blindness' and other symptoms following bilateral temporal lobectomy in rhesus monkey. *American Journal of Physiology*, **119**, 352–353.

Knights, A. & Hirsch, S. R. (1981) 'Revealed' depression and drug treatment for schizophrenia. *Archives of General Psychiatry*, **38**, 806–811.

Koepp, M. J., Gunn, R. N., Lawrence, A. D., *et al* (1998) Evidence for striatal dopamine release during a video game. *Nature*, **393**, 266–268.

Koob, G. & Bloom, F. E. (1985) Corticotrophin-releasing factor and behaviour. *Federation Proceedings*, **44**, 259–265.

Kopp, B. & Rist, F. (1999) An event-related brain potential substrate of disturbed response monitoring in paranoid schizophrenic patients. *Journal of Abnormal Psychology*, **108**, 337–346.

Kraepelin, E. (1883) *Compendium der Psychiatrie*. Leipzig: Abel.

Kraepelin, E. (1896) Dementia praecox. In *The Clinical Roots of the Schizophrenia Concept* (eds J. Cutting & M. Shepherd), pp. 15–24. Cambridge: Cambridge University Press (1987). Translated from *Lehrbuch der Psychiatrie*, 5th edn, pp. 426– 441. Leipzig: Barth.

Kraepelin, E. (1919) *Dementia Praecox and Paraphrenia* (trans. R. M. Barclay). New York: Kreiger (facsimile edn, 1971).

Kraepelin, E. (1920) Die Ercheinungsformen des Irreseins. *Zeitschrift für Neurologie und Psychiatrie*, **62**, 1–29.

Kraepelin, E. (1921) *Manic–Depressive Insanity and Paranoia* (trans. R. M. Barclay from *Lehrbuch der Psychiatrie*, 8th edn. Leipzig: Barth). Edinburgh: Churchill Livingstone.

Krystal, J. H., D'Souza, D. C., Karper, L. P., *et al* (1999) Interactive effects of subanesthetic ketamine and haloperidol in healthy humans. *Psychopharmacology (Berlin)*, **145**, 193–204.

Kulhara, P., Kota, S. K. & Joseph, S. (1986) Positive and negative subtypes of schizophrenia: a study from India. *Acta Psychiatrica Scandinavica*, **74**, 353–379.

Kumar, R., Marks, M., Wieck, A., *et al* (1993) Neuroendocrine and psychosocial mechanisms in post-partum psychosis. *Progress in Neuropsychopharmacology and Biological Psychiatry*, **17**, 571–579.

Kurland, H. D., Yeager, C. T., Ransom, J. A., *et al* (1963) Psychophysiological aspects of severe behavioural disorders. *Archives of General Psychiatry*, **8**, 599–604.

Kuzis, G., Sabe, L., Tiberti, C., *et al* (1999) Neuropsychological correlates of apathy and depression in patients with dementia. *Neurology*, **52**, 1403–1407.

Lahti, A. C., Holcomb, H. H., Weiler, M. A., *et al* (1997) Regional correlations between ketamine-induced actions on psychosis and regional cerebral blood flow (rCBF). *Schizophrenia Research*, **24**, 167.

Lane, C. J. (1999) *An In Vivo Investigation of Neuronal Function in First Episode Schizophrenia: The Effects of Risperidone on Patterns of Cerebral Metabolism and Symptom Profiles*. PhD thesis, University of British Columbia.

Lapierre, D., Braun, C. M. & Hodgins, S. (1995) Ventral frontal deficits in psychopathy: neuropsychological test findings. *Neuropsychologia*, **33**, 139–151.

Laplane, D., Baulac, M., Widlocher, D., *et al* (1984) Pure psychic akinesia with bilateral lesions of basal ganglia. *Journal of Neurology, Neurosurgery and Psychiatry*, **47**, 377–385.

Laruelle, M., Abi-Dargham, A., van Dyck, C. H., *et al* (1995) SPECT imaging of striatal dopamine release after amphetamine challenge. *Journal of Nuclear Medicine*, **36**, 1182–1190.

Laruelle, M., Abi-Dargham, A., van Dyck, C. H., *et al* (1996) Single photon emission computerized tomography imaging of amphetamine-induced dopamine release in drug-free schizophrenic subjects. *Proceedings of the National Academy of Sciences USA*, **93**, 9235–9240.

Ledoux, J. E. (1995) In search of an emotional system in the brain: leaping from fear to emotion and consciousness. In *The Cognitive Neurosciences* (ed. M. S. Gazzaniga), pp. 1049–1061. Cambridge, MA: MIT Press.

Le Melledo, J. M., Bradwejn, J., Koszycki, D., *et al* (1998) The role of the beta-noradrenergic system in cholecystokinin-tetrapeptide-induced panic symptoms. *Biological Psychiatry*, **44**, 364–366.

Lepage, M., Habib, R. & Tulving, E. (1998) Hippocampal PET activations of memory encoding and retrieval: the HIPER model. *Hippocampus*, **8**, 313–322.

Lesch, K. P., Mayer, S., Disselkamp-Tietze, J., *et al* (1990) Subsensitivity of the 5-hydroxy-tryptamine 1A (5HT$_{1A}$) receptor mediated hypothermic response to ipsapirone in unipolar depression. *Life Sciences*, **46**, 1271–1277.

Levy, D. L., Smith, M., Robinson, D., *et al* (1993) Methyl phenidate increases thought disorder in recent onset schizophrenics, but not normal controls. *Biological Psychiatry*, **34**, 507–514.

Levy, D., Kimha, R., Barak, Y., *et al* (1996) Brainstem auditory evoked potentials of panic disorder patients. *Neuropsychobiology*, **33**, 164–167.

Levy, M. L., Cummings, J. L., Fairbanks, L. A., *et al* (1998) Apathy is not depression. *Journal of Neuropsychiatry and Clinical Neuroscience*, **10**, 314–319.

Lewis, S. W. (1990) Computerised tomography in schizophrenia 15 years on. *British Journal of Psychiatry*, **157** (suppl. 9), 16–24.

Libet, B., Gleason, C. A., Wright, E. W., *et al* (1983) Time of conscious intention to act in relation to onset of cerebral activity: readiness potential. *Brain*, **106**, 623–642.

Lidberg, L., Tuck, M., Asberg, M., *et al* (1985a) Homicide, suicide and CSF 5-HIAA. *Acta Psychiatrica Scandinavica*, **71**, 230–236.

Lidberg, L., Modin, I., Oreland, L., *et al* (1985b) Platelet monoamine oxidase and psychopathy. *Psychiatry Research*, **16**, 22–27.

Liddle, P. F. (1984) *Chronic Schizophrenic Symptoms, Cognitive Function and Neurological Impairment*. Membership examination thesis, Royal College of Psychiatrists, London.

Liddle, P. F. (1987a) The symptoms of chronic schizophrenia: a re-examination of the positive–negative dichotomy. *British Journal of Psychiatry*, **151**, 145–151.

Liddle, P. F. (1987b) Schizophrenic syndromes, cognitive performance and neurological dysfunction. *Psychological Medicine*, **17**, 49–58.

Liddle, P. F. (1994) Volition and schizophrenia. In *The Neuropsychology of Schizophrenia* (eds A. S. David & J. C. Cutting), pp. 39–49. Hove: Lawrence Erlbaum.

Liddle, P. F. (1995) Inner connections within the domain of dementia praecox: the role of supervisory mental processes in schizophrenia. *European Archives of Psychiatry and Clinical Neuroscience*, **245**, 210–215.

Liddle, P. F. (1998) Schizophrenia – the clinical picture. In *Seminars in General Adult Psychiatry* (eds G. Stein & G. Wilkinson), pp. 272–320. London: Gaskell.

Liddle, P. F. (1999) *The Thought and Language Index* (UBC Schizophrenia Division Technical Report). Vancouver: University of British Columbia

Liddle, P. F. (2000a) Functional brain imaging of schizophrenia. In *The Psychopharmacology of Schizophrenia* (eds M. Reveley & W. Deakin), pp. 109–130. London: Arnold.

Liddle, P. F. (2000b) Schizophrenic syndromes. In *Neurotransmitter Receptors in Actions of Antipsychotic Medications* (ed. M. S. Lidow), pp. 1–16. Boca Raton: CRC Press.

Liddle, P. F. & Barnes, T. R. E. (1990) Syndromes of chronic schizophrenia. *British Journal of Psychiatry*, **157**, 558–561.

Liddle, P. F. & Crow, T. J. (1984) Age-disorientated chronic schizophrenics have a global impairment of intellect. *British Journal of Psychiatry*, **144**, 193–199.

Liddle, P. F. & Morris, D. L. (1991) Schizophrenic syndromes and frontal lobe performance. *British Journal of Psychiatry*, **158**, 340–345.

Liddle, P. F., Friston, K. J., Frith, C. D., *et al* (1992) Patterns of cerebral blood flow in schizophrenia. *British Journal of Psychiatry*, **160**, 179–186.

Liddle, P. F., Mendrek, A., Smith, A. M., *et al* (1999) An fMRI study of fronto-temporal coordination during working memory in schizophrenia. *Schizophrenia Research*, **36**, 225.

Liddle, P. F., Lane, C. J. & Ngan, E. T. C. (2000) Immediate effects of risperidone on cortico-striato-thalamic loops and the hippocampus. *British Journal of Psychiatry*, **177**, 402–407.

Liddle, P. F., Kiehl, K. A. & Smith, A. M. (2001) An event-related fMRI study of response inhibition. *Human Brain Mapping*, **12**, 100–109.

Lieberman, J. A., Jody, D., Geisler, S., *et al* (1993) Biologic correlates of treatment response in first-episode schizophrenia. *Archives of General Psychiatry*, **50**, 369–376.

Lindstrom, L. H. (1985) Low HVA and normal 5HIAA CSF levels in drug free schizophrenia patients, compared to healthy volunteers: correlations to symptomatology and heredity. *Psychiatry Research*, **14**, 265–274.

Linnolia, M., Virkkunen, M., Scheinn, M., *et al* (1983) Low cerebrospinal fluid – hydoxyindoleacetic acid concentrations differentiates impulsive from non-impulsive violent behavior. *Life Sciences*, **33**, 2609–2614.

Lishman, A. W. (1987) *Organic Psychiatry*. Oxford: Blackwell.

Litvan, I., Mega, M. S., Cummings, J. L., *et al* (1996) Neuropsychiatric aspects of progressive supranuclear palsy. *Neurology*, **47**, 1184–1189.

Litvan, I., Cummings, J. L. & Mega, M. (1998a) Neuropsychiatric features of corticobasal degeneration. *Journal of Neurology, Neurosurgery and Psychiatry*, **65**, 717–721.

Litvan, I., Paulsen, J. S., Mega, M. S., *et al* (1998b) Neuropsychiatric assessment of patients with hyperkinetic and hypokinetic movement disorders. *Archives of Neurology*, **55**, 1313–1319.

Liu, D., Dioro, J., Tannenbaum, B., *et al* (1997) Maternal care, hippocampal glucocorticoid receptors, and hypothalamic-pituitary adrenal response to stress. *Science*, **277**, 1659–1662.

Lopez, J. F., Vazquez, D. M., Chalmers, D. T., *et al* (1997) Regulation of 5-HT receptors and the hypothalamic-pituitary-adrenal axis. Implications for the neurobiology of suicide. *Annals of the New York Academy of Sciences*, **836**, 106–134.

Louilot, A., LeMoal, M. & Simon, H. (1989) Opposite influences of dopamine pathways in the prefrontal cortex and septum on the dopaminergic transmission in the nucleus accumbens: an in vivo voltametric study. *Neuroscience*, **29**, 45–56.

Lucas, G. & Spampinato, U. (2000) Role of striatal serotonin$_{2A}$ and serotonin$_{2C}$ receptor subtypes in the control of in vivo dopamine outflow in the rat striatum. *Journal of Neurochemistry*, **74**, 693–701.

Lucey, J. V., Costa, D. C., Blanes, T., *et al* (1995) Regional cerebral blood flow in obsessive–compulsive disordered patients at rest. Differential correlates with obsessive–compulsive and anxious–avoidant dimensions. *British Journal of Psychiatry*, **167**, 629–634.

Luck, S. J. (1995) Multiple mechanisms of visual-spatial attention: recent evidence from human electrophysiology. *Behavioural Brain Research*, **71**, 113–123.

Luck, S. J., Fan, S. & Hillyard, S. A. (1993) Attention-related modulation of sensory-evoked brain activity in a visual search task. *Journal of Cognitive Neuroscience*, **5**, 188–195.

Lupien, S. J., Gaudreau, S., Tchiteya, B. M., *et al* (1997) Stress-induced declarative memory impairment in healthy elderly subjects: relationship to cortisol reactivity. *Journal of Clinical Endocrinology and Metabolism*, **82**, 2070–2075.

Lupien, S. J., Nair, N. P., Briere, S., *et al* (1999) Increased cortisol levels and impaired cognition in human aging: implication for depression and dementia in later life. *Reviews of Neuroscience*, **10**, 117–139.

Lynam, D. R. (1996) Early identification of chronic offenders: who is the fledgling psychopath? *Psychological Bulletin*, **120**, 209–234.

Lynam, D. R. (1997) Pursuing the psychopath: capturing the fledgling psychopath in a nomological net. *Journal of Abnormal Psychology*, **106**, 425–438.

Lynam, D. R. (1998) Early identification of the fledgling psychopath: locating the psychopathic child in the current nomenclature. *Journal of Abnormal Psychology*, **107**, 566–575.

MacClean, P. D. (1975) On the evolution of three mentalities. *Man–Environment Systems*, **5**, 213–224.

Machlin, S. R., Harris, G. J., Pearlson, G. D., *et al* (1991) Elevated medial-frontal cerebral blood flow in obsessive–compulsive patients: a SPECT study. *American Journal of Psychiatry*, **148**, 1240–1242.

Madler, C., Keller, I., Schwendler, D., et al (1991) Sensory information processing during general anaesthesia: effect of isoflurane on auditory evoked neuronal oscillations. *British Journal of Anaesthesia*, **66**, 81–87.

Magarinos, A. M., McEwan, B. S., Flugge, G., et al (1996) Chronic psychosocial stress causes apical dendritic atrophy of hippocampal CA3 pyramidal neurons in subordinate tree shrews. *Journal of Neuroscience*, **16**, 3534–3540.

Maguire, E. A., Burgess, N., Donnett, J. G., et al (1998) Knowing where and getting there: a human navigation network. *Science*, **280**, 921–924.

Maguire, E. A., Gadian, D. G., Johnsrude, I. S., et al (2000) Navigation-related structural change in the hippocampi of taxi drivers. *Proceedings of the National Academy of Sciences USA*, **97**, 4398–4403.

Mahut, H., Zola-Morgan, S. & Moss, M. (1982) Hippocampal resections impair associative learning and recognition memory in the monkey. *Journal of Neuroscience*, **2**, 1214–1229.

Maier, S. F. (1991) Stressor controllability, cognition and fear. In *Neurobiology of Learning, Emotion and Affect* (ed. J. Madden), pp. 155–193. New York: Raven Press.

Maier, W., Lichterman, D., Minges, J., et al (1993) Continuity and discontinuity of affective disorders and schizophrenia. Results of a controlled family study. *Archives of General Psychiatry*, **50**, 871–873.

Malhotra, A. K., Adler, C. M., Kennison, S. D., et al (1997) Clozapine blunts N-methyl-D-aspartate antagonist-induced psychosis: a study with ketamine. *Biological Psychiatry*, **42**, 664–668.

Malizia, A. L., Cunningham, V. J., Bell, C. J., et al (1998) Decreased brain GABA(A)-benzodiazepine receptor binding in panic disorder: preliminary results from a quantitative PET study. *Archives of General Psychiatry*, **55**, 715–720.

Malla, A. K., Norman, R. M. G., Williamson, P., et al (1993) Three syndrome concept of schizophrenia, a factor analytic study. *Schizophrenia Research*, **10**, 143–150.

Manji, H. K. & Lenox, R. H. (1999) Ziskind–Somerfeld Research Award. Protein kinase C signaling in the brain: molecular transduction of mood stabilization in the treatment of manic–depressive illness. *Biological Psychiatry*, **46**, 1328–1351.

Manji, H. K., Bebchuk, J. M., Moore, G. J., et al (1999a) Modulation of CNS signal transduction pathways and gene expression by mood-stabilizing agents: therapeutic implications. *Journal of Clinical Psychiatry*, **60** (suppl. 2), 27–39.

Manji, H. K., Moore, G. J. & Chen, G. (1999b) Lithium at 50: have the neuroprotective effects of this unique cation been overlooked? *Biological Psychiatry*, **46**, 929–940.

Marder, S. R. & Meibach, R. C. (1994) Risperidone in the treatment of schizophrenia. *American Journal of Psychiatry*, **151**, 825–835.

Marengo, J. T. & Harrow, M. (1987) Schizophrenic thought disorder at follow-up. *Archives of General Psychiatry*, **44**, 651–659.

Marin, R. S., Fogel, B. S., Hawkins, J., et al (1995) Apathy: a treatable syndrome. *Journal of Neuropsychiatry and Clinical Neuroscience*, **7**, 23–30.

Marshall, L. A. & Cooke, D. J. (1999) The childhood experiences of psychopaths: a retrospective study of familial and societal factors. *Journal of Personality Disorders*, **13**, 211–225.

Martin, A., Wiggs, C. L., Altemus, M., et al (1995) Working memory as assessed by subject-ordered tasks in patients with obsessive–compulsive disorder. *Journal of Clinical and Experimental Neuropsychology*, **17**, 786–792.

Martin, K. A. C. (1984) Neuronal circuits in the cat striate cortex. In *Cerebral Cortex*, vol. 2 (eds E. G. Jones & A. Peters), pp. 241–285. New York: Plenum.

Martinot, J. L., Allilaire, J. F., Mazoyer, B. M., et al (1990) Obsessive–compulsive disorder: a clinical, neuropsychological and positron emission tomography study. *Acta Psychiatrica Scandinavica*, **82**, 233–242.

Masand, P. S., Anand, V. S. & Tanquary, J. F. (1998) Psychostimulant augmentation of second generation antidepressants: a case series. *Depression and Anxiety*, **7**, 89–91.

Mathias, C. J., Frankel, H. L., Turner, R. C., et al (1979) Physiological responses to insulin hypoglycaemia in spinal man. *Paraplegia*, **17**, 319–326.

Mattay, V. S., Berman, K. F., Ostrem, J. L., et al (1996) Dextroamphetamine enhances 'neural network-specific' physiological signals: a positron-emission tomography rCBF study. *Journal of Neuroscience*, **16**, 4816–4822.

Matthew, V. M., Gruzelier, J. H. & Liddle, P. F. (1993) Lateral asymmetries in auditory acuity distinguish hallucinating from non-hallucinating schizophrenic patients. *Psychiatry Research*, **46**, 127–138.

Maudlsey, H. (1873) *Body and Mind: An Enquiry into their Connection and Mutual Influence, Specially in Reference to Mental Disorders*. London: Macmillan.

Mayberg, H. S., Starkstein, S. E., Peyser, C. E., *et al* (1992) Paralimbic frontal lobe hypometabolism in depression associated with Huntington's disease. *Neurology*, **42**, 1791–1797.

Mayberg, H. S., Lewis, P. J., Regenold, W., *et al* (1994) Paralimbic hypoperfusion in unipolar depression. *Journal of Nuclear Medicine*, **35**, 929–934.

Mayberg, H. S., Brannan, S. K., Mahurin, R. K., *et al* (1997) Cingulate function in depression: a potential predictor of treatment response. *Neuroreport*, **8**, 1057–1061.

Mayberg, H. S., Liotti, M., Brannan, S. K., *et al* (1999) Reciprocal limbic-cortical function and negative mood: converging PET findings in depression and normal sadness. *American Journal of Psychiatry*, **156**, 675–682.

Maziade, M., Roy, M-A., Martinez, M., *et al* (1995) Negative, psychoticism, and disorganised dimensions in patients with familial schizophrenia or bipolar disorder: continuity and discontinuity between the major psychoses. *American Journal of Psychiatry*, **152**, 1458–1463.

Mazure, C. M. & Bowers, M. B. (1998) Pretreatment plasma HVA predicts neuroleptic response in manic psychosis. *Journal of Affective Disorders*, **48**, 83–86.

McCarley, R. W., Faux, S. F., Shenton, M. E., *et al* (1991) Event-related potentials in schizophrenia: their biological and clinical correlates and a new model of schizophrenic pathophysiology. *Schizophrenia Research*, **4**, 209–231.

McClure, R. K. (1999) Backward masking in bipolar affective disorder. *Progress in Neuropsychopharmacology and Biological Psychiatry*, **23**, 195–206.

McCormick, D. A. & Prince, D. A. (1985) Two types of muscarinic response to acetylcholine in mammalian cortical neurons. *Proceedings of the National Academy of Sciences USA*, **82**, 6344–6348.

McDonald, A. J. (1992) Cell types and intrinsic connections of the amygdala. In *The Amygdala: Neurobiological Aspects of Emotion, Memory, and Mental Dysfunction* (ed. J. P. Aggleton,), pp. 67–96. New York: Wiley-Liss.

McDonald, W. M., Tupler, L. A., Marsteller, F. A., *et al* (1999) Hyperintense lesions on magnetic resonance images in bipolar disorder. *Biological Psychiatry*, **45**, 965–971.

McEwan, B. S., Gould, E. A. & Sakai, R. R. (1992) The vulnerability of the hippocampus to the protective and destructive effects of glucocorticoids in relation to stress. *British Journal of Psychiatry*, **160** (suppl. 15), 18–23.

McGrath, J. J. (1992) The neuropsychology of thought disorder. *Schizophrenia Research*, **6**, 157.

McGuffin, P. & Gottesman, I. I. (1984) Genetic influences on normal and abnormal development. In *Child Psychiatry: Modern Approaches* (2nd edn) (eds M. Rutter & L. Hersov), pp. 17–33. London: Blackwell.

McGuire, P. K., Shah, G. M. S. & Murray, R. M. (1993) Increased blood flow in Broca's area during auditory hallucinations in schizophrenia. *Lancet*, **342**, 703–706.

McGuire, P. K., Bench, C. J., Frith, C. D., *et al* (1994) Functional anatomy of obsessive-compulsive phenomena. *British Journal of Psychiatry*, **164**, 459–468.

McGuire, P. K., Silbersweig, D. A., Wright, I., *et al* (1995) Abnormal monitoring of inner speech: a physiological basis for auditory hallucinations. *Lancet*, **346**, 596–600.

McGuire, P. K., Paulesu, E., Frackowiak, R. S. J., *et al* (1996) Brain activity during stimulus independent thought. *Neuroreport*, **7**, 2095–2099.

McGuire, P. K., Quested, D., Spence, S., *et al* (1998) Pathophysiology of 'positive' thought disorder in schizophrenia. *British Journal of Psychiatry*, **173**, 231–235.

McGuire, P., Shergill, S., Bullmore, E., *et al* (2000) Attenuated engagement of areas implicated in verbal self-monitoring in patients prone to auditory hallucinations. *Schizophrenia Research*, **41**, 12–13.

McNaughton, N. (1997) Cognitive dysfunction resulting from hippocampal hyperactivity – a possible cause of anxiety disorder? *Pharmacology and Biochemistry of Behavior*, **56**, 603–611.

Mellman, T. A. & Uhde, T. W. (1989) Electroencephalographic sleep in panic disorder. *Archives of General Psychiatry*, **46**, 178–184.

Mellor, C. S. (1970) First rank symptoms of schizophrenia. *British Journal of Psychiatry*, **117**, 15–23.

Meltzer, H. Y. (1992) Dimensions of outcome with clozapine. *British Journal of Psychiatry*, **160** (suppl. 17), 46–53.

Meltzer, H. Y. & McGurk, S. R. (1999) The effects of clozapine, risperidone, and olanzapine on cognitive function in schizophrenia. *Schizophrenia Bulletin*, **25**, 233–255.

Meltzer, H. Y., Matsubara, S. & Lee, J. C. (1989) The ratios of serotonin$_2$ and dopamine$_2$ affinities differentiate atypical and typical antipsychotic drugs. *Psychopharmacology Bulletin*, **25**, 390–392.

Meltzer, H. Y., Umberkoman-Wiita, B., Robertson, A., *et al* (1984) Effect of 5-hydroxytryptophan on serum cortisol in major affective disorders. *Archives of General Psychiatry*, **41**, 366–374.

Merikangas, K. R., Angst, J., Eaton, W., *et al* (1996) Comorbidity and boundaries of affective disorders with anxiety disorders and substances misuse: results of an international task force. *British Journal of Psychiatry*, **168** (suppl. 30), 58–87.

Mesulam, M-M. (1988) Central cholinergic pathways: neuroanatomy and some behavioural implications. In *Neurotransmitters and Cortical Function* (eds M. Avoli, T. A. Reader, R. W. Dykes, *et al*), pp. 237–260. New York: Plenum Press.

Mesulam, M-M. (1990) Large-scale neurocognitive networks and distributed processing for attention, language, and memory. *Annals of Neurology*, **28**, 597–613.

Miller, E. K., Erickson, C. A. & Desimone, R. (1996) Neural mechanisms of visual working memory in prefrontal cortex of the macaque. *Journal of Neuroscience*, **16**, 5154–5167.

Milner, B. (1966) Amnesia following operation on the temporal lobes. In *Amnesia* (eds C. W. M. Whitty & O. L. Zangwill), pp. 109–133. London: Butterworths.

Mineka, S. & Suomi, S. J. (1978) Social separation in monkeys. *Psychological Bulletin*, **85**, 1376–1400.

Mishkin, M. (1964) Perseveration of central sets after frontal lesions in monkeys. In *The Frontal Granular Cortex and Behaviour* (eds J. M. Warren & K. Akert), pp. 219–241. New York: McGraw-Hill.

Miyata, A., Matsunaga, H., Kiriike, N., *et al* (1998) Event-related potentials in patients with obsessive–compulsive disorder. *Psychiatry and Clinical Neuroscience*, **52**, 513–518.

Mlakar, J., Jensterle, J. & Frith, C. D. (1994) Central monitoring deficiency and schizophrenic symptoms. *Psychological Medicine*, **24**, 557–564.

Moller, H-J., Muller, H., Borison, R. K., *et al* (1995) A path-analytical approach to differentiate between direct and indirect drug effects on negative symptoms in schizophrenic patients. *European Archives of Psychiatry and Clinical Neuroscience*, **245**, 5–49.

Moore, G. J., Bebchuk, J. M., Parrish, J. K., *et al* (1999) Temporal dissociation between lithium-induced changes in frontal lobe myo-inositol and clinical response in manic–depressive illness. *American Journal of Psychiatry*, **156**, 1902–1908.

Morgan, C. A. 3rd & Grillon, C. (1999) Abnormal mismatch negativity in women with sexual assault-related posttraumatic stress disorder. *Biological Psychiatry*, **45**, 827–832.

Morgan, C. A. 3rd, Grillon, C., Southwick, S. M., *et al* (1995) Yohimbine facilitated acoustic startle in combat veterans with post-traumatic stress disorder. *Psychopharmacology (Berlin)*, **117**, 466–471.

Morgan, M. A., Romanski, L. M. & LeDoux, J. E. (1993) Extinction of emotional learning: contributions of the medial prefrontal cortex. *Neurosciences Letters*, **163**, 109–113.

Morice, R. D. & Ingram, J. C. L. (1982) Language analysis in schizophrenia: diagnostic implications. *Australian and New Zealand Journal of Psychiatry*, **16**, 11–21.

Morris, J. S., Frith, C. D., Perret, D. I., *et al* (1996) A differential neural response in the human amygdala to fearful and happy facial expressions. *Nature*, **383**, 812–815.

Morrison, G. & Haddock, G. (1997) Cognitive factors in source monitoring and auditory hallucinations. *Psychological Medicine*, **27**, 669–679.

Mortensen, P. B., Pedersen, C. B., Westergaard, T., *et al* (1999) Effects of family history and place and season of birth on the risk of schizophrenia. *New England Journal of Medicine*, **340**, 603–608.

Mortimer, A. M., Lund, C. E. & McKenna, P. J. (1990) The positive:negative dichotomy in schizophrenia. *British Journal of Psychiatry*, **157**, 41–49.

Moss, H. B, Yao, J. K. & Panzak, G. L. (1990) Serotonergic responsivity and behavioural dimensions in antisocial personality disorder with substance abuse. *Biological Psychiatry*, **28**, 325–338.

Mountcastle, V. B. (1998) *The Cerebral Cortex*. Cambridge, MA: Harvard University Press.

Muller-Preuss, P. (1978) Single unit responses of the auditory cortex in the squirrel monkey to self-produced and loud speaker transmitted vocalizations. *Neuroscience Letters*, **1** (suppl.), S8.

Murphy, D. L., Brodie, W. K., Goodwin, F. K., *et al* (1971) Regular induction of hypomania by L-dopa in bipolar manic–depressive patients. *Nature*, **229**, 135–136.

Musalek, M., Podreka, I., Walter, H., *et al* (1989) Regional brain function in hallucinations: a study of regional cerebral blood flow with 99m-Tc-HMPAO-SPECT in patients with auditory hallucinations, tactile hallucinations and normal controls. *Comprehensive Psychiatry*, **30**, 99–108.

Naranjo, C. A., Tremblay, L. K., Busto, U. E., *et al* (in press) The role of the brain reward system in depression. *Neuro-Psychopharmacology and Biological Psychiatry*.

Neary, D., Snowden, J.S., Northen, B., *et al* (1988) Dementia of frontal lobe type. *Journal of Neurology, Neurosurgery and Psychiatry*, **51**, 353–361.

Nemeroff, C. B. (1996) The corticotrophin releasing factor (CRF) hypothesis in depression: new findings and new directions. *Molecular Psychiatry*, **1**, 336–342.

Netter, P., Hennig, J. & Rohrmann, S. (1999) Psychobiological differences between the aggression and psychoticism dimension. *Pharmacopsychiatry*, **32**, 5–12.

Ngan, E. T. C. & Liddle, P. F. (2000) Reaction time, symptom profiles and course of illness in schizophrenia. *Schizophrenia Research*, **46**, 195–200.

Ngan, E. T. C., Yatham, L. N., Ruth, T. J., *et al* (2000) Decreased 5-HT$_{2a}$ receptor densities in neuroleptic naïve schizophrenic patients: a PET study using [$^{18}$F]setoperone. *American Journal of Psychiatry*, **157**, 1016–1018.

Nishijo, H., Ono, T. & Nishino, H. (1988) Single neuron responses in amygdala of alert monkey during complex sensory stimulation with affective significance. *Journal of Neuroscience*, **8**, 3570–3583.

Niznikiewicz, M. A., O'Donnell, B. F., Nestor, P. G., *et al* (1997) ERP assessment of visual and auditory language processing in schizophrenia. *Journal of Abnormal Psychology*, **106**, 85–94.

Nolfe, G., Serra, F. P., Palma, V., *et al* (1998) Brainstem involvement in obsessive–compulsive disorder. *Biological Psychology*, **48**, 69–77.

Nordahl, T. E., Benkelfat, C., Semple, W. E., *et al* (1989) Cerebral glucose metabolic rates in obsessive compulsive disorder. *Neuropsychopharmacology*, **2**, 23–28.

Nordstrom, A. L., Farde, L. & Weisel, F. A. (1993) Central D$_2$-dopamine receptor occupancy in relation to antipsychotic drug effects: a double blind PET study of schizophrenic patients. *Biological Psychiatry*, **33**, 227–235.

Norman, R. M. G., Malla, A. K., Morrison-Stewart, S. L., *et al* (1997) Neuropsychological correlates of syndromes in schizophrenia. *British Journal of Psychiatry*, **170**, 134–139.

Norman, R. M., Malla, A. K., Cortese, L., *et al* (1999) Symptoms and cognition as predictors of community functioning: a prospective analysis. *American Journal of Psychiatry*, **156**, 400–405.

Northoff, G., Steinke, R., Czcervenka, C., *et al* (1999) Decreased density of GABA-A receptors in the left sensorimotor cortex in akinetic catatonia: investigation of in vivo benzodiazepine receptor binding. *Journal of Neurology, Neurosurgery and Psychiatry*, **67**, 445–450.

Nutt, D. & Lawson, C. (1992) Panic attacks. A neurochemical overview of models and mechanisms. *British Journal of Psychiatry*, **160**, 165–178.

Nutt, D. J., Glue, P., Lawson, C. W., *et al* (1990) Flumazenil provocation of panic attacks: evidence for altered benzodiazepine sensitivity in panic disorder. *Archives of General Psychiatry*, **47**, 917–925.

Nutt, D. J., Forshall, S., Bell, C., *et al* (1999) Mechanisms of action of selective serotonin reuptake inhibitors in the treatment of psychiatric disorders. *European Neuropsychopharmacology*, **9** (suppl. 3), S81–S86.

O'Connor, K., Todorov, C., Robillard, S., *et al* (1999) Cognitive–behaviour therapy and medication in the treatment of obsessive–compulsive disorder: a controlled study. *Canadian Journal of Psychiatry*, **44**, 64–71.

O'Grady, J. C. (1990) The prevalence and diagnostic significance of first-rank symptoms in a random sample of acute schizophrenia in-patients. *British Journal of Psychiatry*, **156**, 496–500.

O'Keane, V., Maloney, E., O'Neil, H., *et al* (1992) Blunted prolactin response to fenfluramine in psychopathy. *British Journal of Psychiatry*, **160**, 643–646.

O'Keefe, J. & Nadel, L. (1978) *The Hippocampus as a Cognitive Map*. Oxford: Clarendon Press.

Oltmanns, T. F. (1978) Selective attention in manic and schizophrenic psychoses: the effects of distraction on information processing. *Journal of Abnormal Psychology*, **87**, 212–225.

Overall, J. E. & Gorham, D. R. (1962) The Brief Psychiatric Rating Scale. *Psychological Reports*, **10**, 799–812.

Pacak, K., Palkovits, M., Kopin, I. J., *et al* (1995) Stress-induced norepinephrine release in the hypothalamic paraventricular nucleus and pituitary-adrenocortical and sympathoadrenal activity: in vivo microdialysis studies. *Frontiers of Neuroendocrinology*, **16**, 89–150.

Pantelis, C., Velakoulis, D., Suckling, P., *et al* (2000) Left medial temporal volume reduction occurs during the transition from high-risk to first-episode psychosis. *Schizophrenia Research*, **41**, 35.

Pantev, C., Makeig, S., Hoke, M., *et al* (1991) Human auditory evoked gamma-band magnetic fields. *Proceedings of the National Academy of Sciences USA*, **88**, 8996–9000.

Papeschi, R. & McClure, D. J. (1971) Homovanillic and 5-hydroxyindoleacetic acid in cerebrospinal fluid in depressed patients. *Archives of General Psychiatry*, **25**, 354–358.

Pardo, J. V., Pardo, P. J., Janer, K. W., *et al* (1990) The anterior cingulate mediates processing selection in the Stroop attentional conflict paradigm. *Proceedings of the National Academy of Sciences USA*, **87**, 256–259.

Pardo, J. V., Pardo, P. J. & Raichle, M. E. (1993) Neural correlates of self-induced dysphoria. *American Journal of Psychiatry*, **150**, 713–719.

Paulesu, E., Frith, C. J. & Frackowiak, R. S. J. (1993) The neural correlates of the verbal component of working memory. *Nature*, **362**, 342–344.

Pearlson, G. D. & Veroff, A. E. (1981) Computerised tomographic scan changes in manic–depressive illness. *Lancet*, **ii**, 470.

Pearlson, G. D., Wong, D. F., Tune, L. E., *et al* (1995) In vivo D2 dopamine receptor density in psychotic and non-psychotic patients with bipolar disorder. *Archives of General Psychiatry*, **52**, 471–477.

Pellow, S., Chopin, P., File, S. E., *et al* (1985) Validation of open:closed arm entries in an elevated plus-maze as a measure of anxiety in the rat. *Journal of Neuroscience Methods*, **14**, 149–167.

Penfield, W. & Rasmussen, T. (1950) *The Cerebral Cortex of Man*. New York: Macmillan.

Peralta, V., Cuesta, M. J. & deLeon, J. (1992a) Formal thought disorder in schizophrenia: a factor analytic study. *Comprehensive Psychiatry*, **33**, 105–110.

Peralta, V., deLeon, M. J. & Cuesta, M. J. (1992b) Are there more than two syndromes in schizophrenia? A critique of the positive–negative dichotomy. *British Journal of Psychiatry*, **161**, 335–343.

Peralta, V., Cuesta, M. J. & Farre, C. (1997a) Factor structure of symptoms in functional psychoses. *Biological Psychiatry*, **42**, 806–815.

Peralta, V., Cuesta, M. J., Serrano, J. F., *et al* (1997b) The Kahlbaum syndrome: a study of its clinical validity, nosological status, and relationship with schizophrenia and mood disorder. *Comprehensive Psychiatry*, **38**, 61–67.

Perugi, G., Akiskal, H. S., Gemignani, A., *et al* (1998) Episodic course in obsessive–compulsive disorder. *European Archives of Psychiatry and Clinical Neuroscience*, **248**, 240–244.

Petrides, M., Alivisatos, B., Meyer, E., *et al* (1993) Functional activation of the human frontal cortex during the performance of verbal working memory tasks. *Proceedings of the National Academy of Sciences USA*, **90**, 878–882.

Petty, F., Kramer, M., Fulton, F. G., *et al* (1993) Low plasma GABA is a trait-like marker for bipolar illness. *Neuropsychopharmacology*, **9**, 125–132.

Pierson, A., Ragot, R., Van Hooff, J., *et al* (1996) Heterogeneity of information-processing alterations according to dimensions of depression: an event-related potentials study. *Biological Psychiatry*, **15**, 98–115

Pinel, P. (1806) *A Treatise on Insanity* (trans. D. D. Davis from *Traitè Medico-Philosophique sur l'Alienation Mentale ou la Manie*. Paris: Richard, Caille & Ravier). Sheffield: Cadell & Davils.

Plotsky, P. M., Owens, M. J. & Nemeroff, C. B. (1998) Psychoneuroendocrinology of depression. Hypothalamic-pituitary-adrenal axis. *Psychiatric Clinics of North America*, **21**, 293–307.

Pogue-Geile, M. F. & Harrow, M. (1984) Negative and positive symptoms in schizophrenia and depression: a follow-up. *Schizophrenia Bulletin*, **10**, 331–387.

Porrino, L. J., Burns, R. S., Crane, A. M., *et al* (1987) Changes in local cerebral glucose utilization associated with Parkinson's syndrome induced by 1-methyl-4-phenyl-1,2,3,6-tetrahydropyridine (MPTP) in the primate. *Life Sciences*, **40**, 1657–1664.

Posner, M. I. & Dehaene, S. (1994) Attentional networks. *Trends in Neuroscience*, **17**, 75–79.

Post, R. M., Susan, R. & Weiss, B. (1992) Sensitization, kindling, and carbamazepine: an update on their implications for the course of affective illness. *Pharmacopsychiatry*, **25**, 41–43.

Postle, B. R., Berger, J. S. & D'Esposito, M. (1999) Functional neuroanatomical double dissociation of mnemonic and executive control processes contributing to working memory performance. *Proceedings of the National Academy of Sciences USA*, **96**, 12959–12964.

Price, L. H., Charney, D. S., Rubin, A., *et al* (1985) Alpha-2 adrenergic receptor function in depression. The cortisol response to yohimbine. *Archives of General Psychiatry*, **43**, 849–858.

Price, L. H., Charney, D. S., Delgado, P. L., *et al* (1991) Serotonin function and depression: neuroendocrine and mood responses to intravenous L-tryptophan in depressed patients and healthy comparison subjects. *American Journal of Psychiatry*, **148**, 1518–1525.

Prichard, J. C. (1835) *A Treatise on Insanity*. London: Sherwood, Gilbert & Piper.

Pulver, A. E. (2000) Search for schizophrenia susceptibility genes. *Biological Psychiatry*, **47**, 221–230.

Purcell, R., Maruff, P., Kyrios, M., *et al* (1998) Cognitive deficits in obsessive–compulsive disorder on tests of frontal–striatal function. *Biological Psychiatry*, **43**, 348–357.

Purdon, S., Jones, B., Stip, E., *et al* (2000) Neuropsychological change in early phase schizophrenia during 12 months of treatment with olanzapine, risperidone, or haloperidol. *Archives of General Psychiatry*, **57**, 249–258.

Pycock, C. J., Kerwin, R. W. & Carter, C. J. (1980) Effects of lesions of cortical DA terminals on subcortical DA receptors in rats. *Nature*, **286**, 74–76.

Pyke, R. E. & Greenberg, H. S. (1986) Norepinephrine challenges in panic patients. *Journal of Clinical Psychopharmacology*, **6**, 279–285.

Quay, H. C. (1988) The behavioural reward and inhibition system in childhood behavior disorders. In *Attention Deficit Disorder*, vol. 3 (ed L. M. Bloomingdale), pp. 176–186. Oxford: Pergamon.

Raine, A., O'Brien, M., Smiley, N., *et al* (1990) Reduced lateralization in verbal dichotic listening in adolescent psychopaths. *Journal of Abnormal Psychology*, **99**, 272–277.

Randall, P. K., Bremner, J. D., Krystal, J. H., *et al* (1995) Effects of the benzodiazepine antagonist flumazenil in PTSD. *Biological Psychiatry*, **38**, 319–324.

Rauch, S. L., Savage, C. R., Alpert, N. M., *et al* (1995) A positron emission tomographic study of simple phobic symptom provocation. *Archives of General Psychiatry*, **52**, 20–28.

Rauch, S. L., van der Kolk, B. A., Fisler, R. E., *et al* (1996) A symptom provocation study of posttraumatic stress disorder using positron emission tomography and script-driven imagery. *Archives of General Psychiatry*, **53**, 380–387.

Rauch, S. L., Savage, C. R., Alpert, N. M., *et al* (1997) The functional neuroanatomy of anxiety: a study of three disorders using positron emission tomography and symptom provocation. *Biological Psychiatry*, **42**, 446–452.

Raz, S. & Raz, N. (1990) Structural brain abnormalities in the major psychoses: a quantitative review of the evidence from computerized imaging. *Psychological Bulletin*, **108**, 93–108.

Redmond, D. E. (1986) The possible role of locus coeruleus noradrenergic activity in anxiety-panic. *Clinical Neuropharmacology*, **9** (suppl. 4), 40–42.

Rex, A., Marsden, C. A. & Fink, H. (1997) Cortical 5-HT-CCK interactions and anxiety-related behaviour of guinea-pigs: a microdialysis study. *Neuroscience Letters*, **228**, 79–82.

Ribary, U., Ioannides, A. A., Singh, K. D., *et al* (1991) Magnetic field tomography of coherent thalamocortical 40-Hz oscillations in humans. *Proceedings of the National Academy of Sciences USA*, **88**, 11037–11041.

Ring, H. A., Crellin, R., Kirker, S., *et al* (1993) Vigabatrin and depression. *Journal of Neurology, Neurosurgery and Psychiatry*, **56**, 925–928.

Ring, H. A., Bench, C. J., Trimble, M. R., *et al* (1994) Depression in Parkinson's disease. A positron emission study. *British Journal of Psychiatry*, **165**, 333–339.

Risch, S. C., Cohen, R. M., Janowsky, D. S., *et al* (1981) Physostigmine induction of depressive symptomatology in normal human subjects. *Psychiatry Research*, **4**, 89–94.

Robertson, G. S. & Fibiger, H. C. (1992) Neuroleptics increase c-Fos expression in the forebrain: contrasting effects of haloperidol and clozapine. *Neuroscience*, **46**, 315–328.

Robertson, G. & Taylor, P. J. (1985) Some cognitive correlates of schizophrenic illnesses. *Psychological Medicine*, **15**, 81–98.

Robinson, D., Woerner, M. G., Alvir, J. M., *et al* (1999) Predictors of relapse following response from a first episode of schizophrenia or schizoaffective disorder. *Archives of General Psychiatry*, **56**, 241–247.

Robinson, R. G. & Szetela, B. (1981) Mood change following left hemispheric brain injury. *Annals of Neurology*, **9**, 447–453.

Robinson, R. G., Boston, J. D., Starkstein, S. E., *et al* (1987) Post stroke depression and lesion location. *American Journal of Psychiatry*, **145**, 172–178.

Robinson, T. E. (1980) Hippocampal rhythmic slow activity (RSA; theta): a critical analysis of selected studies and discussion of possible species-differences. *Brain Research Reviews*, **2**, 69–101.

Rogers, D. (1985) The motor disorders of severe psychiatric illness: a conflict of paradigms. *British Journal of Psychiatry*, **147**, 221–232.

Roland, P. E. (1985) Cortical organization of voluntary behavior in man. *Human Neurobiology*, **4**, 155–167.

Rolls, E. T. (1989) Functions of neural networks in the hippocampus and neocortex, in memory. In *Neural Models of Plasticity* (eds J. H. Byrne & W. O. Berry), pp. 240–265. San Diego: Academic Press.

Romach, M. K., Glue, P., Kampman, K., *et al* (1999) Attenuation of the euphoric effects of cocaine by the dopamine D1/D5 antagonist ecopipam. *Archives of General Psychiatry*, **56**, 1101–1106.

Roy, P. D., Zipursky, R. B., Saint-Cyr, J. A., *et al* (1998) Temporal horn enlargement is present in schizophrenia and bipolar disorder. *Biological Psychiatry*, **44**, 418–422.

Rubin, E., Sackeim, H. A., Prohovnik, I., *et al* (1995) Regional cerebral blood flow in mood disorders: IV. Comparison of mania and depression. *Psychiatry Research*, **61**, 1–10.

Rumelhart, D. E. & McClelland, J. L. (eds) (1986) *Parallel Distributed Processing: Explorations in the Microstructure of Cognition. Vol. 1. Foundations.* Cambridge, MA: MIT Press.

Rybakowski, J. K. & Twardowska, K. (1999) The dexamethasone/corticotropin-releasing hormone test in depression in bipolar and unipolar affective illness. *Journal of Psychiatric Research*, **33**, 363–370.

Rypma, B. & D'Esposito, M. (1999) The roles of prefrontal brain regions in components of working memory: effects of memory load and individual differences. *Proceedings of the National Academy of Sciences USA*, **96**, 6558–6563.

Salisbury, D. F., Shenton, M. E. & McCarley, R. W. (1999) P300 topography differs in schizophrenia and manic psychosis. *Biological Psychiatry*, **45**, 98–106.

Sargent, P. A., Quested, D. J. & Cowen, P. J. (1998) Clomipramine enhances the cortisol response to 5-HTP: implications for the therapeutic role of 5-HT2 receptors. *Psychopharmacology (Berlin)*, **140**, 120–122.

Scerbo, A., Raine, A., O'Brien, M., *et al* (1990) Reward dominance and passive avoidance learning in adolescent psychopaths. *Journal of Abnormal Child Psychology*, **18**, 451–463.

Schacter, D. L. & Wagner, A. D. (1999) Medial temporal lobe activations in fMRI and PET studies of episodic encoding and retrieval. *Hippocampus*, **9**, 7–24.

Schall, U., Schon, A., Zerbin, D., *et al* (1996) Event-related potentials during an auditory discrimination with prepulse inhibition in patients with schizophrenia, obsessive–compulsive disorder and healthy subjects. *International Journal of Neuroscience*, **84**, 15–33.

Schalling, D., Asberg, M., Adman, G., *et al* (1987) Markers for vulnerability to psychopathology: temperament traits associated with platelet MAO activity. *Acta Psychiatrica Scandinavica*, **76**, 172–182.

Schlaepfer, T. E., Pearlson, G. D., Wong, D. F., *et al* (1997) PET study of competition between intravenous cocaine and [$^{11}$C] raclopride at dopamine receptors in human subjects. *American Journal of Psychiatry*, **154**, 1209–1213.

Schlaepfer, T. E., Strain, E. C., Greenberg, B. D., *et al* (1998) Site of opioid action in the human brain: mu and kappa agonists' subjective and cerebral blood flow effects. *American Journal of Psychiatry*, **155**, 470–473.

Schmider, J., Standhart, H., Deuschle, M., *et al* (1999) A double-blind comparison of lorazepam and oxazepam in psychomotor retardation and mutism. *Biological Psychiatry*, **46**, 437–441.

Schneider, K. (1959) *Clinical Psychopathology* (trans. M. W. Hamilton from *Klinische Psychopathologie*. Stuttgart: Georg Thieme, 1950). New York: Grune & Stratton.

Schreber, D. P. (1955) *Memoirs of My Nervous Illness* (trans. I. Macalpine & R. Hunter from *Denkwurdigkeiten eines Nervenkranken*, 1903). London: Wm Dawson.

Schwab, S. G., Hallmayer, J., Lerer, B., *et al* (1998) Support for a chromosome 18p locus conferring susceptibility to functional psychoses in families with schizophrenia, by association and linkage analysis. *American Journal of Human Genetics*, **63**, 1139–1152.

Scoville, W. B. & Milner, B. (1957) Loss of recent memory after bilateral hippocampal lesions. *Journal of Neurosurgery, Neurology and Psychiatry*, **20**, 11–21.

Seeman, M. V. (1996) The role of estrogen in schizophrenia. *Journal of Psychiatry and Neuroscience*, **21**, 123–127.

Selemon, L. D. & Goldman-Rakic, P. S. (1985) Longitudinal topography and interdigitation of corticostriatal projections in the rhesus monkey. *Journal of Neuroscience*, **5**, 776–794.

Selemon, L. D. & Goldman-Rakic, P. D. (1988) Common cortical and subcortical targets of the dorsolateral and posterior parietal cortices in the rhesus monkey: evidence for a distributed neural network subserving spatially guided behaviour. *Journal of Neuroscience*, **8**, 4049–4068.

Selemon, L. D. & Goldman-Rakic, P. D. (1999) The reduced neuropil hypothesis. A circuit based model of schizophrenia. *Biological Psychiatry*, **45**, 17–25.

Selten, J. P., Brown, A. S., Moons, K. G., *et al* (1999) Prenatal exposure to the 1957 influenza pandemic and non-affective psychosis in the Netherlands. *Schizophrenia Research*, **38**, 85–91.

Shakow, D. (1962) Segmental set: a theory of the formal psychological deficit in schizophenia. *Archives of General Psychiatry*, **6**, 1–7.

Shallice, T. (1988) *From Neuropsychology to Mental Structure*. Cambridge: Cambridge University Press.

Shallice, T., Burgess, P. W. & Frith, C. D. (1991) Can the neuropsychological case-study approach be applied to schizophrenia? *Psychological Medicine*, **21**, 661– 673.

Shapiro, S. K., Quay, H. C., Hogan, A. E., *et al* (1988) Response preservation and delayed responding in undersocialized aggressive conduct disorder. *Journal of Abnormal Psychology*, **97**, 371–373.

Sheer, D. E. (1989) Sensory and cognitive 40-Hz event related potentials: behavioural correlates, brain function and clinical application. In *Springer Series in Brain Dynamics 2* (eds E. Basar & T. H. Bullock), pp. 339–374. Berlin: Springer-Verlag.

Sheline, Y. I., Wang, P. W., Gado, M. H., *et al* (1996) Hippocampal atrophy in recurrent major depression. *Proceedings of the National Academy of Sciences USA*, **93**, 3908–3913.

Sheline, Y. I., Sangavi, M., Mintun, M. A., *et al* (1999) Depression duration but not age predicts hippocampal volume loss in medically healthy woman with recurrent major depression. *Journal of Neuroscience*, **19**, 5034–5043.

Shelley, A. M., Ward, P. B., Catts, S. V., *et al* (1991) Mismatch negativity: an index of a preattentive processing deficit in schizophrenia. *Biological Psychiatry*, **30**, 1059–1062.

Shenton, M. E., Kikinis, R., Jolesz, F. A., *et al* (1992) Abnormalities of the left temporal lobe and thought disorder in schizophrenia. A quantitative magnetic resonance imaging study. *New England Journal of Medicine*, **327**, 604–612.

Shiah, I. S. & Yatham, L. S. (1998) GABA function in mood disorders: an update and critical review. *Life Sciences*, **63**, 1289–1303.

Shiah, I. S., Yatham, L. S., Lam, R. W., *et al* (1999) Growth hormone responses to baclofen in patients with mania: a pilot study. *Psychopharmacology (Berlin)*, **147**, 280–284.

Shioiri, T., Oshitani, Y., Kato T., *et al* (1996) Prevalence of cavum septum pellucidum detected by MRI in patients with bipolar disorder, major depression and schizophrenia. *Psychological Medicine*, **26**, 431–434.

Siever, L. J., Uhde, T. W., Limerson, D. C., *et al* (1984) Plasma cortisol responses to clonidine in depressed patients and controls. Evidence for a possible alteration in noradrenergic neuroendocrine relationships. *Archives of General Psychiatry*, **41**, 63–68.

Silbersweig, D. A., Stern, E., Frith, C., *et al* (1995) A functional neuroanatomy of hallucinations in schizophrenia. *Nature*, **378**, 176–179.

Silverstone, P. H., Pukhovsky, A. & Rotzinger, S. (1998) Lithium does not attenuate the effects of D-amphetamine in healthy volunteers. *Psychiatry Research*, **79**, 219–226.

Simon, H., Taghzouti, K., Gozlan, H., *et al* (1988) Lesion of dopaminergic terminals in the amygdala produces enhanced locomotor response to D-amphetamine and opposite changes in dopaminergic activity in the prefrontal cortex and nucleus accumbens. *Brain Research*, **447**, 335–340.

Slater, E., Beard, A. W. & Glithero, E. (1963) The schizophrenic-like psychoses of epilepsy. *British Journal of Psychiatry*, **109**, 95–150.

Smith, E. E. & Jonides, J. (1999) Storage and executive processes in the frontal lobes. *Science*, **283**, 1657–1661.

Smith, E. E., Jonides, J., Koeppe, R. A., *et al* (1995) Spatial versus object working memory: PET investigations. *Journal of Cognitive Neuroscience*, **7**, 337–356.

Solovay, M. R., Shenton, M. & Holzman, P. S. (1987) Comparative studies of thought disorders. I. Mania and schizophrenia. *Archives of General Psychiatry*, **44**, 13–20.

Southwick, S. M., Krystal, J. H., Bremner, J. D., *et al* (1997) Noradrenergic and serotonergic function in posttraumatic stress disorder. *Archives of General Psychiatry*, **54**, 749–758.

Spence, S. A., Liddle, P. F., Stefan, M. D., *et al* (2000) Functional anatomy of verbal fluency in people with schizophrenia and those at genetic risk. *British Journal of Psychiatry*, **176**, 52–60.

Spitzer, M., Weisker, I., Winter, M., *et al* (1994) Semantic and phonological priming in schizophrenia. *Journal of Abnormal Psychology*, **103**, 485–494.

Spitzer, R. L., Gibbon, M., Skodol, A. E., *et al* (1989) *DSM–IIIR Casebook*, Washington, DC: American Psychiatric Press.

Spohn, H. E., Coyne, L., Larson, J., *et al* (1986) Episodic and residual thought pathology in chronic schizophrenics: effects of neuroleptics. *Schizophrenia Bulletin*, **12**, 394–407.

Squire, L. P. (1993) Memory and the hippocampus; a synthesis from findings with rats, monkeys, humans. *Psychological Review*, **99**, 195–231.

Squire, L. R. & Zola-Morgan, S. (1983) The neurology of memory: the case for correspondence between the findings for man and non-human primate. In *The Physiological Basis of Memory* (ed. J. A. Deutsch), pp. 200–268. New York: Academic Press.

Stahl, S. M. (1998) Mechanism of action of serotonin selective reuptake inhibitors. Serotonin receptors and pathways mediate therapeutic effects and side effects. *Journal of Affective Disorders*, **51**, 215–235.

Stalenheim, E. G., Eriksson, E., von Knorring, L., *et al* (1998a) Testosterone as a biological marker in psychopathy and alcoholism. *Psychiatry Research*, **77**, 79–88.

Stalenheim, E. G., von Knorring, L. & Wide, L. (1998b) Serum levels of thyroid hormones as biological markers in a Swedish forensic psychiatric population. *Biological Psychiatry*, **43**, 755–761.

Starkstein, S. E. & Robinson, R. G. (1989) Affective disorders and cerebral vascular disease. *British Journal of Psychiatry*, **154**, 170–182.

Starkstein, S. E., Preziosi, T. J., Berthier, M. L., *et al* (1989) Depression and cognitive impairment in Parkinson's disease. *Brain*, **112**, 1141–1153.

Starkstein, S. E., Mayberg, H. S., Preziosi, T. J., *et al* (1992a) Reliability, validity, and clinical correlates of apathy in Parkinson's disease. *Journal of Neuropsychiatry and Clinical Neuroscience*, **4**, 134–139.

Starkstein, S. E., Mayberg, H. S., Leiguarda, R., *et al* (1992b) A prospective longitudinal study of depression, cognitive decline, and physical impairments in patients with Parkinson's disease. *Journal of Neurology, Neurosurgery and Psychiatry*, **55**, 377–382.

Stein, D. J., Spadaccini, E. & Hollander, E. (1995) Meta-analysis of pharmacotherapy trials for obsessive–compulsive disorder. *International Clinical Psychopharmacology*, **10**, 11–18.

Stein, D. J., Van Heerden, B., Wessels, C. J., *et al* (1999) Single photon emission computed tomography of the brain with Tc-99m HMPAO during sumatriptan challenge in obsessive–compulsive disorder: investigating the functional role of the serotonin auto-receptor. *Progress in Neuropsychopharmacology and Biological Psychiatry*, **23**, 1079–1099.

Steriade, M. & Amzica, F. (1996) Intracortical and corticothalamic coherency in fast spontaneous oscillations. *Proceedings of the National Academy of Sciences USA*, **93**, 2533–2538.

Stern, L., Zohar, J., Cohen, R., *et al* (1998) Treatment of severe, drug resistant obsessive compulsive disorder with the 5HT1D agonist sumatriptan. *European Neuropsychopharmacology*, **8**, 325–328.

Stoll, A. L. & Severus, W. E. (1996) Mood stabilizers: shared mechanisms of action at postsynaptic signal-transduction and kindling processes. *Harvard Review of Psychiatry*, **4**, 77–89.

Strakowski, S. M., Wilson, D. R., Tohen, M., *et al* (1993) Structural brain abnormalities in first-episode mania. *Biological Psychiatry*, **33**, 602–609.

Strohle, A., Holsboer, F. & Rupprecht, R. (2000) Increased ACTH concentrations associated with cholecystokinin tetrapeptide-induced panic attacks in patients with panic disorder. *Neuropsychopharmacology*, **22**, 251–256.

Suddath, R. L., Christison, G. W., Torrey, F., *et al* (1990) Anatomic abnormality in the brains of monozygotic twins discordant for schizophrenia. *New England Journal of Medicine*, **322**, 789–794.

Susser, E., Neugebauer, R., Hoek, H. W., *et al* (1996) Schizophrenia after prenatal famine. Further evidence. *Archives of General Psychiatry*, **53**, 25–31.

Suzuki, M., Yuasa, S., Minabi, Y., *et al* (1993) Left superior temporal blood flow increases in schizophrenic and schizophreniform patients with auditory hallucinations: a longitudinal case study using 13I-IMP SPECT. *European Archives of Psychiatry and Clinical Neuroscience*, **242**, 257–261.

Swann, A. C., Stokes, P. E., Secunda, S. K., *et al* (1994) Depressive mania versus agitated depression: biogenic amine and hypothalamic-pituitary-adrenocortical function. *Biological Psychiatry*, **35**, 803–813.

Swedo, S. E., Schapiro, M. B., Grady, C. L., *et al* (1989) Cerebral glucose metabolism in childhood-onset obsessive–compulsive disorder. *Archives of General Psychiatry*, **46**, 518–523.

Swedo, S. E., Pietrini, P., Leonard, H. L., *et al* (1992) Cerebral glucose metabolism in childhood-onset obsessive–compulsive disorder. Revisualization during pharmacotherapy. *Archives of General Psychiatry*, **49**, 690–694.

Szentogothai, J. (1978) The neuron network of the cerebral cortex: a functional interpretation. *Proceedings of the Royal Society (London) Series B*, **210**, 219–248.

Szeszko, P. R., Robinson, D., Alvir, J. M. J., *et al* (1999) Orbital frontal and amygdala volume reductions in obsessive–compulsive disorder. *Archives of General Psychiatry*, **56**, 913–919.

Tanaka, M., Kohno, Y., Nagagawa, R., *et al* (1982) Time related differences in noradrenaline turnover in rat brain regions by stress. *Pharmacology, Biochemistry and Behaviour*, **16**, 315–319.

Tassin, J-P. (1992) NE/DA interactions in prefrontal cortex and their possible roles as neuro-modulators in schizophrenia. *Journal of Neural Transmission*, **36** (suppl.), 135–162.

Tassin, J-P., Kitabgi, P., Tramu, G., *et al* (1988) Amphetamine injected into the medial prefrontal cortex attenuates the locomotor activating effects of amphetamine in the nucleus accumbens. *Society for Neuroscience Abstracts*, **14**, 662.

Thakore, J. H., O'Keane, V. & Dinan, T. G. (1996) D-fenfluramine-induced prolactin responses in mania: evidence for serotonergic subsensitivity. *American Journal of Psychiatry*, **153**, 1460–1463.

Thiebot, M-H., Martin, P. & Peuch, A. J. (1992) Animal behavioural studies in the evaluation of antidepressant drugs. *British Journal of Psychiatry*, **160** (suppl. 15), 44–50.

Thierry, A. M., Tassin, J. P., Blanc, G., *et al* (1976) Selective activation of the mesocortical dopamine DA system by stress. *Nature*, **263**, 242–244.

Thompson, P. A. & Meltzer, H. Y. (1993) Positive, negative and disorganisation factors from the Schedule for Affective Disorders and Schizophrenia and the Present State Examination. *British Journal of Psychiatry*, **163**, 344–351.

Thomson, A. M. & West, D. C. (1993) Fluctuations in pyramid–pyramid excitatory postsynaptic potentials modified by presynaptic firing pattern and postsynaptic membrane potential using paired intracellular recordings in rat neocortex. *Neuroscience*, **54**, 329–346.

Thomson, A. M., Deuchars, J. & West, D. C. (1993) Single axon excitatory postsynaptic potentials in neocortical interneurons exhibit pronounced paired pulse facilitation. *Neuroscience*, **54**, 347–360.

Tokunaga, M., Ida, I., Higuchi, T., *et al* (1997) Alterations of benzodiazepine receptor binding potential in anxiety and somatoform disorders measured by [123]I-iomazenil SPECT. *Radiation Medicine*, **15**, 163–169.

Tollefson, G. D. & Sanger, T. M. (1997) Negative symptoms: a path analytic approach to a double-blind, placebo- and haloperidol-controlled clinical trial with olanzapine. *American Journal of Psychiatry*, **154**, 466–474.

Tollefson, G. D., Beasley, C. M. Jr, Tran, P. V., *et al* (1997) Olanzapine versus haloperidol in the treatment of schizophrenia and schizoaffective and schizophreniform disorders: results of an international collaborative trial. *American Journal of Psychiatry*, **154**, 457–465.

Traub, R. D., Whittington, M. A., Stanford, I. M., *et al* (1996) A mechanism for generation of long-range synchronous fast oscillations in the cortex. *Nature*, **383**, 621–624.

Tulving, E., Kapur, S., Craik, F. I. M., *et al* (1994) Hemispheric encoding/retrieval asymmetry in episodic memory: positron emission tomography findings. *Proceedings of the National Academy of Sciences USA*, **91**, 2012–2015.

Uchiyama, M., Sue, H., Fukumitsu, N., *et al* (1997) Assessment of cerebral benzodiazepine receptor distribution in anxiety disorders by [123]I-iomazenil-SPECT: comparison to cerebral perfusion scintigraphy by [123]I-IMP. *Nippon Igaku Hoshasen Gakkai Zasshi*, **57**, 41–46.

Uhlenhuth, E. H., Balter, M. B., Ban, T. A., *et al* (1999) International study of expert judgment on therapeutic use of benzodiazepines and other psychotherapeutic medications: VI. Trends in recommendations for the pharmacotherapy of anxiety disorders, 1992–1997. *Depression and Anxiety*, **9**, 107–116.

Uno, H., Tarara, R., Else, J. G., *et al* (1989) Hippocampal damage associated with prolonged and fatal stress in primates. *Journal of Neuroscience*, **9**, 1705–1711.

Vanderwolf, C. H. (1969) Hippocampal electrical activity and voluntary movement in the rat. *Electroencephalography and Clinical Neurophysiology*, **26**, 407–418.

Van Essen, D. C., Anderson, C. H. & Felleman, D. J. (1992) Information processing in the primate visual system: an integrated systems perspective. *Science*, **255**, 419–423.

Van Londen, L., Goekoop, J. G., Zwinderman, A. H., *et al* (1998) Neuropsychological performance and plasma cortisol, arginine vasopressin and oxytocin in patients with major depression. *Psychological Medicine*, **28**, 275–284.

Van Os, J. & Selton, J-P. (1998) Prenatal exposure to maternal stress and subsequent schizophrenia. The May 1940 invasion of The Netherlands. *British Journal of Psychiatry*, **172**, 324–326.

Van Os, J., Jones, P. B., Lewis, G., *et al* (1997) Developmental precursors of affective illness in a general population birth cohort. *Archives of General Psychiatry*, **54**, 625–631.

van Praag, H. M. & Korf, J. (1971) Retarded depression and the dopamine metabolism. *Psychopharmacology*, **19**, 199–203.

van Praag, H. M. & Korf, J. (1975) Central monoamine deficiency in depression: causative or secondary phenomenon? *Pharmakopsychiatria*, **8**, 321–326.

Van Putten, T., Marder, S. & Mintz, J. (1990) A controlled dose comparison of haloperidol in newly admitted schizophrenic patients. *Archives of General Psychiatry*, **47**, 754–758.

Velakoulis, D., Pantelis, C., McGorry, P. D., *et al* (1999) Hippocampal volume in first-episode psychoses and chronic schizophrenia: a high-resolution magnetic resonance imaging study. *Archives of General Psychiatry*, **56**, 133–141.

Vieta, E., Martinez-De-Osaba, M. J., Colom, F., *et al* (1999) Enhanced corticotropin response to corticotropin-releasing hormone as a predictor of mania in euthymic bipolar patients. *Psychological Medicine*, **29**, 971–978.

Vincent, S. R. & Hope, B. T. (1992) Neurons that say NO. *Trends in Neurosciences*, **15**, 108–113.

Vogt, J. L. & Levine, S. (1980) Response of mother and infant squirrel monkeys to separation and disturbance. *Physiology and Behaviour*, **24**, 829–832.

Vollenweider, F. X., Maguire, R. P., Leenders, K. L., *et al* (1998) Effects of high amphetamine dose on mood and cerebral glucose metabolism in normal volunteers using positron emission tomography (PET). *Psychiatry Research*, **83**, 149–162.

von Korff, M., Eaton, W. & Keyl, P. (1985) The epidemiology of panic attacks and panic disorder: results of three community surveys. *American Journal of Epidemiology*, **122**, 970–981.

Walker, E. & Harvey, P. D. (1986) Positive and negative symptoms in schizophrenia: attentional correlates. *Psychopathology*, **19**, 264–302.

Walker, E. & Lewine, R. J. (1990) Prediction of adult-onset schizophrenia from childhood home videos of the patients. *American Journal of Psychiatry*, **89,** 704–716.

Wang, J. F., Asghari, V., Rockel, C., *et al* (1999) Cyclic AMP responsive element binding protein phosphorylation and DNA binding is decreased by chronic lithium but not valproate treatment of SH-SY5Y neuroblastoma cells. *Neuroscience*, **91**, 771–776.

Weinberger, D. R. & Berman, K. F. (1996) Prefrontal function in schizophrenia: confounds and controversies. *Philosophical Transactions of the Royal Society of London B, Biological Science*, **351**, 1495–1503.

Weinberger, D. R., Berman, K. F. & Zec, R. F. (1986) Physiologic dysfunction of dorsolateral prefrontal cortex in schizophrenia. I. Regional cerebral blood flow evidence. *Archives of General Psychiatry*, **43**, 114–124.

Weinberger, D. R., Berman, K. F. & Illowsky, B. P. (1988) Physiological dysfunction of dorsolateral prefrontal cortex in schizophrenia. III. A new cohort and evidence for a monoaminergic mechanism. *Archives of General Psychiatry*, **45**, 609–615.

Weingartner, H., Cohen, R. M., Martello, J. D. T., *et al* (1981) Cognitive processes in depression. *Archives of General Psychiatry*, **38**, 42–47.

Weissman, M. W. (1990) Epidemiology of panic disorder and agoraphobia. In *Clinical Aspects of Panic Disorder* (ed. J. C. Ballenger), pp. 57–68. New York: Wiley-Liss.

Westenberg, H. J. M. & den Boer, J. A. (1988) Clinical and biochemical effects of selective serotonin-uptake inhibitors in anxiety disorders. In *Selective 5-HT Reuptake Inhibitors: Novel or Commonplace Agents?* (eds M. Gaspar & J. S. Wakelin), pp. 84–89. Basel: Karger.

Whittington, M. A., Traub, R. D. & Jefferys, J. G. R. (1995) Synchronized oscillations in interneuron networks driven by metabotropic glutamate receptor activation. *Nature*, **373**, 612–615.

Wik, G., Fredrikson, M., Ericson, K., *et al* (1993) A functional cerebral response to frightening visual stimulation. *Psychiatry Research*, **50**, 15–24.

Wildenauer, D. B., Schwab, S. G., Maier, W., *et al* (1999) Do schizophrenia and affective disorder share susceptibility genes? *Schizophrenia Research*, **39**, 107–109.

Williams, E. B. (1964) Deductive reasoning in schizophrenia. *Journal of Abnormal and Social Psychology*, **69**, 47–61.

Williamson, S., Harpur, T. J. & Hare, R. D. (1991) Abnormal processing of affective words by psychopaths. *Psychophysiology*, **28**, 260–273.

Willner, P., Muscat, R., Papp, M., *et al* (1991) Dopamine, depression and antidepressant drugs. In *The Mesolimbic Dopamine System: From Motivation to Action* (eds P. Willner & J. Scheel-Kruger), pp. 387–410. Chichester: Wiley.

Willner, P., Muscat, R. & Papp, M. (1992) Chronic mild stress-induced anhedonia: a realistic animal model of depression. *Neuroscience and Biobehaviour Reviews*, **16**, 525–534.

Wilson, F. A., Scalaidhe, S. P. & Goldman-Rakic, P. S. (1993) Dissociation of object and spatial processing domains in primate prefrontal cortex. *Science*, **260**, 1955–1958.

Wing, J. K. & Brown, G. W. (1970) *Institutionalization and Schizophrenia*. Cambridge: Cambridge University Press.

Wise, R. A. & Bozarth, M. A. (1985) Brain mechanisms of drug reward and euphoria. *Psychiatric Medicine*, **3**, 445–460.

Wolfe, N., Katz, D. I., Albert, M. L., *et al* (1990) Neuropsychological profile linked to low dopamine: in Alzheimer's disease, major depression, and Parkinson's disease. *Journal of Neurology, Neurosurgery and Psychiatry*, **53**, 915–917.

Wolkin, A., Angrist, B., Wolf, A., *et al* (1987) Effects of amphetamine on local cerebral metabolism in normal and schizophrenic subjects as determined by positron emission tomography. *Psychopharmacology*, **92**, 241–246.

Wolkin, A., Barouche, F. & Wolf, A. P. (1989) Dopamine blockade and clinical response: evidence for two biological sub-groups of schizophrenia. *American Journal of Psychiatry*, **146**, 905–908.

Wolkin, A., Sanfilipo, M., Wolf, A. P., et al (1992) Negative symptoms and hypofrontality in chronic schizophrenia. *Archives of General Psychiatry*, **49**, 959–965.

Wong, D. F., Wagner, H. N., Tune, L. E., et al (1986) Positron emission tomography reveals elevated D2 dopamine receptors in drug-naïve schizophrenics. *Science*, **234**, 1558–1563.

Woodruff, P. W. R., Wright, I. C., Shurique, N., et al (1997) Structural brain abnormalities in male schizophrenics reflect fronto-temporal dissociation. *Psychological Medicine*, **27**, 1257–1263.

World Health Organization (1978) *Report of the International Pilot Study of Schizophrenia.* Geneva: WHO.

World Health Organization (1993) *The Tenth Revision of the International Classification of Diseases* (ICD–10). Geneva: WHO.

Yamaguchi, S. & Knight, R. T. (1993) Association cortex contributions to the human P3. In *Slow Potential Changes in the Brain* (eds W. Haschke, A. I. Roitbak & E.-J. Speckmann), pp. 71–84. Boston: Birkhauser.

Yatham, L. N. (1996) Prolactin and cortisol responses to fenfluramine challenge in mania. *Biological Psychiatry*, **39**, 285–288.

Yatham, L. N., Liddle, P. F., Dennie, J., et al (1999a) Decrease in brain 5-HT$_2$ receptor binding in patients with major depression following desipramine treatment: a positron emission tomography study with [$^{18}$F]setoperone. *Archives of General Psychiatry*, **50**, 705–711.

Yatham, L. N., Shiah, I-S., Lam, R. W., et al (1999b) Hypothermic, ACTH, and cortisol responses to ipsapirone in patients with mania and healthy controls. *Journal of Affective Disorders*, **54**, 295–301.

Yatham, L. N., Liddle, P. F., Shiah, I-S., et al (2000) Brain 5-HT$_2$ receptors in major depression: a positron emission tomography study. *Archives of General Psychiatry*, **57**, 850–858.

Yonkers, K. A., Wrashaw, M. G., Massion, A. O., et al (1996) Phenomenology and course of generalised anxiety disorder. *British Journal of Psychiatry*, **168**, 308–313.

Young, S. N., Smith, S. E., Pihl, R. O., et al (1985) Tryptophan depletion causes a rapid lowering of mood in normal males. *Psychopharmacology (Berlin)*, **87**, 173–177.

Young, L. T., Warsh, J. J., Kish, S. J., et al (1994) Reduced brain 5-HT and elevated NE turnover and metabolites in bipolar affective disorder. *Biological Psychiatry*, **35**, 121–127.

Yuasa, S., Kurachi, M., Suzuki, M., et al (1995) Clinical symptoms and regional cerebral blood flow in schizophrenia. *European Archives of Psychiatry and Clinical Neuroscience*, **246**, 7–12.

Zakzanis, K. K., Leach, L. & Kaplan, E. (1998) On the nature and pattern of neurocognitive function in major depressive disorder. *Neuropsychiatry, Neuropsychology and Behavioural Neurology*, **11**, 111–119.

Zemlan, F. P., Hirschowitz, J. & Garver, D. L. (1986) Relation of clinical symptoms to apomorphine-stimulated growth hormone release in mood-incongruent psychotic patients. *Archives of General Psychiatry*, **43**, 1162–1167.

Zigmond, M. J., Abercrombie, E. D., Berger, T. W., et al (1990) Compensations after lesions of central dopaminergic neurons – some clinical and basic implications. *Trends in Neurosciences*, **13**, 290–295.

Zipursky, R. B., Lim, K. O., Sullivan, E. V., et al (1992) Widespread cerebral gray matter volume deficits in schizophrenia. *Archives of General Psychiatry*, **49**, 195–205.

Zipursky, R. B., Seeman, M. V., Bury, A., et al (1997) Deficits in gray matter volume are present in schizophrenia but not bipolar disorder. *Schizophrenia Research*, **26**, 85–92.

Zucker, D., Taylor, C. B., Brouillard, M., et al (1989) Cognitive aspects of panic attacks. Content, course and relationship to laboratory stressors. *British Journal of Psychiatry*, **155**, 86–91.

# Further reading

## Structural and functional neuroanatomy

Duvernoy, H. M. (1991) *The Human Brain: Surface, Three Dimensional Sectional Anatomy and MRI*. Wien, NY: Springer Verlag.

Frackowiak, R., Friston, K. J., Frith, C. D. Dolan, R. J. & Mazziotta, J. C. (1997) *Human Brain Function*. San Diego: Academic Press.

Fuster, J. M. (1997) *The Prefrontal Cortex: Anatomy, Physiology and Neuropsychology of the Frontal Lobe* (3rd edn). Philadelphia: Lipincott-Raven.

Gloor, P. (1997) *The Temporal Lobe and Limbic System*. New York: Oxford University Press.

Mouncastle, V. B. (1998) *Perceptual Neuroscience: The Cerebral Cortex*. Cambridge, MA: Harvard University Press.

## Psychopharmacology

Bloom, F. E. & Kupfer, D. J. (eds) (1994) *Psychopharmacology: The Fourth Generation of Progress*. New York: Raven Press.

## General neuroscience

Kandel, E. R., Swartz, J. H. & Jessel, T. M. (2000) *Principles of Neural Science* (4th edn). New York: McGraw-Hill.

## Classic texts in psychiatry

Bleuler, E. (1911) *Dementia Praecox or the Group of Schizophrenias* (trans. J. Zinkin. New York: International Universities Press, 1950).

Cleckley, H. (1988). *The Mask of Sanity* (5th edn). Augusta: Cleckley.

Kraepelin, E. (1919) *Dementia Praecox and Paraphrenia* (trans. R. M. Barclay). New York: Kreiger (facsimile edn, 1971).

Kraepelin, E. (1921) *Manic–Depressive Insanity and Paranoia* (trans. R. M. Barclay from *Lehrbuch der Psychiatrie*, 8th edn, Leipzig: Barth). Edinburgh: Churchill Livingstone.

## Mental disorders

Cooke, D. J., Forth, A. E. & Hare, R. D. (eds) (1998) *Psychopathy: Theory, Research, and Implications for Society*. Dordrecht: Kluwer.

Goodwin, F. E. & Jamison, K. R. (1990) *Manic Depressive Illness*. New York: Oxford University Press.

Hirsch, S. R. & Weinberger, D. R. (eds) (1995) *Schizophrenia*. Oxford: Blackwell.

Noyes, R. & Hoehn-Saric, R. (1998) *The Anxiety Disorders*. New York: Cambridge University Press.

## Clinical and laboratory neuroscience Internet sites

Hyperbrain, University of Utah (http://www-medlib.med.utah.edu/kw/hyperbrain/main.html). Brain atlas, neuroanatomy glossary and neuroanatomy text.

Mind and Brain Laboratory, University of Nottingham (http://www.nottingham.ac.uk/psychiatry/research/mindbrainlab/). Current research in the laboratory of the author of this book.

Neuroguide (http://www.neuroguide.com/). A searchable index of neuroscience resources, covering neurobiology, neurology, neurosurgery, psychology, psychiatry and cognitive neuroscience.

The Digital Anatomist Project, Washington University (http://sig.biostr.washington.edu/projects/da/). Online interactive brain atlases.

# Index